The Business of Critical Care:

A Textbook for Clinicians Who Manage Special Care Units

William J. Sibbald, M.D.
Chief, Program in Critical Care
Professor, Department of Medicine
The University of Western Ontario;
Coordinator, The Richard Ivey
Critical Care Trauma Center
London Health Sciences Centre
Victoria Campus
London, Ontario, Canada

Thomas A. Massaro, M.D., Ph.D.
Professor of Pediatrics and
Business Administration
Harrison Foundation Professor
of Medicine and Law
University of Virginia;
Associate Dean for Clinical Resources
Director of Medical Affairs
Attending Physician Pediatric
Intensive Care Unit
University of Virginia Medical Center
Charlottesville, Virginia

Diane M. McLeod, B.A., B.S.W.
Editorial Assistant
London Health Sciences Centre
London, Ontario, Canada

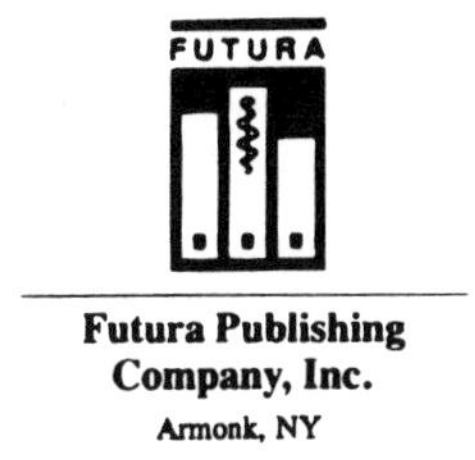

Futura Publishing Company, Inc.
Armonk, NY

Library of Congress Cataloging-in-Publication Data

The business of critical care : a textbook for clinicians who manage special care units / [edited by] William J. Sibbald, Thomas A. Massaro.
p. cm.
Includes bibliographical references and index.
ISBN 0-87993-623-1
1. Intensive care units—Administration. I. Sibbald, William J. II. Massaro, Thomas A.
[DNLM: 1. Critical Care—standards. 2. Intensive Care Units—organization & administration. 3. Hospital Units—standards. 4. Quality Assurance, Health Care—standards. WX 218 B979 1995]
RA975.5.I56B87 1995
362.1'74'068—dc20
DNLM/DLC
for Library of Congress 95-40718
CIP

Published by
Futura Publishing Company, Inc.
135 Bedford Road
Armonk, New York 10504

LC #: 95-40718
ISBN # 0-87993-623-1

Printed in the United States of America.

Printed on acid-free paper.

Dedication

To our wives and children, without whose support our ability to explore the new and exciting challenges of practicing Critical Care Medicine in a rapidly changing environment wouldn't be possible.

WJS
TM
June 1995

Contributors

Steven M. Ayres, M.D.
Director, International Health Programs
Dean of Meritus, School of Medicine
Virginia Commonwealth University/Medical College of Virginia
Richmond, Virginia

E. Richard Brownlee II, C.P.A., B.B.A., M.B.A., Ph.D.
Professor of Business Administration
The Darden Graduate School of Business Administration
University of Virginia
Charlottesville, Virginia

James E. Calvin Jr, M.D.
Associate Professor of Medicine
Rush Medical College
Director, Critical Care Unit
Ruch Presbyterian St. Luke Medical Center
Chicago, Illinois

Douglas Cocks, Ph.D.
Chief Economist
Eli Lilly and Company
Indianapolis, Indiana

Morris Cohen, M.D., M.B.Bch
Director of Neonatal Medicine
Codirector Perinatal
Newark Beth Israel Medical Center
Newark, New Jersey

Albert A. Driedger, M.D., Ph.D.
Professor of Diagnostic Radiology and Nuclear Medicine
Professor of Oncology
Lecturer of Medicine
University of Western Ontario
Director LARGhealth
Department of Nuclear Medicine
Victoria Hospital
London, Ontario, Canada

Charles G. Durbin Jr, M.D.
Professor of Anesthesiology and Surgery
Medical Director of Surgical Intensive Care Unit
University of Virginia Health Sciences Center
Charlottesville, Virginia

Jeannette A. Eberhard, B.Sc., M.B.A.
Associate Scientist
Victoria Hospital Research Institute
Victoria Hospital
London, Ontario, Canada

Malcolm Fisher, M.B., Ch.B., M.D.
Head, Intensive Therapy Unit
Chairman, Management Committee
Royal North Shore Hospital
Sydney, Australia

Shawn Gilhuly, B.A., B.Comm., M.H.A.
Administrative Manager
Chatham Public Hospital
Chatham, Ontario, Canada

Alexander B. Horniman, M.B.A., D.B.A.
Professor of Business Administration
Darden School of Business
University of Virginia
Charlottesville, Virginia

Philip Jacobs, Ph.D.
Professor, Public Health Science
University of Alberta, Edmonton
Edmonton, Alberta, Canada

Thomas A. Massaro, M.D., Ph.D.
Professor of Pediatrics and Business Administration
Harrison Foundation Professor of Medicine and Law
University of Virginia
Associate Dean for Clinical Resources
Director of Medical Affairs
Attending Physician Pediatric Intensive Care Unit
University of Virginia Medical Center
Charlottesville, Virginia

David R. Massell, B.Sc., M.D.
Assistant Professor of Medicine
University of Western Ontario
Medical Director, Cardiac Care Unit
Victoria Hospital
London, Ontario, Canada

Brenda L. Morgan, R.N., CNCC(c), B.ScN(cand)
Nurse Educator
Critical Care Trauma Center
London Health Sciences Centre
London, Ontario, Canada

Tom Noseworthy, M.D., M.Sc., M.P.H.
Professor, Public Health Science
University of Alberta, Edmonton
Edmonton, Alberta, Canada

Deborah J. Nyman, M.B., B.S.
Department of Anesthesia and Critical Care Medicine
Hadassah Hebrew University Medical Center
Jerusalem, Israel

Joseph E. Parrillo, M.D.
Section of Critical Care Medicine
Section of Cardiology
Rush-Presbyterian-St. Luke's Medical Center
Chicago, Illinois

William J. Sibbald, M.D., FRCP, C.H.E.
Chief, Program in Critical Care
Professor, Department of Medicine
The University of Western Ontario
Coordinator, The Richard Ivey
Critical Care Trauma Center
London Health Sciences Centre
London, Ontario, Canada

Edward D. Sivak, M.D.
Chief, Division of Pulmonary and Critical Care
Professor of Medicine
State University of New York, Health Science Center
Syracuse, New York

Charles L. Sprung, M.D., J.D.
Professor of Medicine, Critical Care Medicine
The Hebrew University of Jerusalem
Director, Intensive Care Unit
Hadassah University Hospital
Jerusalem, Israel

W. Leigh Thompson, Ph.D., M.D., Sc.D.
Professor of Medicine
Indiana University
Indianapolis, Indiana
President and CEO
Profound Quality Resources
Charleston, South Carolina

Walter Wadlinton, A.B., L.L.B.
James Madison Professor of Law
University of Virginia Law School
Professor of Legal Medicine
University of Medical School
University of Virginia
Charlottesville, Virginia

Sandy Whittall, R.N., B.A., B.ScN., M.B.A.
Manager, Emergency Care Services & Adult Critical Care
London Health Sciences Centre
London, Ontario, Canada

Laurence G. Wolfson, B.A., M.H.Sc
Lecturer, Health Care Management
Faculty of Business Management
Fanshawe College
Coordinator, Community Services
Mental Health Care
London Health Sciences Centre
Victoria Hospital Corporation
London, Ontario, Canada

Jack E. Zimmerman, M.D.
Professor of Anesthesiology and Medicine
George Washington University
Co-Director, Intensive Care Unit
George Washington University Medical Center
Washington, D.C.

Preface

"Life is short, the art long, opportunity fleeting, experience treacherous, judgment difficult."

Hippocrates, *Aphorisms*

The question is: Was Hippocrates talking about, medicine or financial planning?

For Hippocrates, it was probably medicine. For today's health care professional, it might be both medicine and finance.

Financial issues in medicine are no longer segregated to be dealt with only by hospital administrators in administrative suites or accountants in business offices or secretaries at front desks. Today, every single health care worker must be involved in the economics of what he or she does. In addition, each person must understand the economic warnings implicit in Hippocrates' statement: opportunity is fleeting, experience can be treacherous, and judgments are always difficult.

As President and Chief Executive Officer of a medical college that has a tertiary care hospital as part of the institution, I have been distinctly conscious of the economic pressures pressing in from all sides. Many different levels of government funding must be maintained. Contributions to our Foundation must be solicited. Contracts with insurance companies and HMOs must be negotiated. Grant funding must be aggressively sought. The list goes on.

In this type of economically charged environment, the practice of medicine will be affected. Paradoxically, critical care medicine is one of the most expensive medical services in any hospital; yet before now it has been one of the least examined in economic terms. Drs. Sibbald and Massaro have done the profession a service in this volume by collecting articles by outstanding authors on the economics and business of critical care medicine. The authors contained herein have a truly international perspective and provide both clinical and managerial expertise to this critical issue.

The organization of *The Business of Critical Care* first provides an overview of the health care industry in terms of economics. It then moves to cover specific issues related to critical care treatment in the hospital setting. Few economic stones are left unturned including an especially important one from my perspective as an educator—the cost of educating students and residents in the ICU setting.

As a pulmonologist and critical care physician, I have spent my entire professional clinical life in the intensive care environment. I have witnessed tremendous medical advancements and now many more lives are being saved in ICUs. However, at what cost?

In an editorial I wrote on an article by Gyldmark in *Critical Care Medicine*, I pointed out that her review of nearly 20 years of ICU cost studies demonstrated that there is a major problem in the consistency and quality of ICU cost studies, which severely hampers quality research and economic planning. I concluded that clinicians and researchers in the field of critical care must be willing to adopt standardized approaches to cost accounting questions in ICUs and produce studies that are valid not only in and of themselves but in comparisons with other studies. We cannot move forward and understand costs and savings if we cannot first set basic standards for comparison.[1]

In a second editorial in *Critical Care Medicine*, I reviewed a fascinating study by Noseworthy and colleagues, which examined the economics of ICU patients in a large, urban Canadian hospital. This study examined all costs related to ICU patients and concluded that in order to develop strategies aimed at cost containment, it is first necessary to undertake a thorough examination of cost drivers. Based on this article, I offered five recommendations for the profession to achieve a balanced approach to economics in the ICU.

(1) Collect clinical and economic outcomes and ethical data.
(2) With professional societies, develop practice parameters based on the above data.
(3) Use that data to resist purely economic arguments to limit care.
(4) Also, use that same data and guidelines, when projected outcomes justify limiting care, to then proactively limit care.
(5) Continue—with a marked increase in emphasis—the health care workers' role as patient advocate.[2]

Using valuable information such as the information gathered in this volume, health care professionals can protect the integrity of the medical system in place while still reacting to the real and demanding social and economic issues of our society.

To my knowledge, Hippocrates never had to manage a patient in an intensive care unit. Yet, he still predicted what all of us health care professional must face in pursuing the art of medicine in the ICU: opportunity is fleeting, experience can be treacherous, and judgments are always difficult.

References

1. Bone RC: Editorial—Economic Analysis of the Intensive Care Unit: A Dilemma. *Crit Care Med* 1995;23:805.
2. Bone RC: Editorial—Medicine and Mephistopheles. *Crit Care Med* (In Press).

Contents

Chapter 1

An Introduction to the Business of Critical Care Medicine

William J. Sibbald, M.D., FRCP, CHE

The 1990s have been a time for radical change in health care delivery. The rapidity with which this change process emerged in the last decade has been challenging for health care providers and planners alike. The most important issue now facing health care is the struggle to maintain quality service in the face of declining revenues. At the same time, expectations are that health care utilization and costs will increase, since the population is aging, technology continues to expand treatment options, and society has high expectations of its health care systems. Thus, health care costs are significantly out of balance with existing revenues. In this climate, health planners remind us that the status quo is not acceptable and that change and change management are the operative philosophy in health care. Physicians and other health care providers who can't adapt or who are unwilling to change, are at risk of being excluded from the reorganized health care delivery system.

What are some of the more significant changes that have occurred

From: Sibbald WJ, Massaro T (eds.): The Business of Critical Care: A Textbook for Clinicians Who Manage Special Care Units. © Futura Publishing Co., Inc., Armonk, NY, 1996.

and will continue to symbolize health care for the immediate future? Prior to the 1980s, "health care leaders" analyzed, debated, and planned for our health care systems. Employing what has been referred to as a "medical model", health care provision principally reflected the treating of illness, generally by physicians who assumed the role as the patient's primary advocate. Throughout the 1980s, a different approach emerged, slowly at first, but one that is now fundamentally a part of health care planning and delivery. Increasingly, discussions on health care policy devolved to include broader public representation, defined as a "collective" or "stakeholder" process.[1,2] Health care stakeholders are all members of the public affected by specific health care policy. From the appointment of the public to discussion groups on health care planning, to the level of planning committees for regional restructuring, to the increasing involvement of the public on hospital boards, there is evidence for growing stakeholder participation in both the definition and operationalization of health policy. This expanding stakeholder involvement has paralleled emergence of the notion that health care should emphasize a "wellness" or preventative model, by a health care team that has expanded to include many professionals other than the physician. Nurse practitioners and allied health care workers are increasingly empowered by the regulatory authorities to participate in areas of the delivery of health care which was previously the domain of only the physician.

There have been other changes introduced into health care to manage the current economic pressures. With lessons from industry over the last three decades demonstrating that poor quality results in avoidable increases in costs, continuous quality improvement (CQI) has become an increasingly important feature of health care delivery. Here, the notion is that improving quality in health care will both reduce costs and improve outcomes.[3,4] The CQI philosophy is not difficult to understand—if we can establish systems to measure our current practice, we can then determine how well we are doing by comparison to "best practice" examples in health care. If comparison, the concept of benchmarking, shows the possibility of improvement, actions can then be instituted to create change and thereby improve the care process.

A good quality program now combines lessons from both industry and the health services research communities. Outcomes measurement is fundamental to CQI activities and uses aggregate databases with origin in the health services research community. Here, patient outcomes include functioning described by physiology, physical terms, mental or psychological terms, social terms, and other health related quality of life areas. *Process* improvement and organization-wide continual improvement are more industry based, therefore, relatively new to application in health care. Process improvement involves defining the set of activities that transform inputs (patients with health care needs, equipment, etc.) into outputs (including information, diagnoses, and treatment decisions) that are associated with outcomes realized by patients and others who are affected by the care.

At the same time that the CQI process evolved to help minimize the costs of health care, "down-sizing" of health programs has become a way of life for many of the traditional components of the health care system, particularly at the hospital level. In North America, an increasing emphasis is now placed on shifting health care utilization to the community, while rationalization and regionalization of hospital beds threatens the very existence of some hospitals. The end result of this process is a greater accountability for a patient's health care support at the family level. One wonders whether the quality evaluation process has been adequately built into these system wide changes, to determine if these actions are accomplished without diminishing care quality from the patient's perspective. Importantly, what about the cost effectiveness of this approach. The answer depends on the perspective one takes. From the hospital's perspective, early discharge to the care of the family clearly saves money. From society's perspective, however, this approach may not be the most cost effective because of the costs borne by the family for assuming responsibility for home care.

The need for fundamental change in health care delivery systems is driven by an economic imperative. The 1970s and early 1980s were a time of remarkable growth in the infrastructure of health care in most countries, as the various systems comprising health care delivery (the health care insurers, the pharmaceutical and medical device industry, medical schools, etc.) sought to provide the improvements in diagnosis and treatment that an expanding science had provided. However, when the impact of national debts on the economic planning models of most western countries assumed prominence in the 1990s, political leaders and health care planners agreed that the poorly planned (?uncontrolled) growth of health care in the 1980s must give way to a more fiscally responsible approach. It was quickly understood that more was being spent on caring for the sick than ever before, yet major gains in (quality) life expectancy were not easily demonstrable. The conclusion was unmistakable—the amount of a country's wealth spent on health care had to be indexed to a measure of annual economic performance, and more explicit expenditure targets were set.

"Managed care" in the United States, primarily through insurance carriers, was the result of a failed attempt by government to both control

Table 1

Reduce "Unnecessary" Spending
increase outcomes-based research
encourage practice guidelines
strategic planning in regionalized models
shift away from hospital-based care
strategic planning using regionalized models
Prevent Spending/Reduce Costs
close hospitals
reduce hospital budgets
exert more control over physician fees
limit physicians entering practice
reduce medical school enrolment
reduce/remove residency training positions
restrict MD immigration
reduce wages of health care workers
develop less expensive alternate care workers

health care costs and simultaneously expand health care delivery to the many in this society who were incompletely covered by existing private and public health insurance plans. At the same time, important characteristics of the managed care process emerged in health care jurisdictions where government traditionally underwrote health care costs through national health insurance plans. In Canada, for example, government instituted regionalization and rationalization programs. "Medically unnecessary" procedures were increasingly removed from the health insurance plans, as the "universal" coverage system was no longer affordable. A process of aggressive utilization review was introduced to reward hospitals who perform well in terms of cost effectiveness, while penalizing poor performing hospitals by reducing their global budgets. Other examples of strategies to control costs in health care are listed in Table 1.

This emphasis on health care costs is not unique to North America. In the United Kingdom, Europe, and many other countries, health care planners are facing the same issues—how to maintain quality care in the face of excess inflation in the health care sector and declining revenues for health care services delivery. Interestingly, however, the responsibility for the tough decisions required to reduce health care expenditures has been increasingly devolved to stakeholder groups as the primary insurers have attempted to insulate themselves from (politically difficult) front line decision making.

With such changes, and the economic imperative behind them, it is not surprising that successful health care providers are those now being schooled in more innovative business planning models. Successful health care leaders are learning the importance of combining a clinical background with experience and education in various management curricula. There are now professional organizations devoted solely to health care management, for example, The College of Physician Executive. Business schools are increasingly offering courses targeted to the health care professional who wishes more understanding of the business and management side of organized medicine. Even traditional medical societies are increasingly providing their members with curricula that deals with the business of medicine.

Health care professionals with an interest in health care management are now learning that there are three components of our health care systems: (1) the structure of the delivery system; (2) the operating processes within the system; and (3) the outcomes of health care delivery. They are also taught the importance of building an "evaluation" mechanism into any system developed to provide and improve care. Other "change terminology" has become an everyday component of the physicians' vocabulary. Our often cumbersome expressions of the past are now giving way to management jargon, for example, terms such as down-sizing (or is it right-sizing), managed care, regionalization and rationalization, generic health care providers, health care centers (rather than hospitals) . . . the list is endless! The delivery of health care has been and will continue to change and new skill sets are prerequisite for the physician to survive in this environment.

> "Change means movement. Movement means friction. Only in the frictionless vacuum of a non-existent abstract world can movement or change occur without that abrasive friction of conflict."[5]

Management and Critical Care

Critical care has been defined as "..a multidisciplinary field concerned with patients who have sustained, or are at risk of sustaining, acutely life-threatening, single or multiple organ systems failure due to disease or injury. Critical care seeks to provide for the needs of these patients through immediate and continuous observation and intervention so as to restore health and prevent complications."[6] Because of the recognized high cost of providing critical care services,[7] this hospital unit is particularly vulnerable to the changes in health care that are envisioned for the next decade.

Beginning in the 1950s when technology became available to provide assisted ventilation, the growth of critical care paralleled advances in technology that have permitted the support of patients with organ failure. In this context, critical care provides two unique services to its patients: (1) life-support, the use of specialized technology in patients with life-threatening single or multiple organ systems failure; and (2) monitoring of patients considered at high risk of developing a critical illness thereby, (hopefully) reducing the likelihood of such an adverse occurrence.

Critical care is now a significant component of the services provided by acute care hospitals. Understanding the nature and magnitude of change in critical care over the last decade is fundamental to understanding why health care costs are increasing. From a modest beginning, the hospital's intensive care unit (ICU) has grown into a substantial service with a concomitant and dramatic increase in both utilization and cost. Critical care resources are disproportionately utilized by our aging population, while new drugs and life-support technologies are expanding available treatment options for otherwise life-threatening conditions. An increasing acceptance of organ transplants makes this an increasingly used therapy and expanding treatment options for cardiovascular disease are further increasing utilization.

The financial impact of providing critical care services cannot be over emphasized. Crude estimates have placed the daily cost of ICU care from two to five times that required for care at the general ward level.[7] As much as one-third of a hospitals resources may be devoted to caring for critically ill or injured patients.[7] It is, however, arguable that the modern ICU, including most of its technology, has evolved without objective evidence of benefit to either the patient or society. Despite its resource intensity, few attempts have been made to evaluate the ICU, that is, to systematically link these costs with patient outcomes. However, opinion is that the modern ICU has at least three benefits: (1) a reduction in avoidable morbidity and mortality; (2) the saving and prolongation of lives of good quality; and (3) an increase in the patients' well-being. What is truth? Unfortunately, evidence is increasingly required to justify new and expanded programs and we are of the opinion that there is indeed little evidence documenting the efficacy of critical care units (CCUs). This is not to say that efficacy of the ICU doesn't exist, just that it hasn't been adequately demonstrated.

An increasing imbalance between the demand for health care services and the supply of health care resources will mean that the relatively unrestrained expansion of ICU services in the previous two decades will be impossible to sustain. As in health care generally, there are three possible responses to the growing imbalance between ICU care resources and costs.[8] First, hospitals aggressively analyze ways to increase their critical care revenue through both traditional and nontraditional revenue sources. Second, implicit rationing of health care services is increasingly used to deal with budget shortfalls, through the adoption of both rules and constraints.[9] Finally, considerable emphasis has been placed on identifying methods to achieve improved efficiency, presumably thereby to deliver better quality services at reduced costs.[10]

Because of its high expense, change will be particularly focused in the ICU. "It is time for a rigorous effort to establish what procedures produce beneficial outcomes under what conditions—and to eliminate stark instances of over-utilization."[11] Technology assessment and quality improvement are traditional ways to improve efficiencies. Health care technology has been defined as all of the instruments, equipment, drugs, and procedures used in health care delivery, as well as the organizations supporting delivery of such care.[8] The key to this definition is its scope. Not only are agents and devices considered technology, but also the programs we implement. Thus, a hospital's critical care services can be viewed as a distinct health care technology just as easily as a new drug or diagnostic test. Technology assessment is the process of designing and conducting investigations to evaluate and render judgment on the technology being assessed. The goal of health care technology assessments is to establish the criteria for efficacious, effective and efficient care of the patient. *Efficacy* studies are investigations that examine the probability of benefit to patients in a defined population from a medical technology applied for a given correctly diagnosed, medical problem under ideal conditions of use. These studies address the question of whether the technology can produce clinical improvements. *Effectiveness* evaluations examine the probability of benefit to individuals in a defined population from a medical technology applied for a given medical problem under average conditions of use. These investigations are far more pragmatic, asking whether the implementation of the technology does indeed result in clinical improvements.

CQI in the CCU is another means of reducing costs by improving efficiencies. It is the extraordinary costs in critical care that make this an ideal area to examine innovative methods to establish CQI as an ongoing hospital commitment. However, successful implementation of robust CQI programs in the ICU has been hampered by a number of issues, including inconsistent physician participation, failure to account for implementation costs, lack of appropriate data systems, and failure to return to success to the source unit. Particular frustration faced by critical care professionals interested in CQI is the lack of robust, available, and accessible databases that provide the necessary benchmarking information. One can be optimistic about the benefits of CQI, yet such optimism has not yet been transferred into real gains in the majority of ICUs.

What does this all mean to the critical care professional? With this rapid change in health care delivery comes uncertainty and fear. The traditional securities are jeopardized. Even the terminology has changed—patients are now clients, the physician is just one of a patient's many health care providers, the hospital is a health center, and choice means managed care. In this complex and changing environment, the critical care professional increasingly requires skills in business and management to ensure the resources necessary to provide good care. New knowledge and skills in business are required to successfully advocate for resources for the patient in health care systems increasingly driven by bottom line costs. The astute critical care professional needs to understand hospital budgeting, utilization review and management, and how to organize a teaching program and physician coverage schedules. Other skills increasingly required include how to participate and manage team building, how to assess medical technology, and how to manage ethical and legal issues relating to the care of the critically ill patient.

This text reviews some of the knowledge base behind the business skills we believe are required by critical care professionals in their daily activity, that may have been overlooked in their earlier training. Using a broad range of skill sets from both the traditional health sector and academic business faculties, our objective is to provide the practitioner with an introduction to the changing face of business in critical care. Our contributors have focused on the concept of managing . . . not only the management of change, but also the management of budgeting, planning, evaluations, research, and education, among other topics. We hope the reader will enjoy this text, which concerns the principles of the business of medicine that is increasingly are an important part of our professional lives. The modern ICU is a hospital resource with a high level of activity, expenditure, and risk exposure, thus, it is particularly vulnerable to the changes in health care envisioned over the next decade. Hopefully, some of the lessons in this chapter will prepare the professional with the skills required to help the ICU survive the uncertain future.

References

1. Agass M, Coulter A, Mant D, et al: Patient participation in general practice: who participates? Br J Gen Pract 1991;41:198–201.
2. Crawshaw R, Garland MJ, Hines B, et al: Oregon health decisions—an experiment with informed community consent. J Am Assoc 1985;254: 3213–3216.
3. Berwick DM: Continuous improvement as an ideal in health care. N Engl J Med 1989;320:53–56.
4. Ellwood P: Special report: Shattuck lecture. Outcomes Management 1988; 318:1549–1556.
5. Alinsky S: Rules for Radicals, "The Purpose". New York, Random House, 1971, p. 21.
6. Parillo JE, Ayres SM, eds: NIH Consensus Development Conference Statement on Critical Care Medicine. Baltimore, MD, Williams and Wilkins, 1984, pp. 277–289.
7. Berenson RA: Intensive care units (ICUs): clinical outcomes, costs, and decision making. Health Technology Case Study 28, Prepared for the Office of Technology Assessment.
8. Sibbald WJ, Inman KJ: Problems in assessing the technology of critical care medicine. Int J Technol Assess Health Care 1992;5:227–243.
9. Strauss MJ, LoGerfo JP, Yeltatzie JA, et al: Rationing of intensive care unit services. An everyday occurrence. JAMA 1986;255(9):1143.
10. Luce M: Improving the quality and utilization of critical care. Quality Review Board February, 1991;42–47.
11. Calisano JA. Health care chaos. New York Times Magazine 1988;44:44–48.

Chapter 2

From Clinician To Manager

Malcolm Fisher, M.B., Ch.B., M.D.

Medical treatment traditionally occurred in hospitals in a model similar to the armed services. The front line troops of doctors and nurses performed the tasks that were the raison d'etre of the organization, and the logistic support group provided the tools necessary for the task.

There were only four major deficiencies in this system: major decisions were often made very removed from the front line and without input from those who worked at the front line, there was a minimum of accountability for the actions of those at the front line, and the system was excessive and wasteful. The division lead to reduced appreciation of each other's problems. The major advantages were that people performed the tasks for which they were trained.

We have entered the era of accountability and rationing. Current thinking is that to improve the accountability of the medical profession, and, therefore, the efficiency of the health system and the value obtained in health care spending, the traditional lines of demarcation be-

From: Sibbald WJ, Massaro T (eds.): The Business of Critical Care: A Textbook for Clinicians Who Manage Special Care Units.

tween management and medicine must be dissolved. The advantages of this to health care workers is input at a higher level. The disadvantages are that it requires new skills and tasks for which the health care professional is untrained. The possibility of the Peter Principle is strong. The Peter Principle is that people rise in an organization until they reach a level where they are incompetent, and fail to progress further. The second disadvantage is that it takes people away from the tasks that they trained for and derive their job satisfaction from.

There is also a covert advantage to the controllers of finance. As rationing becomes a more prominent agenda item, the involvement of the clinician, whose traditional role is to do everything possible for the individual patient irrespective of cost, places the clinician in a position of being part of the rationing process rather than its antagonist.

If accountability and cost saving are the major goals of the changes in the role of clinician and manager there is probably a better way to do it, but we have not discovered that yet. There is no question in the 1990s however, that the traditional medical head of department, who achieved the position because of clinical skills and credibility, can no longer function effectively without acquiring some management skills. In an era of rapid change there are immense advantages in acquiring those skills at a more rapid rate than the traditional trial and error methods.

How Does One Learn To Be a Manager?

There are essentially three ways. The first is from the profusion of management texts that are available. An actual foray into such texts usually leaves the clinician convinced that all they describe is common sense, and to a degree this is true. The majority of such texts are related to industry, and there are serious questions regarding how well industrial models and practices relate to hospital practices; the only way to resolve such questions is to apply the principles and see if they work.

The second method is to attend courses, particularly those that are orientated towards health care. These have the obvious advantage of a health care focus, and a second advantage in that they enable discussion of the content with other clinicians.

The third is to visit top clinician managers and to seek advice and guidelines. Such people are best identified by asking colleagues who they admire as medical managers and best utilized by asking specific questions relating to problems in one's own department.

As with one's medical practice, the major factors in success are the institution of a continuing education program for oneself, utilizing all the available resources. In management, as in medicine, ideas, orientation, and the minutiae of processes change, but the basic principles remain constant. The goals of medical management are to have one's staff performing effectively and happily, to be efficient, to have quality outcomes, and to obtain the resources needed to perform all the above.

Getting Started

A Personal Job Description

The clinician who wishes to become an effective manager must first look hard and critically at one's own function and goals. The questions are simple: What do I want in terms of clinical practice and managerial practice? How much time am I to allocate to each? What are my immediate 5 and 10 year personal goals? These questions must be addressed prior to taking on the challenges of management. Devolving management to clinicians is usually not associated with increased costs as it is an additive task. Taking the responsibility for a large department without power, incentives, and administrative support, particularly financial, is to fall into a bureaucratic confidence trick. It is useful to think of departmental management as divided into punitive and incentive management models. In the *punitive* model, the clinician is required to run a department, produce results, and save money without the power or the ability to receive rewards for the effort. Some return of, or ability to use saved money, (and actually control the spending as well as the saving) leads to an *incentive* model that is essential in the achievement of true autonomy and satisfaction.

Time allocation is vital. The effective clinician manager becomes more and more in demand in the institution, and, therefore, runs the risk of compromising the clinical functions from whence came the credibility that made the clinician a desirable manager.

The Mission Statement (See Chapter 14)

This is the second important step. A mission statement defines the goals of your department and should cover customer focus, quality, and emphasize the department's strengths, in addition to the clinical goals.

The Strategic Plan (See Chapter 14)

This process enables the manager to define the goals. It involves identifying the strengths and weaknesses of the department, and outlining strategies to develop the strengths and resolve the weaknesses. The plan should be written to include a time frame and plan for resolution, and identification of the resources and help that are needed for resolution.

In determining the strategic plan, a modified "1-minute problem solver" is helpful. The problem is clearly defined at the top of an A4 sheet of paper. In the top half of the page, the reasons it is a problem are defined. On the bottom half of the page the potential solutions are listed. If a clear solution is not apparent by the bottom of the page the problem either cannot be solved now or cannot be solved without help. In the first instance it may be best to shelve the problem until changed circumstances return it to the agenda.

The key parameters, such as outcomes or staff turnover, in which progress will be measured, must be identified during strategic planning.

Leadership

The good manager is a leader. A credible leader increases the performance of the staff. In the health care system, clinical credibility is important in the staff's perception of the manager, and the importance of the concept of "management by walking around" is greater than that of industry. The manager needs to be in the department communicating with the staff, and needs to, through committee or working party, give the staff input to and a role in management. This emphasizes the worker as part of the team and allows the devolvement of tasks to others who gain skills, responsibility, and the ability to solve one's own and others' problems. This role of the leader in enabling the staff to achieve personal growth and development is vital for their job satisfaction and a low staff turnover. The manager who is regularly at the coal face an often identify changes that will have a cost impact prior to their appearing in budget reports.

The manager who is seen to have the interests of staff as a priority is also in a strong position to deal with mistakes and conflict. The manager has responsibility for the overall environment and the happiness of the work force, but must realize that he or she has a minimal capacity to deal with unhappy individuals. It is not unusual for such individuals to be unhappy in general, and to use the work place as a scapegoat for their failure to control their lives. One unhappy individual may take others with them and be extremely disruptive. Such people should have the effects of their disruptive behavior explained; be given an opportunity to speak; be offered an opportunity to receive help in rectifying the problem; and if resolution does not occur rapidly, be encouraged to seek alternative employment.

A credible leader can deal with mistakes without incurring the anger of the person responsible. The mistake and its actual or potential consequences should be outlined as soon as possible after the event without spectators or listeners. The person responsible is given an opportunity to respond and then the manager should make positive remarks about the person's value and worth to the department. The incident is then closed. Such interactions should be neither hostile, angry, nor aggressive. The manager's role is to restore the person's self esteem and confidence, not to make the person feel bad or guilty—most people do that for themselves.

Information is Power (See Chapter 8)

An effective manager must have an effective database that provides information about activities, workload, and outcomes. There will be other databases in a hospital measuring the department's activities and they are less likely to be accurate than a dedicated departmental one as they are instituted by people with minimal familiarity with the real activities of the department. The manager must understand the weaknesses and potential errors in all databases that cover the department's activities.

Ownership of the information must be controlled. It is a golden rule that people who request information regarding the department's activities do so because they cannot get it any other way and are unlikely to be requesting that information to find ways of giving you more resources. Carefully consider the request for hidden agendas and ask specifically what it is for. It may be better to suggest the information cannot be obtained in the immediate future so the threat goes away.

Saving Money

The effective manager will always have a potential saving up his or her sleeve. The important practical points about cost savings are that there is no point in saving money until those savings can be identified and a reward obtained, and that too many strategies should not be introduced at once. The demand from above will be for repeated savings efforts. A good example is in the reduction of laboratory tests. Unless the cost of the department's tests is identifiable, all a reduction will achieve is a cost saving in the department of the provider. Therefore, this is a potential saving to put on hold until it can be identified as a department saving.

Your Own Money

As budgetary restraints tighten, the acquisition of a substantial departmental fund is important so that growth and function can be maintained even when over budget on hospital allocations. There are many potential sources of revenue, including patients, relatives, industry, drug trials, training of people from industry, and public appeal. A strategy for such acquisition of wealth should be part of the strategic plan and people who can assist in this are sought and enlisted. To assist with this, and to obtain some protection if budget restraints threaten the department, relationships with the media should be established. The provision of material for news and stories in favorable times gives the unit a public profile and creates powerful media allies who will return favors in times of crises.

Manage Up: Lead Down

An important management principle of the 1990s is that those below a manager in the organization are led, involved, and given responsibility and the opportunity for career development. The major group that need to be managed are those above the manager in the organization. This involves a change in attitude by which this group are to add resources and implement the manager's solution to problems and initiative, not solve the problems themselves. Problems can be better identified and solved close to the work force.

Involvement In Processes

With the constraints of time allocation it is important to be involved in the greater activities of the hospital, to understand the processes, problems, and drivers of those who hold the money, assist them in their dilemmas to obtain good will, and to have some control over the department's future at a higher level.

It is important to choose wisely where one's activities are directed. Hospitals tend to have cumbersome and duplicated committee structures, partly to enable many people to participate and feel ownership. Such committees should be avoided. Committees should be selected as those that make decisions or have the capacity to influence the activities of the department. They can be delegated. Delegation of tasks to key department members enables protection of clinical time and allows other members to contribute and feel part of the process and able to influence their destiny.

Conclusion

Health workers need to acquire management skills to become effective, have some control of their destiny, and to ensure that bureaucracies are aware of the consequences of their financial dealings with patients. This has been a neglected part of medical teaching, that may in part have placed health care under threat from political manipulation of finances. Management is about people, money, efficiency, and efficacy. As clinicians turned managers, we have started late, and therefore must move rapidly.

Chapter 3

The Evolution of Scientific Medicine: Delivering Critical Care in a Humane and Cost Effective Manner

Stephen M. Ayres, M.D.

The newest medical specialty, critical care medicine, emerged during the last three decades of the twentieth century and represents a dramatic application of the scientific revolution that began more than a century ago. Not long ago, physicians watched helplessly as life hung in the balance between those forces promoting life and those leading to death. But at long last, the memorable portrait of the physician sitting at the bedside of a child through the long night, waiting for either recovery or death, became a historic memory. Step by labored step the drama unfolded and, at some moment in the very recent past, an extremely ill individual could be said to profit more by medical action than by medical inaction.

The promise of health care in the US has been fulfilled in large measure and the results would certainly have surprised those nineteenth century Victorians who debated the worth of science. Today, 71% of Americans can expect to live to the age of 70; only 32% could

---

From: Sibbald WJ, Massaro T (eds.): The Business of Critical Care: A Textbook for Clinicians Who Manage Special Care Units. © Futura Publishing Co., Inc., Armonk, NY, 1996.

reach that age in 1900; only 20% of those who lived through the first year of life in 1900 could expect to live to 70, while almost 70% of those who survive infancy will live to enjoy their seventies today.[1] Much of this improvement in health status can be attributed to the almost exponential growth of scientific knowledge, in general, and to the application of that knowledge to the maintenance of health and the treatment of disease. This increase in survivorship has been almost linear and was achieved for much of the century with little increase in cost. The acceleration of health costs began in the late 1960s as per capita total health expenditures in the US rose from $346 per American in 1970 to $2,124 in 1988[2] and more than $3,000 in 1991 (real dollars). It is projected to rise to more than $5,000 by the year 2000.

The Politics of Health Care Reform

A review of the socio-economic issues surrounding the practice of critical care medicine—one of the most costly and successful demonstrations of new medical technology—is particularly important at this time because of health care reform in the US. It seems likely that President Clinton's victory was, in part, due to his espousal of more radical changes in the way health care is delivered than his opponent. Health care has been an important public policy issue in many countries, but defied serious consideration in the US until 1991 when the debate finally reached the political boiling point with the unexpected election of Harris Wofford to a seat in the US senate. Wofford campaigned on the inability of the Bush administration to develop a coherent national health care policy and his selection sent a message to both presidential candidates. The presidential campaign of 1992 and the economic recovery plans of both major candidates revolved around the problems of the American health care system. The federal government hesitated to endorse the Canadian style global budget implicit in the Oregon proposal, perhaps, in part, because Democratic vice presidential candidate Al Gore had written an article disapproving of that approach.[3] Both candidates seemed anxious to blend a more informed marketplace with appropriate regulation of insurers and physicians. Their representatives converged on Paul Ellwood's living room in Jackson Hole, Wyoming to seek advice and to learn what middle ground might be found to derail the inflationary spiral of health care costs. Could "managed competition,"[4] they wondered, preserve the pluralistic American system and somehow contain the nation's insurers, hospitals, physicians, and a vast array of related entrepreneurs that some have compared to the baggage train that inevitably followed the armies of yesterday into combat?

President Clinton was warned that the American medical melange of public and private health coverage managed by hundreds of profitable insurance companies, which enriched health care professionals and the "medical arms establishment" while shielding most Americans from the true cost of health care, could not be easily corrected. Cosmetic or incremental change could easily lead to unexpected and undesirable consequences and supporters might collapse if the public became confused or frightened over major change. The worst fears of those committed to sound health reform were realized as the president presented a technically sound but politically unrealistic plan, and a hundred million dollar war chest ridiculed it mercilessly and made any chance of reform impossible.

Fear of special interests, including organized medicine, caused the president, the first lady, and their top advisors to adopt a technically "perfect" plan fashioned by political health policy gurus (or "wonks" as they became known). It was a risky choice because it delayed the political choices for over a year and played into the opposition's contention that it had been presented as a take it or leave it proposal.

The general public never had an opportunity to weigh alternative approaches to achieving universal coverage and cost containment. Persuasive commercials played up the effects of a more equitable distribution of health care costs among taxpayers and emphasized the strengths of the existing system without describing the confusing and choice depriving consequences of the existing managed care environment.

The President's goal was to provide health care coverage to all Americans and to reduce the average rate of growth of health care costs, which had averaged 10% per year for many years. His advisers believed that cost containment techniques could allow the one trillion dollars expected to be spent on health care in 1995 to be across the entire population with little more than a 10% increase in cost for the first year. Clinton had promised to veto any bill that did not deliver universal coverage and much of the press coverage dealt with whether he would keep his word. A numbers game ensued with critics wondering whether the plan would increase the number of insured Americans from 87% to 95% or higher, while the most significant issues were whether the most vulnerable of the public, the 60% of the uninsured who were below 200% of the poverty level, would receive immediate help. Providing subsidies for them would lead to 94% coverage. Beginning with women and children below 200% and the remainder below 100% would also be a reasonable beginning, especially if the public health system was improved and extended. Discussions of these options were rarely reported.

Influential health care theorists wondered whether Clinton would select the single-payer or Canadian-type system proposed in the Wellstone bill, the then centrist "managed competition" approach or the less radical plan based on health insurance reform and the development of voluntary purchasing consortium system for small businesses.

The heart of the Clinton plan was the creation of health care purchasing consortia (HIPCs) or alliances as they soon were renamed. All employees in companies with < 5,000 employees were required to participate in these state organized, consumer directed public trusts. These purchasing consortia had been discussed for many years and were the key element of the managed competition proposals. They collected similar insurance premiums from all of their subscribers but distributed them to a group of "accountable health plans" (AHPs) on the basis of the health status of the people they enrolled. Younger and healthier people would thus pay higher premiums than they had previously—a return to community rating—while the elderly would have to absorb the costs of maternal and child care for families during their reproductive years. The plans were "accountable" because they were required to report the outcomes of their treatments, the health of the people they served, and satisfaction to these people described. The plans were all expected to offer the same basic benefits so that plans could compete on the basis of covered benefits but not on quality or cost. Basic benefits packages typically provide preventive and primary care, medical and surgical services, and mental health and dental care. Individuals can purchase additional coverage if they wish. Only basic benefits would be subsidized for those below the poverty line. The abortion issue was raised frequently by special interest groups and the administration signaled that it would not permit the issue to obstruct acceptance of their plan. Reproductive health coverage for abortion and in vitro fertilization is included in many present day health insurance policies. The administration plan would probably have excluded them from the then basic package but made them available under a separately purchased insurance rider.

As contentious as the purchasing was the recommendation that health care costs for working Americans be funded by an employer tax or mandate. Seventy-four percent of all Americans are offered insurance through their place of work; 66% of workers enroll in these employer based plans and building on this base seemed less radical than other funding solutions such as an individual mandate or general tax. Many small businesses, however, cannot afford to provide health insurance so that 60% of employees in firms employing ten or less workers are uninsured. Opponents of the Clinton plan predicted the collapse of large numbers of small businesses with widespread loss of jobs. A detailed analysis of other funding approaches and attention to the plight of the small business employer with remedies such as folding health insurance and workers compensation into a single system was drowned out by a flood of partisan rhetoric. Small businesses have real problems and an attractive solution might have been a measured antiregulatory stance considering the impact of health insurance, workers compensation, EPA, OSHA, and taxes on the profitability of small business.

The proposal of budgetary restraint implemented through a national health board, which would deal mainly with the cost of health care, was opposed by many as the beginning of rationing and a form of socialized medicine. Budget restraints in the form of annual negotiation of insurance premium or capitation rates is widely practiced by the spectra of a national budget "cap" similar to those used for years by many other countries was an easy target for those opposed to the plan. While purchasing consortia, employer mandate, and global budgetary restraint were the key elements of the Clinton plan, the detailed and lengthy proposal also dealt with many other significant issues such as graduate medical education, support of research, and promotion of public health which had been neglected for years.

Alternates to the Administration Plan

The political battles that followed the introduction of the administration plan never led to adoption of a compromise proposal, even though a number of other plans were introduced for congressional consideration. Amazingly, all but the McDermott-Wellstone plan were based on managed competition. None of the legislative plans were as comprehensive as those of the president and most attempted insurance reform, administrative simplification, and malpractice reform.

Senator John Chaffe's (R-RI) had been a major supporter of health care reform for many years and his Health Equity and Access Reform Today plan was initially the only Republican offering. It called for managed competition and required states to establish purchasing alliances for employers with fewer than 100 employees. Employers were required to make group insurance available to all employees, without exclusions, but were not required to pay any of the cost. Individuals, however, would be required (individual mandate) to purchase insurance some time before 2005. Employers were explicitly required to maintain existing level of premium financing. Subsidies for the poor were to be phased-in but were initially limited to households with incomes below 90% of poverty and would be gradually broadened to families with incomes up to 240% of official poverty thresholds by 2000. Subscribers could select a standard or catastrophic benefits plan; an independent commission would be formed to design the standard benefits package. Care for the unemployed poor would be funded by restructuring Medicaid and limiting its growth. Deductibility would be limited to an average of the lower 50% of plans in area.

The last months of the 103rd Congress was mired in politics as Republicans determined that any health care plan would be viewed as a victory for the President. Once again, health care reform failed as special interests, particularly the insurance industry, convinced the public that the matter was too complex, a crisis did not exist, and any change would be unacceptably expensive. The mid-term election of 1994 swept Republicans into control of the House of Representatives and Senate and many believed that Clinton's support for health care reform was an important reason for their victory. Health care reform faces an uncertain future, but the increase in costs of federally supported programs like Medicare and Medicaid may force the congress to place health care reform on the table once again.

The Development and Control of High Technology

Physicians caring for seriously injured or ill people use a good deal of expensive equipment and this seemingly insatiable thirst for more and more technology has been cited by many as one of the major reasons for the rapid increase in health care costs. Change in the way care is given to these patients could be an early target for health care reformers because it is so expensive. Some observers have taken aim at medical research, and even suggested a moratorium on research in the mistaken belief that scientific advances inevitably increase health care costs. An important historical paradigm, however, demonstrates how science can and will decrease the cost of health care. Poliomyelitis was frequently fatal because of medullary involvement and the reality that the failure to breathe was synonymous with death. The introduction of the negative pressure whole body ventilator or "iron lung" by Drinker and McKhann in 1929 saved many lives, as communities acquired hardware and professional expertise. The first acute care units arose in Scandinavia in the early 1950s to centralize the use of these respirators and similar clusters of respirators arose in the US. The large number of respirators necessary was illustrated in a recent edition of the *Journal of the American Medical Association.*[5] It republished the article and added a striking photograph showing more than 50 iron lungs in a Los Angeles County hospital during a poliomyelitis epidemic in the 1950s. The economic problems of long-term care for ventilator dependent patients were frequently solved by sideshow techniques. Vans carrying a "man (or woman) in the iron lung" traveled from town to town and charged admission to wide-eyed youngsters and adults. Billions and billions of dollars would be necessary today for the care of these unfortunate patients, had not biomedical science developed and implemented effective immunization for the prevention of the disease.

Critical care, in its various forms, plays a central role in the access to medical care for millions of Americans who have experienced it, as well as for those who may, in their lifetime, depend upon it for the management of life-threatening injury or disease. Because it is a dramatic display of medical intervention at its best, critical care runs the risk of being viewed in terms that would conceptualize it as an end in itself. The truth is that it is part of a medical system that is expected to contribute its share of service for the welfare of the entire society. As part of the fabric of medical care, critical care has all of the strengths and weaknesses, and is subject to all of the criticisms and changes that characterize the health and medical effort in this last period of the twentieth century. Simply because the stakes and costs for this sort of care are so high, ill-considered changes could seriously damage the American health care effort, while carefully planned and rational changes in the way such care is delivered could improve the quality and decrease the cost of medical care, in general.

The Conflict Between Science and National Policy

Most governmental leaders and other non-scientists have always had difficulty in understanding how best to make science serve humankind rather than the reverse. This is no better observed than in the unschooled cry for rationing when the answer really lies in rational thought. Rationality, not rationing, should be the guidepost for the development of a sensible health care policy. The inability of the general public and its leaders to deal with the present day fruits and poisons of science may be better understood by briefly recalling past conflicts between science and culture. Culture during the Renaissance was, in the words of Matthew Arnold, the knowledge of "the best that has been thought and said in the world."[6] In other words, a classic education. The works of Copernicus (1543), Harvey (1628), Galileo (1604), and Newton (1687), long criticized by the Church, were generally ignored by the defenders of a classic education. Science seemed much too practical for educated men to consider, cried the humanists, who much preferred reflective theory to anything that smacked of action. The rift between scientists and non-scientists was off and running. University scholars did not believe that the physical sciences belonged in a curriculum aimed at producing educated men, even though men like Thomas Henry Huxley, the defender of Darwin, argued that "Science and Culture" should support each other and that "neither nations nor individuals will really advance, if their common outfit draws nothing from the stores of physical science."[6] Huxley's advice went unheeded and the gulf between scientists and non-scientists continued to widen as science moved onwards in a dizzying display of ever increasing knowledge. It persists to this day in many circles and was celebrated as a problem of "Two Cultures" in C.P. Snow's controversial 1959 Rede Lecture.[7]

Part of the problem in integrating science and public policy may be the difference in the way knowledge is acquired by the two branches of human thought. Scientific information seems to grow at an almost exponential and expanding rate, while the public response to such new information appears cyclic in nature. The cultural and societal response to news about human evolution, environmental contamination, or the appearance and spread of the human immunodeficiency virus is reserved, suspicious, and even downright hostile. In consequence, after periods of little change, cyclical sea-shifts in culture appear to occur as scientific theory is attacked by one group and defended by another. The ebb and flow of human history have been observed by many. Emerson[8] believed it to be due to the rivalry between conservatism and innovation. Henry Adams, the grandson of President John Quincy Adams,[9] thought that a 12-year cycle characterized by the centralization and diffusion of national energy described the historical evolution of the American republic. Arthur Schlesinger wrote in terms of 30-year cycles based on conflicts between "public purpose and private interests."[10] While the regularity, the timing, and the cause of social cycles is unclear, their existence seems certain. Adams was one of the first to recognize the rapid growth of scientific knowledge when he pointed out in 1904 that the coal output of the world had "doubled every 10 years between 1840 and 1900 in the form of utilizable power," and that scientific knowledge, in general, had increased at about the same rate. He proposed a "Law of Acceleration" and suggested that the "new American—the Child of incalculable coal-power, chemical power, electric power, and radiating energy, as well as new forces yet undetermined—must be sort of a God compared with any former creation of nature. At the rate of progress since 1800, every American who lived into the year 2000 would know how to control unlimited power."[11]

The Emergence of the Biomedical Sciences and Critical Care

Adam's century, the nineteenth century, began with the exsanguination by intentional bleeding of the first president of the US in a misguided effort to save his life and ended with the bedrock of biomedical science. Rene Laennec invented the stethoscope in 1816, Crawford Long developed anesthesia in 1843, Oliver Wendell Holmes identified the infectious nature of puerperal or childbirth fever in 1842, Charles Darwin wrote *The Origin of Species by Means of Natural Selection* in 1858, Louis Pasteur and Robert Koch discovered bacteria in the 1870s, and Wilhelm Conrad Roentgen pioneered the clinical use of radiation in 1895. In 1920, Banting and Best discovered insulin and in 1929, Werner Forssmann, experimenting upon himself, performed the first cardiac catheterization. In 1938 Fleming discovered penicillin. Penicillin became generally available in 1942; the cost for one million units was $200.00 and later decreased to $1.50. Modern medicine can be said to have begun in the 1940s, during the second World War.

The physiologic basis of critical care medicine began in the mid-nineteenth century. Adams spoke, of course, about the growth of the physical sciences and of the technology of engineering. He may not have known that at almost the same time hundreds of thousands were dying in the American Civil War, the great French physiologist, Claude Bernard, was formulating his idea that humans lived within a fluid matrix or "milieu interieur" and that "the constancy of the milieu interieur is the primary condition for free and independent life."[12] Flushed as he was with pride over the acceleration of physical science, Adams could not have known how the primitive state of the biologic sciences destined many of those who fell in battle in the great wars of his century to die of relatively insignificant injuries.

Seventy years after Bernard's formulation of the "milieu interieur", Walter B. Cannon, Professor of Physiology at Harvard, introduced the term "homeostasis" to describe the "coordinated physiological processes" that maintain a steady state for most systems. His studies into the "ways in which these self-regulatory agencies operate to preserve constancy of the fluid matrix" set the stage for the development of therapeutic methods aimed at promoting homeostasis. They form the basis for the pathophysiologic approach to serious illness and qualify Cannon to be called "The Father of Critical Care." His book, *The Wisdom of the Body*[13] told how he and his colleagues in France in 1917 found that a reduced blood pressure led to a decreased bicarbonate concentration (measured as the only available test, the CO_2 combining power). Fifty years before the widespread use of lactate measurements to estimate cellular oxygenation, his studies showed that "the alkali reserve rarely falls below normal . . . until the systolic pressure is less than 80 mmHg. Furthermore, just as in the experiments performed at Dijon, the greater the reduction of the blood pressure below that critical level, the greater is the fall in the alkali reserve." And 60 years before the concept of supply dependent oxygen consumption became widely discussed, his colleague, Aub, found that in experimental shock, basal metabolism (oxygen consumption) fell 18.5% and 33%, respectively, when the blood pressure was reduced to 70 and 60 mmHg.

Much of the present practice of critical care is rooted in experiences gained in the two World Wars, the Korean, and the Vietnam war. Wiggers et al.,[14] in a series of papers published between 1942 and 1945, showed that experimental bleeding of 4% of an animal's body weight produced irreversible shock if restoration of blood volume was delayed. At about the same time, Cournand et al.[15] studied human traumatic shock at Bellevue Hospital. They used right atrial catheterization to obtain mixed venous blood to calculate cardiac output by the Fick principle and established the principles that undergird modern hemodynamic monitoring.

Although Dandy had opened a small unit for postoperative neurosurgical patients at Johns Hopkins Hospital in 1927, Safar's special care unit at the Baltimore City Hospital in the 1950s was probably the first real "intensive care unit" (ICU).[16] The subsequent observation that resuscitation was possible only if a trained team of professionals, armed with endotracheal tube and defibrillator, arrived on the scene within several minutes, led to the emergence of the coronary care unit and institutionalized the involvement of internists in critical care units (CCUs). Proof of the importance of the critical care concept was the organization of the Society of Critical Care Medicine and the Association of Critical Care Nurses in 1971. By 1992 "virtually all acute care hospitals had at least one ICU" and Groeger et al.[17,18] were able to compile information on 32,850 ICU beds in 2,876 separate ICUs in 1,706 American hospitals.

The Cost of Critical Care

The cost of caring for extremely ill persons is high. The Office of Technology Assessments Study[19] reported that the total hospital costs for patients who spend any time in an ICU during hospitalization ranged from 28%–34% of total hospital costs. Parno et al.[20] carefully studied hospital charges and long-term survival in 558 ICU and 124 non-ICU patients admitted to a large community medical center in Massachusetts. The authors found that while 9.5% of total hospital admissions to the 950 bed general hospital required intensive care, those patients accounted for 30% of hospital charges. Only 14% of total hospital charges for this 9.5% of patients was related to care within the ICU itself. Hospital care in the US comprises close to 40% of all health care costs. Total health care cost in 1993 will be close to $900 billion and the cost of caring for the critically ill will be in excess of $100 billion. The National Institutes of Health, in response to soaring costs, held a Consensus Development Conference held in 1983 to study critical care outcomes, costs, and decision-making. It was published in 1984 by the US Office of Technology Assessment and emphasized the need to continually evaluate and improve the critical care "system."[21]

In pursuit of this goal, the Society of Critical Care Medicine has sought to study the actual delivery of critical care. Groeger et al.[17,18] studied the 4,233 of the total 6,837 American hospitals that were believed to have CCUs. A response rate of 38.7% enabled them to analyze activities in 2,876 separate ICUs in 1,706 hospitals and to obtain a "snapshot" of activities in a single working day. An idea of the ICU contribution to total health care costs was revealed by their observation that 98.8% of all ICUs provided ECG monitoring, 97.8% mechanical ventilation, 96% pulse oximeters, and 95.8% invasive arterial blood pressure monitoring. Average occupancy rate was 84% and 58% of the patients were over 65. While a substantial number of units were under utilized, an average of 11% of critical care patients were awaiting transfer to a lower level of care. The study also showed, not surprisingly, that about half of all patients in ICUs have one of three diagnoses: ischemic heart disease; respiratory failure; or admission for postoperative evaluation. It also documented problems in both access to care and cost. The study reveals a marvelous system of island-like units that can do a great deal for each patient but rarely refer to one another; < 10% of patients in an average unit are referred from another hospital. Were hospitals unwilling to transfer or did potential recipient hospitals erect barriers? The concept of networking seems foreign and suggests that other factors are at work in the unwillingness of physicians to transfer patients to other facilities.

Paul Ellwood, the physician-health care analyst whose home in Jackson Hole, Wyoming has become a Mecca for those involved in health care reform, coined the term "Outcomes Management" in his 1988 Shattuck Lecture:

> "Outcomes management is a technology of patient experience designed to help patients, payers, and providers make rational medical care-related choices based on better insight into the effects of these choices on the patient's life."[22]

Roper and colleagues[23] at the Health Care Financing Administration attempted to operationalize the Ellwood approach by describing an "effectiveness initiative." Traditionally, medical effectiveness measures the efficacy of medical interventions in actual practice, while medical appropriateness deals with the use of an intervention in a given clinical situation evaluation. Roper chose to collapse both terms and use the term "effectiveness" in a broad manner.

The Effectiveness of Critical Care

Recent studies have shown that the quality of critical care varies widely from hospital to hospital.[24] More than 15 years ago, Senator Abraham Ribicoff,[25] in an important essay entitled "The American Medical Machine" told of patients dying in ICUs because of clogged tracheostomy tubes or accidentally disconnected respirators. Engelhardt and Rie[26] described a $13 million court award to the survivors of a healthy 27-year-old trauma victim who was accidently disconnected from a respirator. The court, in reaching its verdict, was influenced by evidence that only three nurses were available for the care of seven patients, even though the patient required one-to-one nursing care. Neither a medical director nor an administrative policy dealing with census/staff relationships were in place.

Knaus et al.[24] retrospectively measured the severity of illness and mortality rates in 13 American hospitals. Mortality rates varied from 59%–158% of predicted. The authors suggested that those ICUs with the lowest death rates had certain important characteristics: they followed standard approaches or "protocols" and did not permit each physician to develop a completely unique treatment plan for each patient; a medical director with considerable authority for managing admission and discharge policies and for coordinating the care of individual physicians was present; a high level of educational achievement was present for critical care nurses; a strong collegial relationship existed between nurses and physicians. A prospective pilot project organized by the American Association of Critical Care Nurses[27] studied an ICU that demonstrated the same elements identified by Knaus et al.[24] The mortality rate for 192 patients was 51% of predicted. New complications were not observed and both staff and patient satisfaction was high. The ability of specially trained critical care physicians to lower mortality rates in ICUs was shown by two recent studies. Reynolds et al.[28] reported that the mortality from septic shock decreased from 74% to 23% when specially trained physicians supervised care. Brown and Sullivan[29] found a 52% decrease in ICU deaths when a full time critical care specialist was recruited and coordinated the care of the patient's physician.

The Effective and Appropriate Practice of Critical Care

On November 13 and 14, 1989, The Foundation for Critical Care sponsored a forum, *Critical Care in the United States: An Agenda for the 1990's*. Close to 40 people from a wide variety of backgrounds participated in eight small group sessions and a final summary conference used computed based methodology to develop a group consensus. Thirty-one percent of the participants were physicians, 17% nurses, 24% hospital administrators and policymakers, and 28% were in none of these categories, but included individuals with broad interests in health matters such as economics, health insurance, or consumerism. The groups were first challenged to define "quality critical care" and then to identify the problems that might prevent delivering that care to the critically ill and injured. The Forum concluded that substantial major improvements in life expectancy and enhanced quality of life for all Americans could be achieved without incurring substantial additional costs if the access to critical care and the management of the critically ill or injured patient were better organized.

Access to Care

The attendees concluded that rapid access to hospital emergency rooms and ICUs is vital, since there is good evidence that the greatest likelihood for survival after critical illness or injury occurs when an individual promptly receives care appropriate for the specific clinical situation.[30] The "strategic arms race between hospitals" as one participant in the Forum put it, has prevented the rational development of a system providing universal access to critical care. Most hospitals without CCUs, or those with units unable to care for the sickest patients, are not integrated into a transportation network. An individual with a life-threatening illness in a rural setting probably would not survive in certain situations. An individual in a large urban area might also fail to survive a potentially survivable situation since, in most cities, the individual would be taken to the closest hospital, whether or not that hospital had emergency facilities appropriate to the individual's needs. Disincentives for the immediate transportation of patients to hospitals able to care for their problems include financial incentives for referral of insured patients, the desire of physicians for certain types of patients, and the inability of boards of trustees to represent societal rather than individual hospital concerns. Hospitals frequently refuse to care for patients without insurance, even though they report extremely high profit margins. *Virginia Business*[31] reported, for example, that a local hospital associated with a national for-profit network posted a 105% return on equity while limiting its uninsured patients to 0.1%; a nearby Catholic hospital, in contrast, earned 9.4% on its equity and saw 15 times as many charity patients as the for-profit hospital. The federal government is opposed to "dumping" and cost shifting but appears to tolerate both.

Similar levels of prehospital care should be available to all Americans. There seems to be no rational explanation for the presence of well trained paramedics in one geographic location but not in another. Standards exist for paramedic training in some states but not in others. Since the states vary widely in their commitment to the support of social services, minimal federal guidelines for training and certification should be developed. The cost of an integrated hospital transportation system would pay for itself because inappropriate or delayed care is itself extremely expensive. The costs of a patient languishing in a coma for months following serious injury could probably pay for one or two ambulances! An untapped resource for prehospital care exists in the many fire departments throughout the US. Firemen and women make ideal paramedics and should receive such training and certification.

Improving Effectiveness

There is evidence that the process or manner of providing critical care is an important determinant of survival.[24,27] The level of collaboration between physicians and nurses and the organization of human resources, rather than the technical capability of individual practitioners, seems to determine outcome. The better the management of human resources, the better the outcome, independent of resources. On-site physician and nurse leaders ensure that patient needs are matched in the availability of resources by the implementations of sound admission and discharge policies. Effective clinical managers triage patients and attempt to resolve conflict among health practitioners, particularly among physicians. In many units, physician managers are managers in name only and do not triage, make decisions, or resolve conflicts. Nurses are forced, in the absence of a working medical director, to make moment-to-moment decisions that determine patient outcome. A collaborative nurse-physician relationship usually suggests that physician leadership is present within the units on a reliable and regular basis. The most successful units seem to carefully utilize nurse resources. Clerical tasks, such as seeking laboratory reports, managing patient records, certain housekeeping tasks, and making a variety of phone calls, are performed by individuals other than nurses.

The Forum suggested that physician behavior is widely regarded as reducing the efficiency of a hospital and its ICU. While hospitals have elaborate nursing hierarchies, the physician governance structure is incomplete. There is a political difficulty in encouraging physicians who admit patients to ICUs to view them as communal resources that should be managed rationally and for the entire community, not for the individual patients. Financial disincentives influence physician behavior. Surgeons want immediate access to operating rooms and critical care beds for elective surgery so that patients do not seek care in other facilities or with other surgeons. Competition among physicians is a serious health care issue. Many players in the American health care system act only for their own self-interest. As a result, many patients in CCUs today can be safely discharged to other hospital units while others urgently needing admission are denied access.

Improving Appropriateness

Understanding the type of patients admitted to ICUs is important, since the costs generated by individual patients vary widely. Postoperative patients fill many ICU beds17,18 but frequently consume substantially less resources than do other ICU patients. A small group of patients with limited prognosis account for more than half the total costs in some units but, although Zimmerman et al.[32] found that most patients with DNR orders actually die in ICUs, it is frequently difficult to determine the optimal unit occupant in advance. Step-down units for patients who require less than the usual ICU care are necessary for patients who are either recovering from critical care or those who are too ill to benefit from critical care. Step-down units are frequently not appropriately reimbursed so that hospitals tend to keep patients in ICUs for longer periods of time than necessary. Regionalization of units optimize quality and cost but has not worked well in the US because of patient and physician preference, hospital competitiveness, territoriality, and the prestige associated with offering high-technology care. Indeed, many hospitals willingly lose money on certain services viewing them as "loss leaders."

CCUs constantly face the problem of caring for patients with little chance of survival. While the autonomy of patients and their surrogates in making medical decisions must be respected, physicians must not shirk their own responsibility to make difficult medical decisions. Questions over what constitutes "futile care" must be strongly influenced by the professional staff. Futile care extends beyond whether immediate physiologic improvements can be achieved. Treatment is also futile if it cannot alter the underlying disease state or significantly improve the patient's condition or prognosis.[33] While age is sometimes important in determining the appropriateness of care, recent studies have shown that age alone is not a major determinant of the outcome of critical care.[34] Conflicts over the refusal of the physician to deliver what he or she believes to be futile care on the one hand, or to participate in assisted suicide on the other hand, are increasing and trouble health professionals in most ICUs. Howard Brody's most useful comment that:

> "We cannot resolve these moral tensions by making one side of the tension disappear. Instead we must learn to live with these tensions within a pluralistic society. This requires more reliance on negotiation, compromise, and practical reasoning, and less on abstract ethical theory."[35]

The writing of "do not resuscitate" orders or the termination of life sustaining treatment systems does not mean the discontinuation of all care. Life sustaining measures must give way to care aimed at easing the dying process. There are no intrinsic differences between categories of treatment such as CPR, ventilatory support, vasopressors, insulin, antibiotics, and the provision of hydration and nutrition by artificial means in terms of decisions to withhold or withdraw therapies. There is an important difference between active euthanasia and relief of pain and suffering. If narcotics are not supplied in sufficient quantities, the ICU can become a "torture" chamber. Important from a philosophic and theological standpoint is the "intent" of using narcotics. The dose necessary to control pain and relieve suffering is usually not lethal, but the patient should use whatever dose is necessary in order to remain comfortable. The legal principle has been called the "double effect." The intent of the narcotic dosage is to control pain; the death of the patient, if it occurs, is an unintended "double effect." Spending time with the dying patient is as important as the use of drugs. Reimbursement policies do not compensate for the time spent in talking with patients. The suffering associated with the dying process may be better eased by the presence of supportive family and health professionals than by the use of drugs. Obviously, the family must be able to visit at all times and participate in the care of their loved ones.

How to Improve the Delivery of Critical Care

The Forum attendees believed that a significantly better critical care system could be achieved without substantial increase in cost. Such a system would require the rationalization of care and its linkage to reimbursement. All agreed that the delivery of health care in the US today is excessively expensive because of the lack of a national health policy. Reimbursement policies, fear of litigation, and physician behavior are the major reasons for the inability to match patient need with hospital resource.

Fear of litigation is cited as a major reason for failing to develop rational admission and discharge policies. Hospital administration and its legal counsel are frequently extremely conservative and tend to act more in the hospital's interest rather than in the interest of the individual patient. While the physician is motivated by the needs of each patient and the physician's own self-interest, hospitals tend to give priority to the hospital's self-interest, setting up an intense dialectic that contributes to high cost and less than ideal quality of care. The participants did not know of an instance where a successful malpractice action had been sustained for either discontinuation of futile treatment, or for transfer of a patient from an ICU, although a lawsuit was made against an ICU which was so overcrowded and understaffed that a patient, who was believed to have a good chance of survival, died from accidental disconnection of a ventilator.[26]

Current reimbursement policies foster the misuse of care and fail to provide care for those most in need. The closing of trauma programs and the opening of multiple open heart surgical programs is an example of reimbursement driving resource development. The disease related grouping for cardiac surgery is quite lucrative and many hospitals prefer to care for an insured cardiac surgical patient rather than a penniless gunshot wound victim. The consequence of these misplaced incentives is revealed in the study of Groeger et al.[17,18] While there were 145 cardiothoracic units and 54 burn units in the "surgical" category, there were only 17 trauma units. Is this the optimal number of trauma units actually required or could the issue of payer mix have influenced the decisions of hospitals to pick cardiac or burn centers over trauma units? The physician payment system provides perverse incentives for the performance of procedures rather than for the delivery of organized and effective care. In addition, some hospitals and physicians attempt to maximize revenues by breaking down charges into a group of separate charges (unbundling).

The Impact of Health Care Reform on the Delivery of Critical Care

Even though systematic health care reform in the US failed, the American health care system continues to undergo massive change as market forces are unleashed and fortunes are made by managed care entrepreneurs. The raw power of unbridled capitalism has already led to considerable frustration among practitioners and the general public and provides an informative glimpse at two competing approaches to health care delivery.

The two quite different approaches, the regulatory approach and the free market approach, are presently under consideration. Either approach requires substantial political courage and may test whether the country is ready to tackle a problem that has been ignored for decades. Kenneth Thorpe, a professor of health policy and administration at the University of North Carolina and now a member of the Clinton health care team, has outlined requirements of the two models.[36] The regulatory model requires: (1) the definition of a legal body to determine how to structure a global health care budget that holds spending growth to that of general inflation; (2) introduction of national fee schedules, capitation rates, or physician salaries; (3) control of $266 billion in costs related to the pharmaceutical and other health care industries; (4) regulation of balance billing; and (5) regulation of technological innovation. The market oriented approach attempts to make consumers knowledgeable and cost conscious purchasers of health care. It would require: (1) restriction of the federal tax deduction subsidy; (2) that everyone purchase health insurance with public subsidy for the purchase of insurance for low-income individuals and families; (3) regulation of the health insurance market by the federal government; and (4) enrollment of all health providers and consumers into competing organizations or plans.

Since the US is racing down the pathway of ever more intrusive managed care while other countries are adopting many of its tenets, intensivists must fall back on their well honed experiences with carefully managed ICUs.

The Competitively Managed CCU

The organizational problems in American CCUs described above and their high cost make them targets for change under either model of reform. Care in ICUs should be managed by physician and nurse leaders who must make certain that unit resources are allocated in the most efficient ways possible. The large employers and public sponsors envisioned in the model of *Managed Competition* envisioned by Enthoven and Kronick[4] could support systems for critically ill and injured patients that would facilitate their rapid transport to tertiary or level III CCUs. Patient access and disposition would be closely guided by admission and discharge criteria and care stratified by admission to units able to provide appropriate levels of care.

Care for individual patients must be governed by protocols tailored to individual patient needs. Intensivists might profitably follow the approach recommended by the American College of Physicians in their health care reform plan. They proposed a sequential process asking three questions of increasing specificity to determine effectiveness: (1) Is a service medically effective? (2) Is the service medically appropriate for a particular group of patients or set of clinical circumstances? and (3) Is the service appropriate and of value to a particular patient?[37] Patients within each unit must be assigned some sort of severity score so that "outcomes management" can become an organizing principle for the unit. Outcomes information should be used to develop and continually refine guidelines and protocols that assist medical decision-making. Outcome evaluations should be tabulated, published, and used as case material for regular conferences that are managed and attended by physicians, nurses, and other health professionals such as physical and respiratory therapists who are in regular attendance in the unit.

Both cost containment and quality care could be enhanced by allowing only physicians trained and experienced in caring for seriously ill patients to care for patients in the ICU, much like the obvious requirement that only trained and experienced surgeons should work in the operating room. This view is supported by a recent study showing that 61% of physicians "were unable to recognize or respond appropriately to a blood gas analysis consistent with arterial cannulation" while 47% were "unable to determine the pulmonary capillary wedge pressure from a clear tracing.[38] A close relationship between ICU specialists and generalist physicians must be established. Both should serve as care coordinators of a reformed system and the generalist must be encouraged to informally follow patients while in the ICU. The generalist can help ICU physicians understand the patient's bio-psycho-social background and values that may influence personal health care decisions. The personal physician can also help the patient and family prepare for continued care following discharge from the ICU and help to decide the necessary medical follow-up care, both in the hospital and after discharge. Nursing staff must be highly trained in critical care and encouraged to work collaboratively with the medical staff and specialty consultants in the ICU.

Appendix

Members of the Foundation for Critical Care Forum were: NS Abramson MD, CJ Armstrong JD, SM Ayres MD, HJ Bachofer, HR Champion MD, HE Chappelear, RE Cranford MD, LJ Dugas Jr, SA Evans RN, H Falck, MSW, PhD, IA Fein MD, AR Fleischman MD, LF Rossiter PhD, R Forssmann-Falck MD, DM Grandstrom RN, BSN, CCRN, M Grant MD, DPH, AN Grenvik MD, PhD, P Holbrook MD, SM Houghland MPA, DL Jackson MD, PhD, PD Jeffrey, RW Landen, H Masur MD, LB McKnew JD, AV Mehling, K Morrison BBA, MBA, CE Perez MBA, P.EMT, HD Reines MD, RA Rettig PhD, C Rushton RN, MSN, L Searle RN, NJ Shoemaker RN, MN, MA Strosberg PhD, DD Trunkey MD, ED Viner MD, SK White RN, MN, CCRN, CE Windsor, and SJ Youngner MD.

References

1. Vital Statistics of the United States, 1988, Life Tables. Washington, DC, National Center for Health Statistics, Washington, D.C. March, 1991, p. 12.
2. Levit K, Lazenby H, Letsch S, et al: National Health Spending 1989. Health Affairs 1991;10:119.
3. Gore A, Jr: Oregon's Bold Mistake. Academic Medicine 1990;65:64–65.
4. Enthoven AC, Kronick R: Universal health insurance through incentives reform. JAMA 1991;265:2532–2536.
5. Drinker P, McKhann C: The use of a new apparatus for the prolonged administration of artificial respiration. I. A fatal case of poliomyelitis. JAMA 1929;92:1658. Reprinted JAMA 1986;255:1743.
6. Huxley TH: Science and Culture (1880), in Science and Education. New York, American Home Library Co., 1902.
7. Snow CP: The Two Cultures. New York, New American Library, 1964.
8. Emerson RW: The Conservative (1841), Essays and Lectures. New York, The Library of America, 1983.
9. Adams H: History of the United States of America During the Administration of Thomas Jefferson and James Madison (1891). Prentice-Hall, 1963.
10. Schlesinger AM Jr: The Cycles of American History. Ch. 2. Boston, Houghton Mifflin Co., 1986.
11. Adams H: The Education of Henry Adams. Ch. 34. Boston, MA, Massachusetts Historical Society, 1918.
12. Bernard C: Lectures on the phenomena of life common to animals and plants. Bailliere, Paris, 1878; transl. by Hoff HE, Guillemin R, Guillemin L, pg 84: American Lecture Series, Charles C Thomas, Springfield, Ill, 1930.
13. Cannon W: The Wisdom of the Body. Ch. 1. New York, Norton & Co, 1932.
14. Wiggers CA: Physiology of Shock. Ch. 51. New York, The Commonwealth Fund, 1950.
15. Cournand A, Riley RL, Bradley SE, et al: Studies of the circulation in clinical shock. Surgery 1943;13:964–995.
16. Safar P, DeKornfeld T, Pearson J, et al: Intensive care unit. Anesthesia 1961; 16:275–284.
17. Groeger JS, Strosberg M, Halpern N, et al: Descriptive analysis of critical care units in the United States. Crit Care Med 1992;20:846–863.
18. Groeger JS, Guntupalli KK, Strosberg M, et al: Descriptive analysis of critical care units in the United states: Patient characteristics and intensive care utilization. January 1993.
19. Berenson RA. Office of Technology Assessment, United States Congress: Intensive care units (ICUs): clinical outcomes, costs and decision-making, November 1984.
20. Parno RP, Teres D, Lemeshow S, et al: Hospital charges and long-term survival of ICU versus non-ICU patients. Crit Care Med 1982;10:569–574.
21. Parillo JE, Ayres SM, eds: Major Issues in Critical Care Medicine Consensus Conference. Baltimore, Williams & Wilkins Co., 1984.
22. Ellwood PM: Shattuck Lecture-Outcomes management: A technology of patient experience. N Engl J Med 1988;318:1549–1556.
23. Roper WL, Winkenwerder W, Hackbarth JD, et al: Effectiveness in health

care: An initiative to evaluate and improve medical practice. N Engl J Med 1988;319:1197–1202.

24. Knaus WA, Draper EA, Wagner DP: An evaluation of outcome from intensive care in major medical centers. Ann Intern Med 1986;104:410.
25. Ribicoff A: The American Medical Machine. New York, Saturday Review Press, 1972.
26. Engelhardt HT, Rie MA: Intensive care units, scarce resources, and conflicting principles of justice. JAMA 1986;255–1164.
27. Mitchell PH, Armstrong SA, Simpson TF, et al: American Association of Critical-Care Nurses demonstration project: Profile of excellence in critical care nursing. Heart and Lung 1989;18:219–237.
28. Reynolds HN, Haupt MT, Thill-Baharozian MC, et al: Impact of critical care physician staffing on patients with septic shock in a university hospital medical intensive care unit. JAMA 1988;252:2023–2027.
29. Brown JJ, Sullivan G: Effect on ICU mortality of a full-time critical care specialist. Chest 1989;96:127–129.
30. Trunkey DD: Trauma. Scientific American 1983;249:28–35.
31. Bacon JA: Move over Florence Nightingale. Virginia Business May 1990; 76–88.
32. Zimmerman JE, Knaus WA, Sharpe SM, et al: The use and implications of do not resuscitate orders in intensive care units. JAMA 1986;255:351–356.
33. Youngner SJ: Who defines futility. JAMA 1988;260:2094–2096.
34. Chelluri L, Pinsky MR, Grenvik ANA: Outcomes of intensive care of the "oldest-old" critically ill patients. Crit Care Med 1992;20:757–761.
35. Brody H: Assisted death: A compassionate response to a medical failure. N Engl J Med 1992;327:1384–1388.
36. Thorpe KE: Cost containment and national health care reform. In Brecher C (ed): Implementation Issues and National Health Care Reform. (conference proceedings) New York, NY, Josiah Macey, Jr. Foundation, 1992, pp. 77–100.
37. Scott HD, Shapiro HB: Universal insurance for American health care: A proposal of the American College of Physicians. Ann Intern Med 1992;117: 511–519.
38. Iberti TJ, Fischer EP, Leibowitz AB, et al: A multicenter study of physicians knowledge of the pulmonary artery catheter. JAMA 1990;264:2928–2932.

Chapter 4

Understanding and Managing Change in Critical Care Medicine

Thomas A. Massaro, M.D., Ph.D.

Intensive care units (ICUs) are committed to managing clinical change. Most people who gravitate toward ICUs enjoy the pace and the sense of accomplishment that comes from working in an active, rapidly changing environment. Although improvements we introduce and champion are the most satisfying, a full discussion of the management of change must include situations where the changes are being imposed from the outside without endorsement or consent. Unfortunately for medicine in general, and for critical care units (CCUs) in particular, this is the prevailing situation today; most special care directors are forced to manage in a reactive or defensive mode in contrast to the proactive or growth mode of the past. Table 1 provides an outline of the evolutionary process through which we are moving. We are changing from a world where a solo practitioner was dominant to one where care is delivered in a network by large groups of physicians and other caregivers. Although networks are generally larger than the groups we

From: Sibbald WJ, Massaro T (eds.): The Business of Critical Care: A Textbook for Clinicians Who Manage Special Care Units. © Futura Publishing Co., Inc., Armonk, NY, 1996.

Table 1
Health Care Evolution

Conceptual Model	Financial Focus	Provider Structure
Autonomy	Elements of Care	Individual Practitioner
Assessment and Accountability	Episodes of Care	Group Practice, PHO
Risk Sharing	Covered Lives	Network

are familiar with, the approach does not present a conceptual problem for intensivists because, as has been discussed earlier, critical care medicine has been at the forefront of team based practice. But we may encounter problems with the risk sharing aspects of the new world. ICUs by their nature deal with higher than normal risk situations.

Table 2 outlines some of the transitions that are occurring in our environment as part of the evolution outlined in Table 1. The two changes most significant for the intensive care community are the concern over the expansion of high technology and the pressures to keep as many patients as possible out of the hands of specialists and special units. Virtually every industrialized country in the world is examining its level of commitment to high-technology medicine. ICUs are clearly involved in that reevaluation. We may argue that as generalists for the sickest patients, intensivists working in appropriately staffed units provide more cost effective care than multiple specialists operating without integration. However, we are not well equipped to demonstrate that scientifically with meaningful outcome data. Thus, unless we become quite proactive in telling our story, we will likely be viewed by society as just another group of specialists and an expensive one at that.

In this environment, the capacity for understanding and managing change is an important strategic asset. This chapter examines the change

Table 2
Reordering of Priorities

New Priorities	Old Priorities
Outpatient Care	Inpatient Services
Capital Investment	Growth of Personnel
Generalists	Specialists
Technology Control	Technology Expansion

process, how it is perceived, why it is often resisted, and finally, offers suggestions regarding how ICU managers can be most effective in the often difficult situations in which they find themselves.

Elements of Change

There are at least three levels of the change process that a manager must consider. At the highest or most global level there are environmental factors that reflect the external realities of the situation. This includes the market forces, competitive demands, government regulation, and technology advances that influence the organization. In most circumstances these pressures may originate and remain outside of the manager's sphere of influence. However, to be successful in the management of change, even if one cannot control one's environment completely, the rational manager should have a vision or mental model of the external environment and the direction in which it is going. A sophisticated manager should be able to test various options or solution alternatives against that vision.

The next level of change includes those organizational issues that limit or determine the institutional responses. The effective manager has some limited control over these factors that include the allocation of resources available; the leadership characteristics of the senior executives involved; and the governance or decision-making processes. To complement their vision of the external environment, change managers also need a mental model of their own organization with its strengths and weaknesses in order to persevere.

The final level of change management represents those individual behaviors over which managers presumably have the greatest control, i.e., the planning process, implementation schedule, and follow-through capabilities. However, the manager's options and ultimate potential can be limited due to resistance of the individuals involved, especially because of their personal responses to the initiatives. Thus, in the final analysis, change management becomes another case of people management, complicated at times by the negative or adverse perceptions associated with the direction in which the change proceeds.

In a dynamic world, a manager has the option of accepting the changes imposed from the outside, i.e., acting upon attempts to channel and, when possible, control the change processes. Fundamental to influencing the change process is understanding where you would like to be. To be effective, one must have a sense of direction. Many people find it convenient to develop that sense through a Strengths-Weaknesses-Opportunities-Threats (SWOT) analysis. Issues and ideas are arranged in the four categories according to whether they are positive or negative, optimistic or pessimistic. This process can be very insightful, and when done in a group (either the entire caregiving team or a representative group of clinical leadership), can be an important aspect of development of the shared vision, which is key to managing change in a team oriented organization. From the SWOT analysis, one can develop a set of long-term goals and strategies, usually defined in shorter-term measurable objectives. Each of these objectives should have measurable (quantifiable when possible) outcomes and an associated timetable that can be followed. Tasks and responsibilities should be defined and recognized. Successes should be documented and celebrated.

Assumptions and Perceptions

Change is a modification of behaviors or thought processes that occurs as a result of new information or an increased understanding of existing information. We process and integrate new information by relating it to our perception of existing reality. Our reality, in turn, is defined by our experiences and by the intellectual framework that integrates our experiences into a coherent world view. This framework is derived from the set of assumptions or paradigms we hold. These provide mental models of our external reality, against which new information can be tested. Developing, modifying, and accepting mental models of both the external environment and the internal organizational structure is a major part of the role of a manager. The phrase "reality testing" indicates a comparison between new input and the existing mental models that we believe to be true.

The structure and, at times, the rigidity of our beliefs operate as filters that influence how we interpret new information. We always perceive our world through our assumption filters. The process may lead to an incomplete or very inaccurate view of the external reality. "Seeing the world through rose-colored glasses" suggests a filtering that provides at the minimum an incomplete and, at worst, an inaccurate view of the external reality.

There are different levels of assumptions. Operational assumptions influence our daily practices and provide guidance for routine functioning. At a second or deeper level are the structural concepts that help organize our operational assumptions. At the deepest level we have a set of core values that reflect what is fundamental to our interpretation of reality.

The change process can impact directly on our assumption sets. When it challenges structural concepts or core values it can be an especially painful one. Learning, the process of accepting change, requires that our assumptions be modified. As we learn, we add to our assumption sets, but simultaneously we may also replace previously held assumptions or beliefs. The loyalty or commitment to the ideas that are being superseded in a learning situation often manifests itself as resistance to the new idea or behavior. The strength of the resistance reflects the intensity of belief in the challenged assumption, that is directly proportional to the time, energy, and significance of the assumption to our personal and professional identity.

When the assumptions at the core values level are challenged, there is a deep sense of loss. Both individuals and institutions are saddened when previously held beliefs can no longer be sustained. Our behaviors follow the grieving process described by Elisabeth Kubler Ross. When confronted with changes we perceive to be noxious, most of us first deny then get angry. Next we can try to bargain. When this fails we respond by showing organizational depression (low morale) and only then do we begin to accommodate the change and move forward. Organizational grieving appears to follow the relatively extended time frame (2–5 years) that applies in individual grieving situations as well.

Changes in Health Care and Critical Care Medicine

Medicine has never been static. Change has occurred at a considerable pace throughout the 20th century. For years, most changes were technology based: penicillins replace sulfas; MRIs replace CT scans; transplants revive failing organ systems. These are modifications of our operational assumptions. They impact on the way we perform our daily tasks but challenge few basic beliefs.

Many elements in medicine resisted when governments entered the insurance business because this was inconsistent with their assumption of how medicine should be practiced. But hospitals and caregivers accommodated the new system and prospered under it. It is likely that we will eventually prosper perhaps in a different way under the new boundaries being imposed on us but the effort to reach that point will be significant.

Management Implications

One of the most important parts of managing change in an organization like an ICU is developing a shared vision. As simple as it sounds, one of the biggest problems we face is lack of clarity and common understanding of presumably simple terms. It is easier to communicate and share ideas when everybody accepts the same vocabulary. Although we

Table 3

MISSION	The enterprise's **mission** is a general statement of the purpose and nature of the enterprise. Each enterprise can be characterized by a single mission.
OBJECTIVE	An **objective** is a broad, longer-term result that the enterprise wishes to achieve to support its mission. The planning horizon for an objective is generally between five and ten years.
STRATEGY	A **strategy** is the means by which an objective is achieved. Each objective must be supported by a strategy.
GOAL	A **goal** is a special target the enterprise wishes to reach at a specific point in time. Each goal of the enterprise supports a single strategy (and, thus, a single objective). A strategy, on the other hand, is likely to be supported by many goals.
CRITICAL SUCCESS FACTOR	A **critical success factor (CSF)** is a factor that has a major influence on whether the enterprise will achieve a particular objective or goal. Some planners may prefer to distingush between positive CSF's (called **facilitators**) and negative CSF's (called **inhibitors**). A goal or objective influenced by a facilitator will be at risk if the facilitator *does not* successfully occur, while a goal or objective inhibitor will be at risk if the inhibitor *does* occur.
PLAN	A **plan** is a schedule of actions to be taken to implement the strategies and deal with the critical success factors. It constitutes a detailed, step-by-step action list to attain specific goals.
PERFORMANCE MEASURE	A **performance measure** is an indicator that shows the progress of an action against the plan. It indicates the extent to which the goal it measures has been reached. Each performance measure monitors a specific goal or objective and may be influenced by many CSFs.
INFORMATION NEED	As **information need** is an unstructured statement describing a type of information required by an organizational unit to meet its objectives and support its functions.

Source: A Guide to Information Engineering Using the IEF, 1988, Texas Instrument Corporation.

presumably speak the same language, a significant amount of confusion occurs over different interpretations of commonly used words. Table 3 is an attempt to define terms as steps in the development of a common vision for reengineering the technical process. These are relatively simple terms, but a glossary can begin to get much more complicated when it starts including the more value laden terms like quality, dignity, and respect that we use so frequently, but that may have very individualized meanings for different people.

Understanding the change process through the assumptions framework coupled with an appreciation of the Kubler Ross stages of change leads us to believe that the present initiatives will require time, patience, and energy. Change requires us to think and act quite differently, and, thus, can be a difficult process requiring considerable dialogue at the assumption framing level. Only through a willingness to challenge and reframe assumptions at a very profound level will the change process be effectively managed. To modify and adjust basic beliefs, we need to articulate a clear vision of the change process, using commonly accepted vocabulary. The process of building a shared vocabulary helps identify the assumption sets that may be challenged. But through continued effort, communication, and vision, teams can make great progress towards accepting new ideas, new processes, and new ways of doing things. In short, we can learn to manage change.

Chapter 5

The Health Care Industry: An Overview

Tom Noseworthy, M.D., M.Sc., M.P.H., Philip Jacobs, Ph.D.

Size and Scope of the Industry

Health care in western nations is no longer a practice or profession, it is a vast industry. Although normally defined as being comprised of health care producers, a broader definition of the industry to include health care insurers is more appropriate, given the inextricable link between the provision of health care and its funding.

Providers within the health care industry offer a wide variety of services with varied modes of delivery including, but not limited to, private physician services, acute care services, long-term care, home care, technical, and support services. The provision of these services occurs in varied settings, including general hospitals, ambulatory care

From: Sibbald WJ, Massaro T (eds.): The Business of Critical Care: A Textbook for Clinicians Who Manage Special Care Units.

units, and patient homes. Indeed, almost every where one goes these days, it is possible to encounter some facet of the health care industry.

Providers vary significantly in their organizational characteristics. These include: corporations selling shares on major stock exchanges; private surgical suites; physician and professional offices organized as small cottage industries; and nonprofit or charitable institutions. These organizations vary in the degree of intensity of care they provide. The service array encompasses primary personal contact and "high-touch care" to intensive care and high-tech intervention, monitoring, and support. Irrespective of the manner in that these services are identified, they are accompanied by some type of reimbursement or health insurance coverage. Thus, the industry has two major product lines—health care provider services and insurance. This makes the organization incredibly complex.

Economic Organization

To understand the economic organization of the health care industry, it is helpful to illustrate the flow of money and services, and the roles played by each of the major economic units.[1] Figure 1 presents the traditional health care market, as it existed in the US prior to the introduction of health maintenance organizations (HMOs) and preferred provider organizations (PPOs) in the early 1980s, and as it existed in Canada prior to the introduction of national hospital insurance in

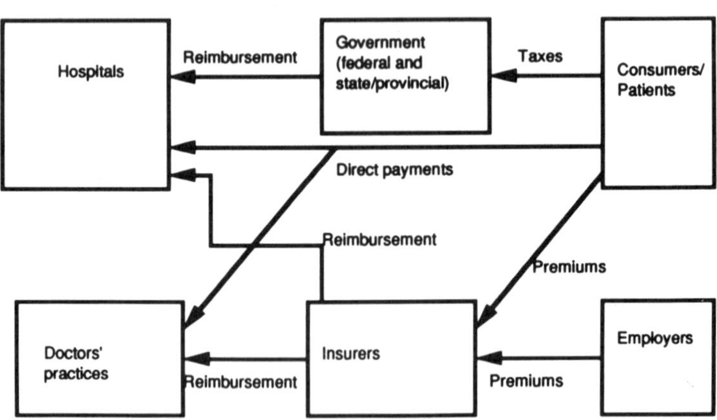

Figure 1. "Traditional" health care market.

1961. Funds were provided by taxes and premiums. Financial intermediaries such as governments and insurance companies provided coverage to consumers. These insurers reimbursed providers (hospitals, physicians' practices, etc.), for services. In such a system, there was a mixture of private and public health insurance and financing while the provision of care was largely private (non-government), though much of the hospital care was non-profit.

Not all consumers were insured in Canada before Medicare and coverage for physician services was introduced in 1971. This is true in the US to this day with some 37 million people lacking health insurance. This does not mean, of course, that the uninsured patients receive no care. There remains considerable cross-subsidization from local government agencies, hospitals, programs, and providers. In the US, not all of the insured have full or first-dollar coverage while in Canada they do. Many US patients also have insurance policies that include variable out-of-pocket or direct pay provisions. A proportion might be paid through deductibles or co-payments. Today, there are a wide variety of co-payment features in the US, though it is believed that such payments deter care, necessary or otherwise, often to the disadvantaged and most vulnerable and disease-prone populations.[2]

Traditionally, hospitals have been paid on a per diem basis and doctors on a fee-for-service basis. In 1983, the US Health Care Financing Administration commenced hospital payments for those over 65 years of age on a per case basis, with a defined fee for each case type. Cases were grouped by Diagnostic Related Groups or DRGs. Physician practices were largely reimbursed on a fee-for-service basis. Of prime importance was the fact that all services were funded on a per service, unit basis. That is, an individual unit of hospitalization, or an individual physician visit or service received separate payment. This unit-payment basis was felt to create an incentive for providers to expand the volume of services (procedures, visits, hospitalizations) although the level of the fee, as well as the basis for payment influenced the degree to which supply has expanded.

In 1961, the Canadian government passed the landmark Hospital Insurance Diagnostic Services Act that provided for hospital coverage, and in 1966 the Medical Care Act, that formed the basis for virtually complete coverage and government financing of hospital and essential medical services by 1971. These acts set up a framework for the transfer of funds from the federal to the provincial governments. In 1984, the federal government annunciated five principles to be followed: universality, accessibility, comprehensiveness, portability, and public administration. Each province was charged the responsibility of organizing

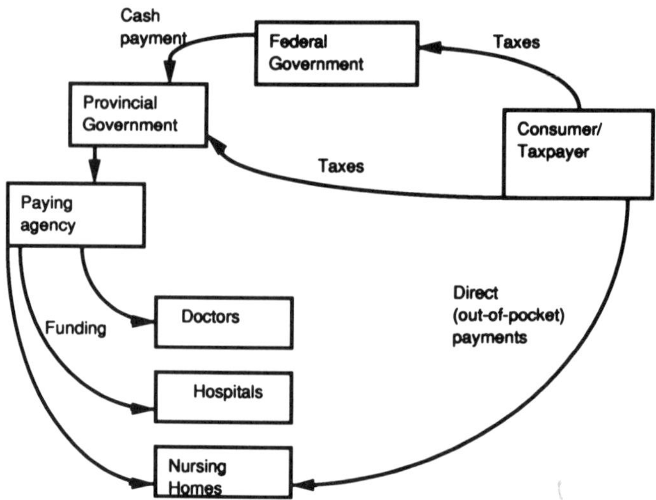

Figure 2. Canadian health care system.

its health insurance or Medicare program. Funds transferred were, very roughly, one-half the total provincial expenditures on hospital and medical care services. Each province administered its own programs, yet the provision of care was maintained in private hands. Not surprisingly, federal concerns mounted as a consequence of the escalating expenditures and its responsibility of 50%. The basis of federal-provincial cost sharing agreements has changed and has become more restrictive in the federal contribution.

Figure 2 illustrates the economic structure of the health care industry in Canada. Tax payers pay both federal and provincial taxes and the federal government, in accordance with the principles of the Medicare program, transfers funds to the provinces, as well as allowing the provinces a share of federal income taxes collected. Provincial governments are responsible for operating the health insurance programs, much like state governments and the Medicare programs in the US. Provincial governments have a single department or commission designated as the paying agency, and this department negotiates and administers physician fees and determines hospital and nursing home funding. Public health functions remain the ultimate responsibility of provincial health departments, although they may delegate some functions to local health units.

Hospitals have been funded on the basis of global operating budgets since 1961, but several provinces, such as Alberta and Ontario have been moving to a case-mix based funding system, with funding adjustments being determined by ADRG (adjacent DRG) or RDRG (refined DRG) weights. Presently, the system continues to fund physicians on a per visit or service basis. The principal change in the Canadian system as a result of national health insurance has been the "insurance" function, that has evolved to a single-payer model with the provincial government being that payer. The system has, as a consequence, become much less fragmented and, arguably, some would say less bureaucratic.

Although the Canadian and American health care systems started with similar organizational structures, the two approaches have evolved quite differently. The American system began to change dramatically in the early 1980s, at which time new payment approaches were introduced. Prepaid care, that later became known as HMOs presented a change in the basis of payment from the service unit to the enrollee. As shown in Figure 3, the HMO receives a fixed annual premium for each enrollee for which, in turn, it is responsible for the provision of all health care services. If the HMO hires and employs its physicians and owns its hospitals, as for example Kaiser Permanente, then it has the potential of reducing its cost through enhanced efficiencies in managing the service intensity and utilization of services. HMOs monitor the provision of care by doctors and introduce incentives for reductions in hospitalization and surgery, the major forms of expense. Thus, the

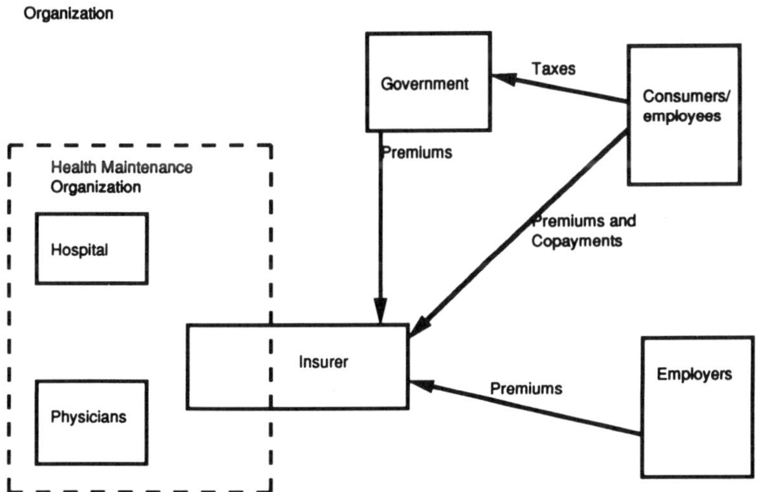

Figure 3. Flows related to a health maintenance organization.

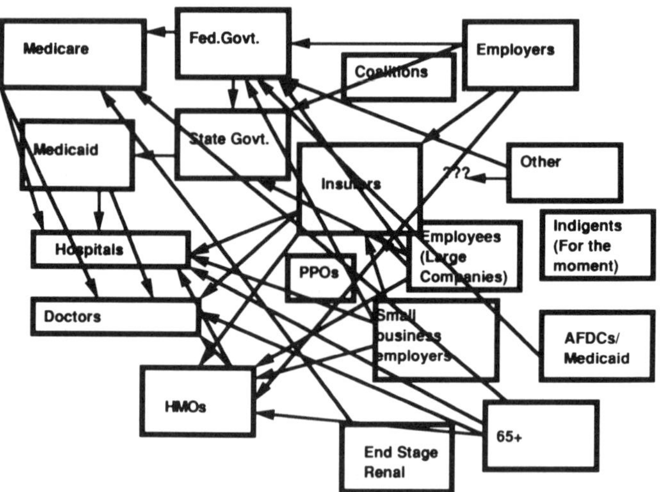

Figure 4. The United States health care system (a simplified version. c. 1990).

insurance and care provision functions have merged, with resultant savings through utilization management.

Prepaid care has become quite popular since the early 1980s. Problems with the US health care system have, nonetheless, escalated largely because of fragmentation in the system. While DRG payment has encouraged providers to reduce cost, it has discouraged cross-subsidization of care for the indigent, as this practice merely adds to average cost. There has been growing inducement for providers to cut cost, and for insurers to cover the cost of only their own insurees. Furthermore, there has been a proliferation of models of prepaid care.

PPOs, in effect middlemen, seek providers who will render services at favorable rates. Coalitions of premium paying businesses and employers also seek out favorable rates. This "each for his own" milieu has resulted in a bewildering array of payers, providers, consumers, and middlemen, in the midst of which are vast numbers of uninsured. Figure 4 presents a simplified caricature of the US health care system of today.

Economic Cost of the Health Care System

By any standard of measure, health care is a major industry and one of the largest employers in both the US and Canada. In terms of total dollars, the US spent $666 billion in 1990, while Canada spent $48 billion. These figures represent $2,566 for each person in the US and $1,869 in Canada.

The main feature of health care resource consumption in both countries, though more so in the US, has been its spectacular growth! No conventional indicator better illustrates this than health care cost as a percent or gross national product (GNP), a measure of a nation's wealth or total economic output, in the form on all goods and services produced. This ratio illustrates the degree to which health care expenditures have "displaced" resources from other uses. This is especially true given that the GNP of both countries has been growing through the 1970s and 1980s. As illustrated in Figure 5 in 1990, the ratio of health care costs to the GNP was about the same in both countries, 7.3% in the US and 7.1% in Canada. By 1980, the proportion was 9.2% in the US and 7.5% in Canada. However, by 1990 the ratios diverged with 12.2% in the US and 9% in Canada. By US comparisons, the Canadian picture appears to be one of spectacular success, especially since it has been achieved with virtually full health care coverage yet with moderate queuing. But, by international standards, especially in comparison with western Europe, Canadian performance has been less impressive. It is

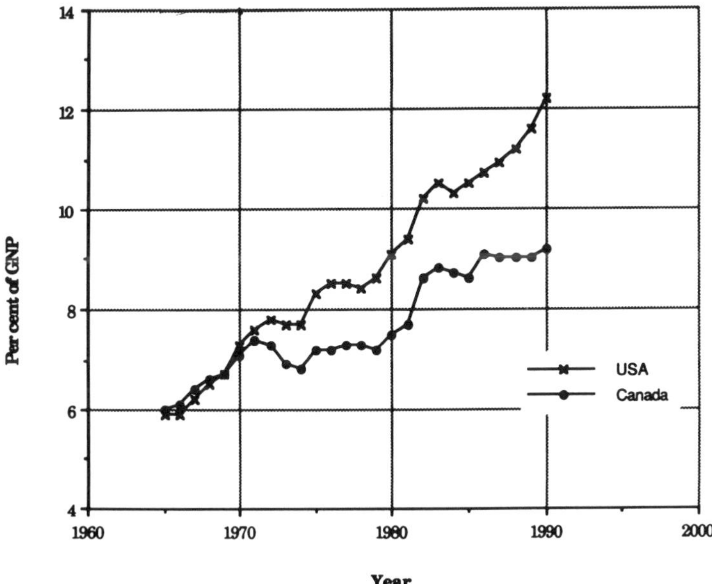

Figure 5. Health care costs as a percent of GNP, Canada and the United States.

the US that is the outlier in this regard. Given that these costs are being attained with far less than universal health insurance coverage, it signals a serious problem indeed in the US health care system.

Input to the Production of Health Care

The health care industry, and in particular the hospital sector, engage highly specialized and expensive resources. These resources consume significant dollars for both production as well as maintenance.

The labor services of physicians, nurses, therapists, technicians, and support staff represent an enormous "human capital". Indeed, the training of these individuals in many instances cannot be dissociated from the production of health services. For example, surgeons and critical care physicians are largely trained on the job and provide health services that accompany their training. This complicates accounting for health care costs from the perspective of human capital.

Although health care is regarded as being highly labor intensive, with the labor being of a highly skilled nature, it is not the case as it is in other endeavors that the labor has been substituted for other resources (equipment, materials). In many activities including intensive care, labor, capital, and other resources are "complementary" to one another, meaning that as one increases it is necessary to add the others as well. In some high-tech industries, equipment substitutes for labor. Contrariwise in the health care industry, high-technology equipment usually must be accompanied by high-tech labor. Expensive drugs and devices may accompany other high-tech inputs as well. The net result is that the resources for much of hospital care, have become increasingly more expensive. This is not true in all of health care. For some services, such as surgery, less intensive ambulatory care has become an acceptable or preferred substitute for inpatient care. Significant economic savings have resulted.

Output of the Health Care System

The size and scope of the health care industry is vast, yet this represents only one component of the strategy for procuring health in the population. The determinants of health are substantially broader than addressed by the health care system and include biological, behavioral, sociocultural, and environmental indicators. In reality, the health

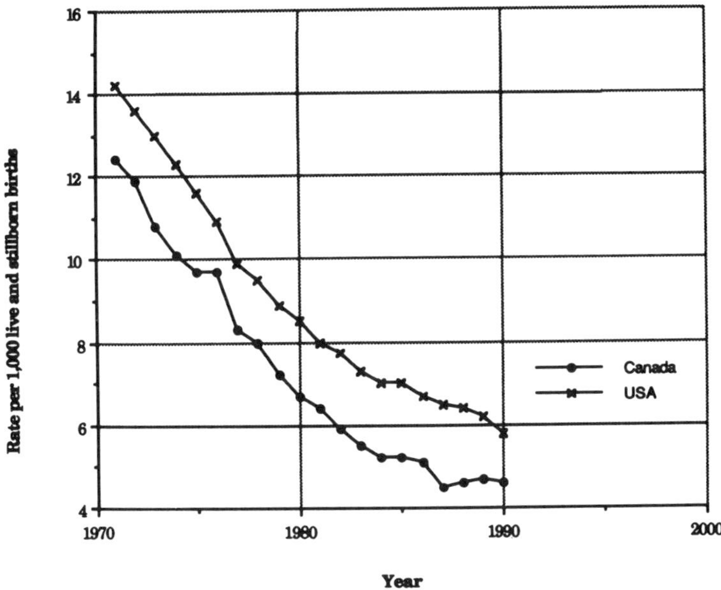

Figure 6. Neonatal mortality rates, Canada and the United States.

status of a nation is often measured in terms of life expectancy or infant mortality, largely because these data are readily available (Figure 6). The limitations of these data are evident.

Within the population, as mortality is reduced, morbidity is enhanced through the salvaging of a larger population from which some are destined to chronic illness. Measuring morbidity, be it sickness or impairment, is a formidable challenge, particularly given the broader determinants and definition of health. It should be no surprise, as a consequence, that industrialized nations may produce limitless information on the output from their health delivery systems. Yet, there remains insufficient information upon which to judge the comparability of the health of one nation as compared to that of another. Given that the output is ill-defined, it is impossible to assess whether the expenditures of one nation are more justifiable or of value than those of another. Variations in approach and perceived value limit conclusions on optimal organization of services or delivery of care.

Notwithstanding this enigma, there is an additional reality. The role of medicine and health care in enhancing the public health is both finite and, in some instances, modest. Regardless of the importance we assign to modern advances in health care, much of the decline in world mortality seen in the past three centuries is not directly attributable to medical science, but rather to reduced poverty, enhanced education, improved sanitation, cleaner water supplies, and better nutrition. This is not to say that advanced technology in medicine has not produced benefit or has no place. It does exemplify the stark reality that within the larger context of health, health care as we know it and medical practice specifically produces marginal benefit at substantial cost.

Recognizing the enormous cost of health care, there is an advocacy for the view that more attention ought to be paid to health promotion and the prevention of disease. Using an analogy, hospitals and intensive care units (ICUs) devote virtually their entire resources toward rescue of drowning victims, with little attention to preventing those potential victims from falling in the river in the first place. The logical extension of this argument, that remains to be proven of course, is that future resource allocation to hospitals should be constrained in favor of economic and social interventions that promise a greater, cheaper, or proximate potential for preserving health. However, it must be emphasized that the economic case for many health promotions and preventive interventions has not been fully established. Despite this, many believe that more lives would be saved through social and economic reform than enhancements to the health industry. For some, this may be a theoretic argument. Pragmatically, there is a mandate to deal with the patients who have succumbed to disease and affliction. To do otherwise would be irresponsible. For instance, we must provide trauma services for the victims of automobile crashes. In doing so, however, it is unfathomable not to assign and enforce a reasonable speed limit as a complimentary approach for the preservation of health. Contending that prevention must take precedence over diagnosis and treatment is illogical, these are compliments not substitutes. Contrariwise, it may be argued that to diagnose and treat but not to prevent will result in cost escalation with only marginal returns in benefit to the public health. The challenge, of course, is to strike an appropriate balance.

Hospitals: The Principal Stakeholders

Organization of the provision of medical care dates to several centuries B.C. Hospitals as sites for the delivery of health care, however, did not come to North America until 1527, in Mexico City. The first hospital in Canada was founded in Quebec in 1635. In 1751, the Pennsylvania Hospital, in Philadelphia, became the first permanent hospital for civilians in continental US. Today, acute care hospitals represent the costliest and most visible component of the health delivery system in industrialized nations. Some 40% of the health care budget in North America is consumed by hospitals.

In the US, following World War II, the federal government encouraged construction, expansion, and refurbishment of hospitals by providing grants under the Hill-Burton Act. An aggressive building program ensued. In Canada, though the post-war building program was much less substantial than in the US, the rate of hospital cost growth was impressive, on average some 13% per annum between 1969 and 1986.

Governments both in Canada and the US have attempted to control the cost of hospitals using a multiplicity of means. Perhaps best known is the DRG system in the Medicare population, introduced in 1983. This sort of approach to reimbursement has spread to other parts of the US and Canadian health systems. Two Canadian provinces have adopted payment systems based on funding formulae believed to approximate the severity-predicted cost of patients.

The consequence of reimbursement systems for hospitals in both countries has been the potential encouragement of volume-driven, as opposed to volume-managed, philosophy of care. The by-product has been enhanced competition among hospitals, with inevitable financial consequences, mergers, regionalization of services, closures, and innumerable other reactions, by no means all negative. Regrettably, the policy shifts have been largely reactive, as opposed to deliberately planned within the context of strategic health policy.

At a superficial level, hospitals in the US and Canada are quite comparable. However, Canadian hospitals have more admissions, more outpatient visits, and more inpatient days per capita than hospitals in the US. Surprisingly, Canadian hospitals spend less.[3] This appears to be related to lower administrative costs. Hospital administrative costs in the US are greater than twice that of Canada.[4] In fact, if US hospitals had the same spending pattern as Canadian hospitals, in 1985 the annual savings would have exceeded $30 billion.

Hospitals as Businesses

Canadian hospitals assumed federally administered, single-payer funding as of 1961. This was the predecessor to the universal care system, under the Medical Care Act introduced in 1966. By 1971, all provinces participated in the system in which physician fees and hospital costs were captured. In 1984, the Canada Health Act reaffirmed the federal government's commitment to deter user fees and extra billing.

US hospitals have not encountered the single-payer model found in Canada. Contrariwise, there is an enormous and competitive industry of third party payers. Hospitals negotiate contracts for service or standardized costs for certain bundles of care. A reasonable summary of the present appears to be that in both Canada and the US, despite differences in the structure and organization of the health delivery systems, increasingly hospitals are being paid an amount for what they do that does not vary despite the hospital's cost. Conceivably, both systems aspire to ultimately paying hospitals for how cost effectively they provide services, a reorientation from output to outcome.

In several industrialized nations, principally the US, the past two decades have seen the emergence of for-profit, private hospitals. Often, these facilities are a component of a large network of hospitals, well suited to compete for a share in the health care market. Claims for greater efficiency for the investor-owned hospitals are not well substantiated. While it may be true that investor-owned hospitals may generate higher before tax net income for investors, this is largely a result of enhanced charges, as opposed to reduced operating expenses. Given the competitive nature of today's hospitals, to the observer there may be little difference evident between for-profit and not-for-profit hospitals. The principal distinction, is the owner of the profits—the investors, or the hospital board of the public institution.

Hospitals as Caregiver

Hospitals, of course, do not practice medicine but are centers for the coordination of an expansive health care team, the members of which have more or less direct patient contact. As a means of organizing care for patients, hospitals are labor intensive and have as their largest cost centers as nursing services. Since the development of hospitals, the nursing profession has largely confined its activities to hospitals. Contrariwise, except for academic medical centers, most of the medical profession does not limit practice to hospitals. In fact, hospitals may be viewed as physicians' workshops. Nonetheless, physicians are solely responsible for admission and discharge, and virtually all orders for interventions, diagnostic, and therapeutic activities. Oddly enough, physicians until recently have been largely uninvolved with hospital management.

Prior to prospective payment systems, physicians exerted demand and nurses and administrators responded with supply. Within this context, there was inherent friction, particularly in the face of constrained resources. This is changing. Physicians are taking a more active involvement in hospital management. Furthermore, the reimbursement systems for hospitals are creating incentives to maintain higher occupancy and efficient utilization of hospital services, assuming the services are profitable and/or affordable. Thus, while the hospital itself does not provide care, it organizes the provision of care by others, with greater or lesser commitment and influence in the management of that facility.

The challenges facing the health care industry in hospitals are multiple and complex. The integration of hospitals as businesses and organizations for the provision of care is nonetheless essential. Acute care beds are in lesser demand as patterns of practice and technology reduce the need for inpatient services. Operating margins are decreasing and hospitals are being highly influenced by provincial, federal, and state economics. In the face of this, the consumer public and patients, and in fact their doctors, have high expectations of hospitals. This does not make organization and operation any easier.

Hospital Futures

The ICU and the critical care industry has only emerged within the acute care hospital sector over the past four decades. Nonetheless, at present, critical care maintains the largest budget of all clinical departments in most large hospitals. Some institutions report that 18%–20% of annual operating budget is allocated to the provision of critical care services.[5]

There is very little information on the true cost and growth of intensive care services in North America. Using hospital bed figures, percent occupancy, and cost ratios of ward to ICU beds, it is evident that the aggregate cost of critical care is substantial.[6] From 1969 to 1986, ICU costs represented the fastest growing component of hospital operating budgets. In Canada, it is estimated that utilization increased from 17 to 42 patient days per 1,000; ICU days as a proportion of total hospital days increased from 1%–3%; and the calculated impact on hospital operating budgets was 10%. In the US, in sharp contrast, ICUs by 1986 cost $32.8 billion and represented 0.8% of GNP. Unexplainably, it appears as if ICU utilization as represented by ICU days per 1,000 population in the US may be as much as 2.5 fold that of Canada.

Macroeconomic data of this sort requires careful interpretation. Data collection is not constant between provinces, states, and federal governments. Assumptions and calculations based on assumptions are the only available alternative to actual utilization and cost data. Nonetheless, it may be concluded that intensive care is expensive, the industry is growing at an impressive rate, it represents the largest clinical component of hospital operating budgets, and like most other clinical areas it experiences marked variations in patterns of utilization and clinical behavior.

The DRG system introduced in 1983 has had a significant impact on ICUs. There is expressed concern that the current DRG system appears to be an inequitable means of reimbursement for the patient who receives treatment in the ICU during the hospital stay. Many have warned that full implementation of a DRG-type reimbursement system could severely limit future ICU access. Viewed in the positive, there is an enormous stimulus to pursue cost containment and to implement cost effective measures for services. Ignoring this would be irresponsible.

ICUs, besides being a philosophy and process for the provision of critical care services, are businesses. Managing these businesses with effective management information systems, organizational structures, and teams committed to collaborative interaction, is central to the message of this text.

References

1. Jacobs P: The Economics of Health & Medical Care. Third Edition. Rockville, Maryland, Aspen Publishers, 1991.
2. Beck RG: The effect of co-payments on the poor. J Hum Res 1974;9:19.
3. Redelmeier DA, Fuchs V: Hospital expenditures in the United States and Canada. N Engl J Med 1993;328:772.
4. Woodlandler S, Himmelstein DV, Lewontin JP: Administrative costs in US hospitals. N Engl J Med 1993;38:400.
5. Shepard DS, Ghanotakis AJ: Hospital Costs in Massachusetts: A Report of the Massachusetts Funds Flow Project. Springsfield, VA, National Technical Information Service (HRP-0029335), 1979.
6. Jacobs P, Noseworthy TW: National estimates of intensive care costs in Canada & the United States. Crit Care Med 1990;18:1282.

Chapter 6

Managing Health Care Economics: An Introduction

Laurence G. Wolfson, B.A., M.H.Sc.,
Shawn Gilhuly, B.A., B.Comm., M.H.A.

The objective of this chapter is to introduce the reader to the field of health economics and its relationship to health status and health care. A thorough analysis of health economics, including its methods and applications, is not the goal. An entire book, and a lengthy one at that, would be required to do the topic justice. Rather, this effort will have fulfilled its purpose if it conveys a clear understanding of what health economics is, what it strives to do, the context in which it operates, and how it applies to clinical practice.

Health economics, as with most areas of advanced study, has its own language and terminology. Therefore, at the outset, it seems useful to define a few key terms and principles (Table 1). Of particular importance is the differentiation between health status and health care. This has particular relevance to economic evaluation in the health care arena.

From: Sibbald WJ, Massaro T (eds.): The Business of Critical Care: A Textbook for Clinicians Who Manage Special Care Units.

Table 1
Glossary of Terms

Opportunity Cost	The benefits of alternative choices that are foregone by committing resources to a selected option.
Diminishing Returns	As equal increments of a particular input are added to a process while quantities of other inputs are held constant, beyond a certain threshold, resulting increments of output will decrease relative to input.
Marginal Cost/Utility	Marginal cost is the expense of producing the last unit of output while marginal utility is the good or satisfaction that is derived from that last unit consumed.
Cost Effectiveness Analysis (CEA)	Economic analysis where costs of alternatives are measured in dollars and consequences or outputs are measured in natural units (e.g.,—life years gained).
Cost Benefit	Economic analysis where both costs and consequences of alternatives are measured in dollars due to the heterogeneity of outputs.
Cost Utility	Economic analysis where costs of alternatives are quantified in dollars while measures of consequences take into account utility measures such as quality-adjusted life years (QALY's).

After analyzing the concept of health (or health status) as a state of affairs with multiple determinants, we then turn to an examination of health care—the economic good. Though a commodity, it becomes readily apparent that health care is unique from several perspectives. First, it is a deeply cherished public good, subject to social, political, and economic pressures that evoke public policy responses. Second, it operates in a manner quite unlike the free market ideal of perfect competition. As such, it is a topic of great interest to economists who concern themselves with the selection of choices in the face of limited resources.

The balance of the chapter investigates how health care economic policy might be rethought with a view to maximizing health outcomes. This is accomplished by broadening the conceptual model for understanding health to include determinants that are traditionally thought of as external to health care but that nevertheless, have significant impact on health outcomes. This shift in framework calls for policy options that promote both private and public sector participation that in turn, poses new sets of circumstances for conducting economic analysis.

Health Versus Health Care

What is Health?

"Health is a state of complete physical, mental and social well-being and not merely the absence of disease or infirmity."[1] This World Health Organization (WHO) definition sees health as a resource for everyday life, rather than the objective of living. It is a positive concept that emphasizes social and personal resources, as well as physical capacity. It advocates intervention to improve health along four main dimensions:

1. Adding years to life by reducing premature deaths, thereby increasing life expectancy.
2. Adding life to years by maximizing the development and use of the individual's physical and mental capacity to cope with, contribute to, and benefit from life in a healthy way.
3. Adding health to life by reducing disease and disability.
4. Promoting equity in health by reducing gaps in health status between countries and among groups within countries.

The WHO definition of health is based upon a conceptual framework that is underpinned by three fundamental constructs.

First, is the proposition that to truly understand health we need to incorporate the concept of well-being? This calls for consideration of the host's functionality and quality of life rather than mere elimination and/or containment of the disease processes. This shifts the health paradigm from an illness focus (i.e., avoidance of disease) to one that understands health as being more than the absence of undesirable conditions.

The second tenet of the conceptual framework is acceptance of the premise that health status is multifactorial where many of its determinants lie outside the traditional parameters of the health care system.[2] Indeed, the production and distribution of wealth, development of sanitation systems, public policy, and lifestyle choices all have been directly linked to the overall well being of a given population.

Third, is there appreciation of the importance of the context within which health determinants operate? Thus, the conceptual framework pays heed to the environment for it is here, within this crucible, that the various determinants of health operate and make their presence felt. Furthermore, the determinants interact with the host and each other in ways that are not yet fully understood. In fact, the relationship between determinants may be more important than the determinants themselves.

We will analyze these concepts in greater depth as they form the foundation on which health economics rests.

The Host

A good appreciation of the role of the host is fundamental to understanding health status as well as anticipating the consequences of health care interventions. Analysis of the interactions between the host and factors such as illness, health determinants, and the health care system itself provides important information for assessing health outcomes. To truly comprehend the wellness/illness process, it is necessary to have a thorough understanding of how the host reacts and responds to various stimuli along physical, political, economic, and social dimensions.

Furthermore, differences in perception and outlook can result in situations where the patient's view of illness does not correlate with the care provider's assessment of the disease process. This may account for the fact that different patients, with similar physical ailments, can and do experience substantial variation in symptoms, distress, and loss of functional capacity. For example, in oncology, a substantial body of literature exists that underscores the importance of host coping mechanisms in altering the course of disease progress. Equally impressive is the emerging body of knowledge in social biology that has identified a strong correlation between heightened self-esteem and increased immune function.

Health Determinants

Investigation of the role of non-health care system determinants in influencing overall health status is not new. Twenty years ago, The Lalonde Report "A New Perspective On The Health Of Canadians" attempted to broaden the health policy framework by moving away from near exclusive focus on health care as the means for studying and understanding health status. By categorizing determinants under headings such as Lifestyle, Environment, Human Biology, and Health Care Organization, the Lalonde Report[3] sought to draw attention to these factors and the thesis that their regulation might yield greater improvements in health status than increases in health care system activity. This line of thinking attracted considerable attention and, although much investigation remains to be done in this area, recent studies have identified a variety of non-traditional health status factors such as employment, income, stress, self-esteem, domestic supports, and social isolation.[4] Unemployment, for example, has been implicated as a negative health status determinant by virtue of its effects on social isolation and stigmatization—not to mention income loss.

Environment

The importance of the environment vis-a-vis health status is rather evident in a physical sense—as in the cases of sanitation, clean air, and water. However, other less obvious environments, be they political, economic, or social in nature, also impact on health status. As an illustration, within Southwestern Ontario, injuries, particularly motor vehicle accidents, are among the highest contributors to death rates and even more so to lost person years for those in the 20–39 age group.[5] In light of this fact, the strategic use of public policy, in the form of traffic safety legislation and incentives to promote seat belt use, may well have greater positive impact on health status than the provision of additional health care resources.

In summary, health status is multifactorial. To fully appreciate its nature, attention must be paid to non-health care system determinants and factors. Traditionally, these have been under emphasized and yet they may offer fertile ground for outcome improvement.

Health Care

The tremendous improvements in quantity and quality of life that have been accrued to individuals and societies by virtue of modern health care is well known. It is, therefore, not surprising that there has been widespread belief that the availability and consumption of health care resources is the key variable in determining health status. However, in recent years, within Canada and the United States, as health care costs have grown without commensurate increases in the population's health status, the health care system itself has come under close scrutiny. This has resulted in a general consensus that the health care system is in need of major structural and management reform. Indeed, the need for health care reform was a major topic in the 1992 US presidential election debates and continues to be one of the defining issues of the Clinton Administration.

One particular concern is that much of what is provided within the health care system today is done so without being supported by good scientific rationale. This revelation has not been lost on paying agencies, both public and private, where reaction is perhaps best summed up by the Ontario Premier's Council on Health Strategy, "We know now that increased spending on formal health care in developed economies is not having a corresponding positive impact on health status. At the same time, there is growing evidence that population health status may be significantly influenced by measures taken outside the formal health care system."[2]

Over and above the government's natural inclination towards pursuing such an agenda, given the current economic climate of constrained resources, there is genuine skepticism regarding the justification for many present day health care interventions. Thus, we are beginning to see calls for thorough economic evaluation of new techniques and procedures before their introduction whereas, until recently, new advances and innovations were launched and disseminated freely, by-passing this important step.

Discussion

In this section, we have tried to emphasize that in setting the foundation for a discussion of health economics, it is critically important for the reader to bear in mind the distinction between health status and health care. Appreciation of the difference between these two concepts is crucial to understanding health economics. For while scientific modes of inquiry have undoubtedly increased the knowledge base of clinicians and enabled great advances in health care system interventions leading to real improvements in health outcomes, there has been a cost. It is that the health care system per se has become the vehicle for transmitting and translating advances in medical knowledge into hoped-for health status improvements. This is despite the fact that often, linkage between particular interventions and positive health outcomes is lacking. Furthermore, if we accept the proposition that non-system factors play a key role in determining health status, then it seems fair to conclude that present day models, many of which do not take into account non-health care system determinants, are ill equipped to explain health outcomes adequately. This is important because the manner in which an issue is framed determines the questions that are asked, the kinds of evidence that are given weight and the conclusions that are drawn. Evans[6] notes that this may explain situations where valid data are ignored, as if they did not exist, because the models of the day do not accommodate these new entities and inter-relationships. The result is that the emphasis of health policy has been centered on the provision of health care in spite of the realization that we may be approaching the point where increments in health care offer limited potential for increasing health status.

How Big is Health Care?

Health care expenditures have exhibited steady growth, particularly in the past two decades in North America to the point where many public officials maintain that current levels of health care expenditures are unsustainable.

In 1970, the US spent $74 billion on health care or approximately 7.3% of Gross Domestic Product (GDP). More than 20 years later, it is estimated that the US is spending in the order of $900 billion (13.4% of GDP) per annum, making the American health care system equivalent in size to the seventh largest economy in the world! Expenditures for Medicare (elderly) and Medicaid (indigent) alone consume more than $200 billion per annum, approximately four times the United Kingdom's entire National Health Service budget. It should be remembered that these numbers reflect a situation where 35 million Americans do not have health care insurance plus another 20 million who have levels of coverage that most of us would find wanting.

Even in Canada, with universal health care and expenditures in the range of 8.5% of GDP, public officials are quickly realizing that this level of expenditure may be beyond the electorate's willingness to pay. In Ontario, for example, health care spending makes up one-third of the provincial budget (up from one-quarter 10 years earlier) and is a prime target for cost cutting.

One significant lesson that we can learn from the American and Canadian experiences is that the portion of national income devoted to health care will rise in the absence of a controlling mechanism.[7] Without such a mechanism, economic prosperity may be adversely affected. In addition, the public's ability to fund other priorities may be restricted.

Health Economics

Economics is concerned with the manner in which resources are allocated among competing alternative uses, to satisfy human wants.

Resources may be defined as the inputs used to produce goods and services and can be classified into three major categories: labor, capital, and land. Human wants, on the other hand, are the goods, services, and/or circumstances that a population desires. Wants vary markedly among individuals and change over time.

Scarcity is a fundamental economic truth—that is, there are always more legitimate demands to satisfy than can be accommodated with the resources at hand. This means that choices must be made. As a result of this reality, economists are drawn to three basic questions governing the allocation of resources.

1. What determines the selection and volume of what is produced?
2. What determines how a product/service is produced?
3. What determines how a product/services's output is distributed among society's members?

These questions form the core of economic thought and analysis precisely because they focus on choice. In order to quantify choice, economists use the concept of opportunity cost that may be defined as the value of what available inputs could have produced had they not been selected for the chosen alternative but rather directed toward satisfying the next best (i.e., not selected) alternative. In other words, given that resources are finite, using them for the chosen purpose means that they are no longer available for alternative purposes whose benefits are thereby foregone. The quantification of that missed "opportunity" is the opportunity cost.

Health Care Economics

Scarcity, choice, and opportunity cost provide the framework for economic analysis within the health care sector. Thus, health care economics may be defined as "the attainment of the optimum use or resources for the care of the sick and the promotion of health . . . its task is to appraise the efficiency of the organization of health services and to suggest ways to improve it."[8] Evans[9] sharpens this focus by honing in on the production and consumption of that particular set of goods and services that have been "identified as having a special relationship to health status and to the activities associated with their production and consumption." Evans further states that as with other branches of economics, health care economics "studies the processes and institutions that govern the allocation of scarce social resources to the selected alternatives, the choice of production techniques, the mix of outputs, and the distribution of health care among end users—that is consumers/patients."

Diminishing Returns and Marginality

A key economic principle that applies to health care in much the same manner as for other goods, is that of diminishing returns. The law of diminishing returns holds that if equal increments of a particular input are added to a process while quantities of other inputs are held constant, beyond a threshold, resulting increments of output will decrease relative to additional input. With respect to health care, the law of diminishing returns impacts, in a major way, on determining the allocation of scarce resources.

The law of diminishing returns, by its very nature, concerns itself with marginal costs (and benefits). Marginal cost is the expense of producing the last unit of output while marginal benefit refers to the satisfaction or utility that is derived from consuming that last unit.

Within the health care domain, the law of diminishing returns is in evidence as health status improvements have not been keeping pace with the substantial growth in health care expenditures. For example, health care costs in the US have grown from 7.3% to 13.4% of GDP between the 1970s and the 1990s. At the same time, conventional measures of health status have not detected commensurate improvements. How far along the curve of diminishing returns we find ourselves in Western societies is open to debate. However, there is a consensus of informed opinion that suggests that we have reached a point (at least in the developed world) of diminishing returns. This suggests that it is worth investigating other variables such as income, housing, environment, crime, nutrition, personal habits, and social networks—all of which affect health status. This does not presume that new health care interventions will not be undertaken. Rather, that there may be alternative inputs, including those from outside the formal health care system where the cost/health status ratio may be more favorable.

Before turning to some special economic features of the health care system, a few caveats are in order. First, given the above definition of economics that concentrates on choice in the allocation of limited resources, and given our earlier discussion regarding the difference between health status and health care, it appears that the term "health economics" is, in reality, a misnomer. Rather, what is being discussed is the application of economic principles to the social good of "health care"—hence a more appropriate term would be "health care economics". Second, the connection between health status and health care is complex and anything but straightforward. Third, health care displays idiosyncrasies that make it difficult to apply mainstream economic theory and analysis. As such, key economic constructs such as the laws of supply and demand do not apply in the same manner as in more traditional environments. We now turn to a discussion of these unique characteristics.

Market Anomalies

What makes health care special and, by extension, health care economics? Evans[10] identifies three distinctive characteristics. First is the uncertainty of illness. Illness onset is irregular, often unforeseeable and unpredictable. This makes it extremely difficult to forecast incidence and prevalence rates and, accordingly, planning health care services is a risky business. Second, is the asymmetry of information between health care providers and consumers. Many patients lack even basic information and knowledge regarding indications for treatment and the available alternatives. To make matters worse, consumers/patients are often called upon to make these far-reaching decisions when not feeling well and, at times, in constrained timeframes. Third, is the issue of externalities or external effects. These occur when a third party receives a benefit or incurs a loss without choosing to do so.

Seller Effects

How is health care special from an economist's perspective? Perhaps most striking is the unique manner in which demand for health care services is expressed. All of us are consumers in one context or another. We shop for cars, appliances, clothes, and so on. All the while, there is the inherent assumption of an educated consumer making an informed decision. If a good is priced too highly, the supplier either reacts to market signals by lowering the price, discontinuing the product, or in some other way. However, this does not hold in the health care arena. Here, the product/service is complex and consumers often lack adequate information and knowledge necessary for informed judgments. As a consequence, patients tend to rely on health care providers (most often doctors) to both produce the product/service and to act as consumer agents and advisors. This leads to a scenario where the physician, with superior professional knowledge, both supplies a service and, at the same time, influences the demand for it. Few, if any other industries exhibit this supplier-induced demand anomaly. Also, as mentioned previously, we need to bear in mind that the perspectives and orientations of consumers and producers differ, as in most walks of life. For example, while a patient's prime goal may be freedom from pain, the clinician may also be motivated by a desire for increased knowledge regarding the disease process. In economic terminology, we say that the utility or satisfaction functions of consumers differ from those of providers. This dual role, consumer/patient advisor and supplier of the very same service, is not envisaged by traditional economic theory. Indeed, in confronting this issue, the economics student might well suggest that competition from other sellers would provide an effective counterweight to this concentration of power. However, to date, supplier control of training and licensure requirements has, for all intents and purposes, ruled out this option although the example of the Province of Ontario's recent plans to legalize midwifery in the Province of Ontario may be a harbinger of changes to come.

Insurance Effects

Consumers in most markets are limited in what they can spend on a particular product or service. In health care, with the provision of third party insurance coverage, the burden of payment shifts, so that the load is shared among enrollees. Furthermore, in those jurisdictions where health insurance is financed from the public purse, responsibility for payment is distributed further afield to the taxpayer. Whether or not this is desirable public policy, it does distort the market for health care services in two main ways: moral hazard and adverse selection.

Moral Hazard

Health insurance can be thought of as the pooling of risk from disease and illness. Individuals who hold insurance coverage are shielded from out-of-pocket expenses (with the exception of co-payment charges). Faced with a situation where someone else is paying the expenses, there is a built-in incentive for the patient and/or his agent to demand as much health care as possible. Cost is of little concern to the patient at the point of entry to the health care system due to the lack of direct, out-of-pocket expenses. When combined with a fee-for-service delivery system that rewards high volume production, the result is unrestrained demand for health care services. This is known as moral hazard.

Adverse Selection

Illness is uneven and unpredictable. Moreover, it is involuntary with disabling, or even fatal consequences. As well, the health care consumer, armed with the knowledge that disabling disease can bring about financial hardship, is motivated to purchase insurance, particularly if there is a belief that disease onset is unavoidable or even likely. Conversely, private insurance companies, who wish to maximize profits and increase shareholder value have powerful incentives not to provide coverage to patients who are likely to undergo expensive medical episodes—in other words, to avoid poor risks. Therefore, in the pursuit of business growth and profitability, private insurers attempt to insure only those who are least likely to contract illness and require costly services. This is accomplished by "experience rating" or setting individual premium rates based on a forecast of each potential subscriber's future demand for health services. As well, insurers can deny, or at least restrict, coverage to applicants who have previous or existing medical conditions that are unattractive from an insurer's point of view. These measures, known colloquially as "skimming the cream", can result in health care insurance arrangements that are inconsistent with the societal goal of providing adequate, affordable health services to all.

Externalities

A fourth distinctive economic feature of health care concerns itself with the role of externalities or external diseconomies. Simply put, an externality occurs when a third party receives some advantage or endures some loss due to circumstances outside (external to) his/her span of control. Externalities can be either rewarding (positive) or punitive (negative). Traditional health examples of each include vaccinations that prevent the spread of infectious diseases and pollution/second-hand smoke.

Any legitimate economic appraisal of a health care intervention ought to include an analysis of societal costs and benefits. Often these are hidden, or at least obscure, yet they are real and important. Externalities identify these issues for inclusion in the cost/benefit equation. For example, the existence of a societal group without health insurance poses an additional burden (diseconomy or negative externality) on the taxpayer. The costs of treating these individuals in cases of illness falls on the rest of society who, de facto, assume an additional coverage liability through no fault of their own.

Implications for the Clinician

We have postulated that at a societal level, current measures of health status are only slightly affected by additional health care system inputs. And yet, when the context shifts to an individual situation such as a patient within the intensive care unit (ICU), the equation changes dramatically. On the one hand, from a system perspective, we question the wisdom of providing ever increasing amounts of tertiary health care interventions and yet, when our loved ones are at risk, the apple cart is upset and our skepticism goes flying out the window and we want the interventions. Why the difference?

The apparent paradox can be explained largely by reference to two key social science concepts. The first is Maslow's hierarchy of need that attempts to explain human behavior and motivation in terms of satisfying unmet needs. Maslow suggests that basic survival and biological needs assume primacy and that higher order needs such as self-esteem become effective motivators only after primary needs have been satisfied (Figure 1).

The second concept is that of marginality as discussed previously under the topic of diminishing returns. Intensive care medicine operates at the health care margin, where each additional day survived in the ICU is achieved at considerable cost. What is not articulated nearly as well is that the marginal benefits are also very high as life-saving and sustaining measures are cherished by patients and loved ones. However, at a macro level, this benefit is not apparent.

The implication for health care economics is that when attempting to evaluate the benefits of health care interventions, we need to apply a Maslow-like mindset. For if the environment is tertiary intensive care medicine, then it is inappropriate to evaluate these interventions from a broad, community health status perspective. ICU activities and im-

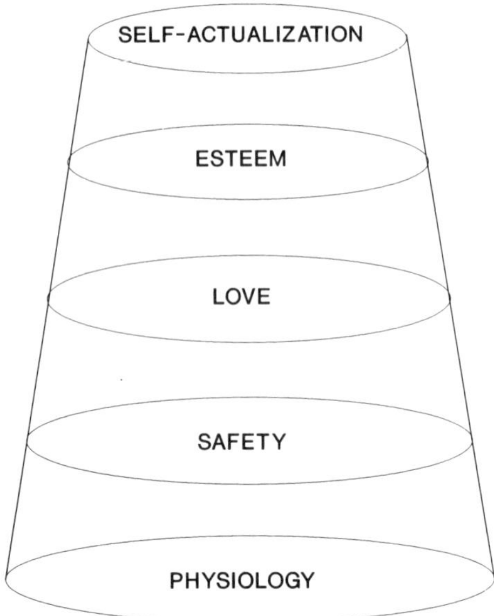

Figure 1. A depiction of Maslow's Hierarchy of Needs.

pacts are almost imperceptible from this vantage point. However, when viewed in detail, at the margin, at the pinnacle of a "Maslow Health Care Hierarchy", a markedly different picture emerges. Here, incremental costs are high, but so are benefits. Thus, the perspective of the front-line intensive care clinician operating at the health care margin is quite different than that of the system evaluator who comes to the discussion with a much more global mindset. One's view is determined, to a large extent, by one's orientation. Indeed, Maslow would likely argue that the very existence of intensive care medicine means that needs requiring less specialized forms of health care interventions are already being met relatively well.

Within the agency role, the intensivist is called upon to advocate on behalf of the patient. In the ICU, however, the patient is often incapacitated, unable to communicate. This leaves the clinician in the unenviable position of trying to guess what the patient's wishes might be. And these are not trivial matters (often life and death situations with attendant ethical considerations). While the input of family members may sometimes be helpful in articulating the patient's interests, this may not be a reliable proxy, given family dynamics and the emotional turmoil that is often associated with intensive care medicine.

Quite apart from the agency role, the intensivist is also expected, albeit implicitly perhaps, to carry out a "gate-keeping" function for the health care system. Assuming that intensive care medicine is costlier than "normal" modalities of care, there is a heightened expectation that only those interventions that are cost effective will be undertaken. As indicated elsewhere, good measures of cost effectiveness are rare in health care, including intensive care. Yet in individual cases, patients (or loved ones) may expect and even demand treatment that may be questionable from a cost-benefit perspective and even in ideal circumstances, where the intervention passes the cost effectiveness test at the "ICU margin", the benefits may not be apparent at a macro system level.

Government Intervention

The preceding analysis of market anomalies suggests that exclusive reliance on the invisible hand of the marketplace to guide the production and distribution of health care is problematic. This is recognized increasingly by a public who supports some form of government intervention in health care. In response, governments have entered the health care field via two main vehicles: regulation and insurance coverage.

Regulation

While there is considerable opposition in some circles to government regulation of health care, it does have its place and even the harshest critics of government intervention would, in all likelihood, approve of it when it comes to issues such as public health and safety, standards for the construction and operation of nursing homes, etc. Indeed, even in the provision of medical services, the result of unbridled free enterprise would allow any individual to set out a shingle with the title "Doctor", charge whatever the market will bear, and rely on caveat emptor for consumer/patient protection. This is hardly a position that most citizens would endorse.

Insurance

As indicated previously, illness onset is uncertain, irregular, and unpredictable. As a result, individuals have an interest in minimizing the financial burden potentially imposed by illness and the resultant need for health services. They do this by purchasing insurance where the goal is to reduce exposure to the negative consequences of sickness by pooling or sharing risk.

A detailed description of the various types of health care insurance coverage is beyond the scope of this chapter. Suffice it to say that there are many different models with varying degrees of coverage. For our purposes, the provision of insurance is an important variable to take into account with regard to economic analysis, particularly its relevance to moral hazard as discussed earlier.

In the next section, we offer some lessons and recommendations that we believe hold promise and generate future benefits for those providing and consuming health services.

Lessons and Recommendations

Shift the Paradigm

First and foremost, we cannot over-emphasize the need to differentiate between health (or health status) and health care. As discussed previously, many important determinants of health status lie outside the purview of the health care system per se. Thus, the framework for understanding health must shift to take account of health determinants such as wealth production and distribution, existence of social networks, lifestyle choice, housing, employment, and education.[4] Until new paradigms are developed that help to fundamentally understand the effects of these factors, there is a risk that emerging data in these areas will not receive the attention that they merit. This is crucial for the future of health care economics for, as the health paradigm shifts, so too does the arena in that health economics questions are posed. To keep pace, health economics will need to broaden its horizons to differentially assess the effects on health outcomes from interventions within as well as external to the formal health care system.

Share the Knowledge

Countries with developed economies differ markedly in how they organize and finance the delivery of health care. One can take heart from the fact that many effective strategies for the provision of cost effective health care are already in place. From the US, there is leadership in the development of output measures, quality assessment tools, and technological innovation. From the United Kingdom come well established primary and preventive care systems. Canada and many Western European nations have demonstrated an ability to provide widespread coverage and yet operate with relatively effective cost controls, and Japan boasts the successful utilization of reasonably priced paramedical personnel. Despite these accomplishments, there appears to be very little attention paid to what seems to work for others, as individual jurisdictions attempt to reform their health care systems without sufficient regard to what they can learn from one another. Rather than trying to discover the elusive magic bullet, a combination of tried and tested measures is likely to yield more positive results.

Include the Consumer

Patient/consumer education is a fundamental goal of our health care system. However, the evidence to date suggests that, to a large degree, it has been an†unrealized one. Yet, progress is being made. Consider the example of surgical intervention for benign enlargement of the prostate where approximately 320,000 cases per annum are reported in the US with substantial incentives to American physicians and hospitals for carrying out this procedure. It is interesting to note the experience of Kaiser Permanente's Denver-based health maintenance organization (HMO) in promoting patient education regarding this procedure. When potential candidates for the surgery (men over the age of 60) view a videodisc explaining the pros and cons of surgery, the operation is performed 45% less often, resulting in cost savings to the plan of approximately $200,000 per year.[11]

While consumer involvement has been a sine qua non in business circles for decades it has been significantly absent within health care circles. But times are changing and there is formal recognition that governance of the health care system needs to be responsive to community health needs and to involve people to a more significant degree in making decisions that have an impact on their health and well-being.[5] Examples like Kaiser's suggest that informed consumer opinion provides important feedback as to whether therapeutic and diagnostic procedures are wanted. Consumer input can provide important clues for predicting future illness as patients' perceptions of their own health may give insights that standard work-ups and questions may overlook.

As well, an informed consumer is a valuable asset in the effort to foster competition in the health care marketplace. Initiatives like that of the American Health-Care Financing Administration (HCFA), where physician and/or hospital success rates for selected procedures are published for public review, introduces a significant new element into the clinical decision-making equation. A valuable second opinion is sought—that of the patient.

Measure Outcomes

Perhaps the most damning indictment of current health care practice is that so much of it has been unevaluated. In Ontario, this has led to the recent, rather sobering assessment that little information exists on health status and considerable research is needed on how to measure and assess health needs.[2] Fortunately, there seems to be universal realization that this state of affairs is no longer acceptable. Under the rubrics of Outcomes Management, Total Quality Management, Continuous Quality Improvement, etc., increasing attention is being paid to questions such as "Are we doing the right things to the right people?" and "What are the effects (outcomes) of our interventions?" Given the magnitude of health care expenditures, this development should not come as a surprise. What is striking, however, is that it has taken so long to come to pass. Only 3-years old, the US based Agency for Health Policy and Research (AHCPR) has launched a number of patient outcomes research teams (PORTs) that attempt to determine the most effective and efficient ways of treating a variety of illnesses including coronary heart disease, pneumonia, diabetes, and lower back pain. The example of lower back pain gives a glimpse of the potential impact that PORTs can have. In the US, lower back pain is the second leading reason for physician visits and has been implicated as a major source of questionable hospitalization where it is estimated that $24 billion (four times the cost of AIDS treatment) is spent treating this problem. Of particular interest is a study of Medicare patients, which found that 70% of the nonsurgical hospitalizations were unnecessary and that practice patterns vary wildly.[11]

Evaluate Technology

The rapid diffusion of technology has been implicated as one of the major sources of cost escalation in health care today.[12] In other industries, the significant outlays that are made in introducing and disseminating technological advances are expected to be offset by efficiencies (i.e., reduced operating costs) that result from the innovation. Not so in health care where technology growth is argued on effectiveness (improved service) rather than efficiency grounds. Indeed, the introduction of new technologies has not reduced health care system operating costs, quite the contrary. However, cost need not be the only consideration. One could argue in favor of health care technological advances on the grounds of clinical efficacy. This line of reasoning maintains that even though technology introduction and dissemination may be costly, it is still worthwhile in light of expected outcome improvements from both quantity and quality of life perspectives. Unfortunately, this linkage has not been demonstrated to a sufficient degree. Rather, there has been widespread demand for new technologies (from health care providers and consumers alike) with little attention paid to quantifying the expected outcome improvements. This has led observers of the health care system to question the wisdom of bringing technological innovation to the health care market place until certain fundamental issues are addressed. Feeny et al.[13] suggest that the following questions be answered prior to technology proliferation.

1. How effective are the new technologies?
2. For what conditions and which patients?
3. Do the expected benefits in improved health justify the costs?

Evans[9] points out that traditionally, in health care, most new technologies are tested for safety, but not efficacy. This is a luxury that we can ill afford as its continuation poses the threat of short-changing other interventions that may be efficacious and cost effective. To avert this danger, empirical studies are required that assess the costs and consequences of introducing new technologies. Furthermore, in analyzing consequences, there needs to be a commitment to measure effects at a health status level. For while technological advances have improved diagnostic techniques, shortened lengths of stay in hospital, etc., the question of whether patients/consumers have benefitted to the point where the costs (including externalities) are justified, has largely been left unanswered.

Drawing upon the work of Birdsall[14] in comparing mortality rates of industrialized and developing nations between 1960 and 1980, Massaro reports that mortality rates in technology-dependent diseases were nearly identical indicating that "the increased technical resources available in the developed nations have not added a great deal to the overall health status of the population."[15] Interestingly, the mortality rate reductions that both industrialized and developing countries experienced during the period, were attributable to improvements in the so-called "poverty-related" illnesses.

The foregoing does not suggest that health care technology is a frill in today's fiscal environment. Rather, given its significance as a health care cost driver, particularly in the intensive care setting, we support the recommendations of Sibbald et al.[16] who argue for the development of guidelines to manage the diffusion of technology within the critical care field. Sibbald cautions that without technology assessment guidelines, mutually agreed upon between government, industry, and the medical community, health care funders will be inclined to limit the introduction and dissemination of health care technology at large rather than focusing on restricting those innovations that do not have proven efficacy to critical care. He suggests that this lack of differentiation potentially puts emerging technologies in critical care medicine (that may merit serious consideration on both clinical and economic grounds) at a disadvantage.

Promote Mix of Private and Public Markets

One promising strategy for controlling health care expenditures without coverage erosion is to combine sensible, incentive-driven regulation with market-based reform. An example of this type of integrative approach is being explored in Holland where a government commission discovered a health care system with little incentive for efficient operation, limited competition, and constrained consumer choice.[17] In response, the Dutch government has committed itself to a system design that blends public and private insurance alternatives. A basic insurance package covering 85% of health care spending will be compulsory. This will likely be provided by a government insurance plan financed by premiums that are geared to income level or, alternatively, by a competing market-based arrangement where interested private carriers set a flat fee. The expectation is that there will be increased competition and decreased regulation, all the while providing a "health care safety net" for economically disadvantaged groups. Of course, one must be wary of adverse selection as private, profit oriented firms seek to minimize risks by avoiding undesirable customers such as AIDS patients despite government mandates that entire communities be insured at equivalent premium rates. Notwithstanding these potential pitfalls, it certainly appears that developed countries have reached the stage where potential resource infusions from the private sector warrant consideration. The excesses of loosely regulated imperfect competition in the US need not be repeated. The German and Japanese experiences demonstrate that compulsory, single-payer public insurance can co-exist with supplementary private insurance. Along these lines, possible policy options that merit consideration include:

1. Stimulation of private sector participation by means of insurance reform that would allow the pooling of risks within a small employer insurance market.
2. Adoption of "all-payer" systems like in Canada where a single-payer (provincial health care plan) exercises monopsony (single buyer) power to offset the market imperfections of supplier-induced demand and fragmentation of third-party insurance coverage.
3. Imposition of co-payment fees. Despite significant amounts of research and investigation, the idea of co-payments for health care, whether in the form of premiums or user charges, remains contentious.

One of the more comprehensive studies regarding co-payments is the Rand Health Insurance Experiment[18] where a large number of subjects (n = 1,000) were assigned to one of six groups that differed according to the amount of co-payment charged. Out-of-pocket fees were not allowed to exceed 15% of income or $1,000 per annum, whichever is lower. The results of the Rand Study are significant and subject to interpretation. On the one hand, the introduction of co-payment charges did in fact reduce utilization by almost 20% with the greatest drop coming from the heavier users of the health care system. On the other hand, Stoddart et al.[19] point out that the charges were about equally likely to deter patients from using both unnecessary and necessary services. This observation seems somewhat at odds with the study's conclusion that despite some minor exceptions, health outcomes remained very similar across groups regardless of the co-payment charge.

Thus, the controversy surrounding the effects of co-payment charges continues. On the surface, it seems reasonable to apply user fees to deter health service utilization by the "worried well", particularly if they could be applied differentially to exclude emergency and urgent services. However, the reader would do well to bear in mind Stoddart's conclusions that user charges:

1. Will almost certainly increase, not decrease, the total cost of the health care system.
2. Are unlikely either to reduce the use of health services significantly, or to discourage unnecessary and only unnecessary use.
3. Serve to shift the benefits and cost of health care with the benefits going increasingly to those who are able to pay for their care and the costs falling increasingly on those who need and use health services.

Market-Based Reform

In order to pursue market-based reform, policy changes are needed that provide incentives for behavior that promotes system goals and objectives. One of the great mysteries of health care organization in the US is its paradoxical incentive structure. On the one hand, cost control and financial integrity are articulated system goals. On the other, health care services have been organized in such a way as to provide virtually no incentive to limit the consumption of health care resources. Clearly there seems to be room for establishing incentives that would foster more efficient usage of scarce health care resources while maintaining consistency with fundamental system goals.

Health care providers in developed countries have shown themselves to be sensitive and responsive to incentives. In some HMOs, capitated payments to physicians are adjusted by as much as 25% (up or down) depending on desirable cost and quality performance as determined by chart reviews, patient satisfaction surveys, utilization data, and physician participation in preventive programs for enrollees.[20,21]

Indeed, there is much room and need in the health care field for promoting desirable behavior by providing positive incentives. Stoddart[19] suggests that if inappropriate patient initiated utilization of the health care system is a real problem then physicians could play a major role in educating patients in self-care and in recognizing situations that call for appropriate use of the health care system. This function is in keeping with the doctor's mandate as patient counsellor yet the physician who practices this way, under current arrangements, is not financially rewarded—quite the contrary.

Sensible Regulation

As discussed previously, regulation has an important and valuable role in health care. Indeed, with private sector participation in health care, the specters of adverse selection and "cream skimming" cannot be ignored. Regulatory mechanisms such as legislation requiring open enrollment and community rating (same premiums to all members in a group) can mitigate these distortions. What is perplexing is that too much regulation is at odds with the goals and objectives of the health care system. For example, in the US, rather than improving equity, well intentioned state regulation of the insurance market has made it extremely difficult for small employers to purchase insurance due to a dizzying array of complex and costly policies and legislation.

Sensible Tax Policy

Reform is needed in the taxation field as well. In what amounts to a piece of baffling public policy, American legislators exempt employer-paid insurance premiums from federal and state income taxes. To a large degree, these premiums are made in support of fee-for-service medicine that gives hospitals and doctors incentives to treat people in the most expensive ways. This amounts to an estimated annual subsidy of $60 billion annually. Moreover, it weakens any interest that consumers might have to shop around for cheaper insurance alternatives.

A more rational approach would be to eliminate this tax subsidy and replace it with tax exemption status for costs incurred within preferred, non-fee-for-service arrangements such as HMOs. These proposals hold promise in the US given the Clinton Administration's commitment to health care reform.

Rationing

We have seen that health care is a commodity. We have also seen that due to a number of idiosyncrasies, it sometimes functions as though it were shielded from market forces. Yet, as an economic good, it cannot and, arguably, should not be immune from the reality of rationing. For rationing is a mechanism by which priorities (i.e., choices in the face of limited resources) are set.

Despite the discomfort it evokes within some medical circles, rationing is very much like a common clinical practice with which physicians will readily identify, the concept of triage. Essentially, rationing is the application of triage principles to the production and consumption of health care resources within a given population. As such, it governs the distribution of a limited resource. Accordingly, we should accept the principle of rationing and move on to the important issues of who makes the tough decisions inherent in rationing and by which criteria. Such thinking is not confined to the hallowed halls of academia, far removed from everyday realities. The Oregon Formula[22] while somewhat revolutionary, constitutes a practical response by a funding authority (i.e., state government) to a very real fiscal dilemma. It seeks to relate the costs of medical procedures to their benefits as measured in quality-adjusted life years (QALYs—Table 1). Treatments are then ranked according to the cost of producing one QALY with the least expensive procedure at the top of the list, then the next least expensive treatment, and so on, down the list. Available health care resources are allocated to covering the costs of treatments in descending "QALY per dollar" order until the cut-off point when the budget is exhausted. All remaining procedures are left uninsured.

The Oregon Experiment is not a panacea. First, at the present time it applies to only a subset of the population—low income individuals and families who qualify for Medicaid support. Second, there are concerns regarding the validity of QALY values that are derived by means of extensive consultation with community groups, clinicians, legislators, and other health care system stakeholders by means of sampling public opinion through telephone interviews. While cost effective and democratic, this method requires members of the public to express views in areas where they may lack knowledge and experience. Third, there is the technical question of the selection of appropriate discount rates to enable "level playing field" comparisons of alternative treatments whose costs and benefits differ in their timing.

Despite these and other issues, the Oregon Formula represents a serious attempt to face the problem of scarce resources squarely and establish health care priorities by a rational assessment of need, outcome, and ability to pay. In essence, it is a rationing exercise with a cost-utility analysis at its heart. Although it calls for difficult, often unpleasant choices, the Oregon Experiment is an illustration of a realistic response to a set of economic circumstances that we are likely to see for the foreseeable future.

Conclusion

Examples like the Oregon Experiment demonstrate vividly the relevance of economics to the delivery of health services. Despite the unique characteristics of the health care market place, it is clear that the application of economic theory and principles has made important contributions to the appreciation of how health services are produced, distributed, and consumed. These efforts should, and will continue. In addition, reorientation to include non-traditional health determinants has the potential to pay handsome dividends in terms of understanding, and ultimately, improving health outcomes. In light of the importance of health care as a social good, the costs of providing it, the level and the fiscal realities that we now face, the need for health economics has never been greater.

References

1. World Health Organization . . . International Health Conference 19 June-22 July 1946. Amendments January 1984.
2. Nurturing Health: A Framework on the Determinants of Health. Premiers Council on Health Strategy, Queens Printer.
3. Lalonde M: A new perspective on the health of Canadians. Information Canada, Ottawa, 1975.
4. Taylor P: Why the rich live longer, healthier. Toronto Globe and Mail. October 16, 1993, p. A1.
5. Working together to achieve better health for all. Southwestern Ontario Comprehensive Health System Planning Commission, 1991.
6. Evans R, Staddart G: Producing Health. Consuming Health Care. Centre for Health Evaluation and Policy Analysis, #90–6, 1990.
7. Barer B, Evans R: Riding North on a South-Bound Horse? Expenditures, Prices, Utilization, and Incomes in the Canadian Health Care System. In Medicare at maturity. Edited by Evans R and Stoddart G, 1986, p. 63.
8. Klarmen H, ed: Trends and Tendency in Health Economics. In Emperical Studies in Health Economics, Johns Hopkins Press, 1970, part I, p. 3.
9. Evans R: StrainedMercy: The Economics of Canadian Health Care. Butterworths, 1984, p. 3.
10. Evans R: Strained Mercy: The Economics of Canadian Health Care. Butterworths, 1984.
11. Faltermayer E: Let's Really Cure the Health Care System. Fortune, March 23, 1992, p. 46–58.
12. Schwartz WB: The inevitable failure of current cost-containment strategies: Why they can provide only temporary relief. J Am Med Assoc 1987;257: 220–224.
13. Feeny D, Gryatt G, Tugwell P: Introduction: Health Care Technology. In Health Care Technology Effectiveness, Efficiency, and Public Policy. Institute for Research on Public Policy. 1986, p. 1.
14. Birdsall N: Thoughts on good health and good government. Daedalus 1989; 118:89–123.
15. Massaro TA: Impact of New Technologies on Health CARe and on the Nations Health. Clin Chem 1990;36:1614.

16. Sibbald WJ, Escaf J, Calvin JE: How can new technology be introduced, evaluated and financed in critical care? Clin Chem 1990;36:1604–1611.
17. Economist. 1991;July 6:3–18.
18. Lohr KN, Brook RH, Kamberg CJ, et al: Use of Medical care in the Rand Health Insurance Experiment: Diagnosis and service-specific analyses of a randomized controlled trail, Medical care, 25 (supp), p. 531–538.
19. Staddart GL, Barer ML, Evans RG, et al: why not user charges? the real issues. Discussion paper. THe premiers council on health, well-being, and social justice. Sept. 1993.
20. Johnsson J: Physician bonus: HMOs reward high-quality care. Hospitals, Novermber 5, 1989, p. 70.
21. Luft HS: How do health-maintenance organizations achieve their savings? Rhetoric an devidence. N Engl J Med 1978; 298:1336–1343.
22. Stevenson R: The Oregon formula: Health economist's dream or Stalinist nightmare? Archives of disease in childhood. 1991;66:990–993.

Chapter 7

Health Economics for Practitioners of Critical Care Medicine

W. Leigh Thompson, Ph.D., M.D., Sc.D., Douglas Cocks, Ph.D.

Critical care practitioners are colleagues with industry in the pursuits of research and education, are customers of industry in the purchase of goods and services, and are vendors to industry of their expert advice and other services. They are special customers as they select, but usually do not pay for, products for their patients. To understand the special nature of these relationships and potential conflicts among them, and the differences between the health care industry and other industries, let us examine some basic principles. The reader should better understand yesterday and today, and be better prepared to predict and adjust to the rapid changes expected tomorrow.

Free Market, Controlled, and Regulated Economies

In a totally planned economy, a central authority controls the production and distribution of goods and services. In the People's Republic

From: Sibbald WJ, Massaro T (eds.): The Business of Critical Care: A Textbook for Clinicians Who Manage Special Care Units. © Futura Publishing Co., Inc., Armonk, NY, 1996.

of China, for example, you would be assigned an abode, school, job, and permission to have one child, but you would be provided access to goods (e.g., drugs) and services (e.g., physician visits) at the suffrance of the state.

In a totally free-market global economy, each member can purchase whatever goods and services she can afford without restrictions on their origin or quality. Entrepreneurs offering a scarce and valuable service (e.g., bone marrow transplantation) or product (e.g., a drug that cured cancer) would expect to be paid more than a vendor offering dross.

In a democratic market economy, regulations are often imposed for the public good, as determined by the representatives of that public. Such controls benefit some more than others, and impose an administrative cost to be borne by the public. Boston limited the number of cattle that could be grazed upon the Commons to protect the food supply. Competition for a common resource was thereby limited, as today one is constrained from starting a private utility. But Boston had to maintain regulations and regulators to count the cattle and penalize excess grazers.

In developed countries there are few restraints on access to health care for patients who pay for goods and services either directly or through private insurance. Many developed countries, such as Canada and the United Kingdom, limit access to government-paid health care by control of practitioners and hospital beds. In many European countries and Japan the price of health care products is controlled.

In the US there are few restraints on access for patients who pay; certificates of need for capital-intensive devices are one attempt at such restriction but they have restrained little the growth of health care technology in the US. Today Philadelphia has more MRI scanners than Canada. Health care resources in the US are abundant but expensive and heterogeneous in distribution.

Health Care Regulation

The regulation of health care is greater than regulation of most market segments. This regulation is unusual in several respects. Health care practitioners are essentially unconstrained after initial licensing. A plumber is required by law to practice procedures approved by a building code; a physician is usually licensed to perform any medical procedure or to administer to an individual patient any chemicals, subject to product liability and malpractice laws and ethical concerns. This form of regulation assumes the practitioners to be learned, the best judges of optimal care for their own individual patients, and to be acting responsibly for the public good. This, on occasion, may seem to place in conflict the physician's primary responsibility for the best care of an individual patient and distribution of scarce resources (such as tax revenues) for the public good.

Unregulated use of health care products stands in stark contrast to the strict regulation of the sale of devices and drugs. The supply side is highly regulated. A practitioner is deemed sufficiently competent to treat an individual patient with any means available, but sale of those means is usually restricted to articles accepted by a central authority. The demand side is relatively unregulated. A surgeon may investigate and promote a unique surgical procedure with little surveillance; an internist or pediatrician could be jailed for similar use of a new chemical. This differentiates services, which are unregulated, from goods, the supply but not use of which is tightly restricted.

The regulation of human pharmaceuticals in the US began early in this century to ensure purity. When a solvent used for sulfanilamide caused fatal kidney damage in many patients, requirements for proof of safety were added. When thalidomide testing in pregnant women resulted in recognizable birth defects, safety rules were tightened further and proof of efficacy was added.

In general it takes 12.8 years to gain first approval of a newly invented drug; the regulatory review time itself is more than 2 years in many countries. The US Food and Drug Administration (FDA) has changed recently to shorten the overall development time by promoting collaboration with manufacturers early in research to effect the most efficient study designs and by accelerating their approval of truly life-saving innovative products.

Japan has similar tough regulatory requirements, especially for products developed outside of Japan that, in general, must be retested in that country. Although there are differences in drug metabolism among the races, many cross-cultural differences may reflect not drug kinetics but cultural differences in diagnosis, therapeutic philosophy, and relative balance of safety and effectiveness. In Japan small doses that cause few side effects are given commonly with frequent physician visits and an emphasis on caring. This contrasts with intensive chemotherapy in the US guided by technocrats who may have little personal rapport with the patient—a different cultural interpretation of the art and science of medicine.

European requirements accept lesser proofs of safety and efficacy, allowing use of new products earlier in Europe than in the US. Partly because of such disparity in requirements among countries, development of the information package sufficient to launch a new drug worldwide is very expensive. The US Congress Office of Technology Assessment estimated the costs of research on drugs first given to humans in 1970 to 1982 to be about US$358 million (in 1990 dollars), but they also showed these costs to be increasing about 10% per year. Adjusting for the much greater requirements of today would suggest a current investment in a drug just beginning clinical trials in 1993 to be about US$1 billion.

That investment, over a long period at very high risk of failure, is recovered from sales. If the intellectual property is expensive, and the product is expensive to manufacture, these costs must be reflected in the price to ensure that the research investment is repaid to allow continuing research. If others are permitted to sell the product, but are not required to invest in the intellectual property that makes it valuable, they are spared the cost of funding research and can obtain the same profit with a lower price.

Regulation of medical devices and diagnostics by the US FDA began more recently and is evolving. Even a small change in a drug molecule requires de novo testing. In contrast, a modification of an approved diagnostic or device often has been approved quickly after testing in a few sites and relatively few patients. This more laissez-faire approach has changed in 1994 to proofs of safety and efficacy that more closely resemble the rigor of pharmaceutical testing, approval, and manufacturing oversight. The US FDA in particular requires manufacturers to prove that they maintain tightly controlled systems that will prevent a defect from occuring. Recent concerns about faulty heart valves and pacemaker leads has heightened attention on quality assurance beginning with good design and continuing through follow-up of patients with implanted devices.

The demand side is changing rapidly. In a fee-for-service system or when a third party pays for health care, choices are made more on expected benefits than costs and marginal improvements are rewarded with premium prices. But, money is running out. In the US we spent approximately US$ trillion on health care in 1995. That is about US$4,000 per capita, though much more for the elderly. Over a lifetime of 75 years, at today's rates, that suggests each new baby or immigrant will consume US$300,000. Overall spending must increase because the US population is growing rapidly, more than 1% per year, and the success of health care is increasing life expectancy and exchanging expensive eldercare for early death. If the 1993 spending on health care per US resident, by age, were applied to the US population in 1911, the expenses for the 1911 population would be on 28% of the 1993 population. So health care success, aging, immigration, and a high birth rate have more than tripled health care spending in one lifetime.

Within the health care market segment, in which goods are tightly controlled, the need for proofs of efficacy and safety has created a free market in the services of therapeutics research by investigators. In this market the price of research services by critical care practitioners is closely coupled with their quantity, quality, and availability.

Health Care Costs

The buyer's cost is the product of quantity and price. In free markets these are related to the wealth of the population of buyers and the utility the buyers expect of the goods or services. Patients are sensitive to price in selection of automobiles or tailors. The same patients become insensitive to price about health care. More is better and the best is none too good. The patient deserves the best and rarely would an insured patient request lesser quality of care at lower cost.

This is described as a moral hazard. Patients who are insured are not conservative in caring for themselves and may take risks they would otherwise avoid. Also, they tend to overuse services and products provided by group indemnification.

Practitioners also are motivated to provide optimal care, and rarely sacrifice a real but small marginal benefit because of its greater cost. Price insensitivity, or inelasticity, is furthered by separation of payment from the service. You pay cash for a shoeshine, but most Americans prepay health insurance and feel that they should *get all they deserve.* Health care practitioners are agents in health economics, but are not efficient agents in restraining costs.

With rapidly expanding science and technology and few restraints on quantity or price, health care has become expensive. The ward of 30 patients with one nurse has become 15 semiprivate rooms with 8 nurses. One generalist physician has become a team of specialists. A neurological examination by a physician with a pin and hammer has become an MRI with scheduling, transportation, accolytes, and augurers at the capital-intensive shrine. How much is helpful to the patient and how much defends against legal assaults? Has the long-term benefit to critically ill patients been enhanced by on line computer monitoring of many variables? By bedside stat laboratories? Is society better served by intensive care of a 700-gram infant, transplantation of a liver to an alcoholic, prenatal care, or smoking prevention programs?

Rationing

In almost all free countries any patient can pay for any legally available medical services or goods. Some restraints may be applied by governments or other insurers on beneficiaries or benefits. The United Kingdom has chosen to restrict benefits, making local decisions on investments in health care facilities that are available for all. The US, in contrast, has limited beneficiaries but with little restraint, in the past, on the quantity or price of services available to those so selected. This has produced the unusual situation in which lavish health care is more readily available free to a person who is poor than to members of the middle class who must pay directly for care.

There are limited strategies that will impact significantly the overall cost of insured health care. The quantity can be restrained by limiting beneficiaries, benefits, or both. These are major social issues. Oregon is attempting to extend coverage of Medicaid-funded health care to more patients by restricting the procedures for which reimbursement is available. The price can be controlled, and we will examine this option in greater detail below. Finally, almost forgotten in many countries, is improvement in the quality and efficiency of care. What is the real utility to an individual patient of expensive but fruitless health care or excessive documentation? Does every vegetative uremic American require hemodialysis? Why does a skilled physician with decades of experience need the assent of a high school graduate to perform a medical procedure? Why can you get immediate cash from an automatic teller with a plastic card but health care reimbursement requires pages of forms, correction of errors, months of concern, and considerable Pinteresque dialogue? Many US practitioners, on contacting Medicare or Medicaid, feel like they are on hold waiting for Godot. Most employ more assistants to treat paper than patients.

Impact of Regulation of Health Care Goods

If services are unrestrained, what are the effects of restriction on availability of health care goods? Some patients with AIDS or cancer disagree with the standards established by health authorities and insurers and argue for less substantial proofs of efficacy and earlier access to new drugs and devices. Such dialogues bring into conflict the individual versus collective utility and the wisdom of the individual practitioner at the bedside versus an expert body considering only abstractions of patients.

The cost of providing new medical products is proportional to the duration and extent of the testing required for their approval. The major pharmaceutical manufacturers in the US spend more on research than does the National Institute of Health (NIH). This annual investment of $12.5 billion is mostly spent on new drugs, of which about two dozen are approved each year in the US. Worldwide the pharmaceutical industry spends about $24 billion on research that is recovered largely from about 50 new drugs approved in the world each year.

Thus each new drug requires an investment of about US $500 million in current cash flow to discover, develop, win approval, launch, and support its use worldwide. Unfortunately, this US $500 million is spent over a very long time as drugs have a longer development cycle than any other major products.[1] From the beginning of a discovery research program until substantial revenues from international marketing takes more than two decades.

Recovery of Investments in Health Care Products

If you were to invest $500 in even payments of $2.08 each month for 20 years, what return would you expect on this investment? In 1991, diversified equity mutual funds had an average return of 26.27% per year.[2] If you were to expect this average return on your $500 investment, you would expect to receive the equivalent of $17,109 at the end of 20 years of constant investment. If you were not to be paid immediately, but in installments, you would expect even more.

The pharmaceutical industry has greater risk than the average equity investment. Few drugs are approved and only about one-fourth recover their research investments.[3] Pharmaceutical firms themselves are risky investments, as illustrated by the many recent mergers and acquisitions. Since 1990, the US pharmaceutical industry has lost about US $120 billion in market value with shares now trading at 1/2 to 2/3 their previous values. Thus Wall Street, in assessing risks, time, and returns, has voted with their wallets to divert investments from new cures to other, less risky, shorter-term endeavors like making guns, cigarettes, alcoholic beverages, or condoms.

The return to the investor-owners in the pharmaceutical industry is conditioned on the profit and quantity of new drugs sold. To increase the quantity, firms vigorously promote new products worldwide in three markets of almost equal size: North America, Europe, and Asia.

Profit is the difference between price and cost. What is the cost of a drug? The molecule itself has little value. It is the information, garnered from research and experience, that adds value to the molecule. Thus the price must be sufficient to pay for the cost of providing the material itself and also providing the information that is the result of the expensive and prolonged research effort. The sale of today's products must support the research needed for the products of 20 years in the future. Foolish indeed would be the discovery research group not planning for the health care of 2010.

Exclusivity and Intellectual Property Rights

Exclusivity in the marketplace is an important determinant of price. After exclusivity expires, other firms may offer for sale molecules that are physically identical to those of the originator without bearing the cost and risk of research to provide the information that makes these molecules valuable. If customers use the information from the originator, but purchase the cheaper goods, the originator's investment in the information is partly lost.

What determines exclusivity? Patent laws protect intellectual property in many countries. Some countries, however, allow copying and exportation of those copies. This has damaged the intellectual property values of books, recordings, and drugs. In practice it is very difficult to stop importation of a drug manufactured by a patent-protected synthetic process in a country that does not honor patent protections.

Exclusivity is shortened by the time needed to discover, develop, and win approval of a new drug. Some devices have development cycles of months, leaving almost the entire 17 years of patent protection in the US. If, after discovery, a drug takes 13 years to win approval for marketing, its period of exclusivity may be almost entirely exhausted. For this reason many new uses of an older product are not fully developed, because the intellectual property of the new information about the product cannot be protected when the product itself can be freely copied. This explains why some excellent ideas for seemingly valuable new uses of an older product are unfunded by the manufacturer.

Many new drugs and devices, with excellent potential benefits, cannot be developed because their exclusivity has not been properly protected. It is important that critical care practitioners recognize the importance of this element before making public disclosures that limit patent rights. In most countries, a patent must be sought before public disclosure such as a scientific presentation, abstract, or paper. In the US, one has an interval of 1 year after disclosure to file a patent, but in most cases worldwide exclusivity is needed to justify the investment in product development.

Academe and Industry Concerns About Disclosure

Academicians are driven to disclose their innovations and are rewarded for their thinking. Industry is rewarded by marketing a valued exclusive product. Academicians resent delays and restrictions on their disclosing innovative findings. Industry fears that supported researchers, students, consultants, or visitors will prematurely disclose data and information that are the property of, in fact the major product of, the research-based pharmaceutical and medical device industry.

Fundamental to collaboration between industry and academy must be agreement on intellectual property and its protection. Industry is generally pleased to bear the cost of patent applications. Industry is also generally pleased to pay royalties for use of valuable intellectual property. The fears of industry about inadvertent loss of exclusivity can be assuaged by strict attention to this principle by investigators and their entire staffs and collaborators.

Consultations with Industry

Industry wishes to pay experts for their advice and opinions. In return, industry expects candid, thoughtful, objective advice. Never err, as a consultant, by telling what you think your employer wishes to hear. Everyone enjoys being told they are perfect, but such consultations are worthless. Remember your papers in school. You may have beamed at the A+ scrawled on the last page, but you learned from the extensive red marks left by a caring mentor.

In many cases you will need to prepare for consultations by review of the literature or materials provided. In each case, try to determine the scope of the consultation expected—should you restrict yourself to the questions asked explicitly or expand into other areas of your knowledge.

As a consultant, accept that all your suggestions will not be implemented immediately. Your thoughtful suggestions and comments should be welcomed and considered, but there are often many other factors and opinions.

Also, be graceful in interaction with other consultants and employees who differ with your opinions. This does not mean you should not speak up. As Arno Penzias, the Nobel Laureate who heads Bell Labs, has said: "When all in a group agree, all minds but one are redundant." Perhaps he was paraphrasing Satchel Paige: "None of us is as smart as all of us."

A second requirement of the consultant is protection of the employer's intellectual property. Some firms prefer exclusive consultants who do not consult with competitors. If through consultation you gain access to confidential information, you must safeguard it thoroughly. Even the attitude of one firm toward certain products or markets is a valuable secret that must not color your discussions with others.

In the US there are strict laws prohibiting private disclosure of information by "insiders" that would impact investment decisions. If you learn of good or bad news about a product or other affairs of a publicly-traded company as a consultant you are an "insider" and you must not disclose that information privately and you, your family, and your associates may not act upon it before it is widely known to the public.

Restraints on Consultations

Some critical care practitioners may be restrained from serving as consultants to industry, to foundations, or to governmental authorities. Many practitioners are members of multiple medical groups including schools, hospitals, clinics, scholarly societies, and other associations. Investigate carefully the restrictions on offering your services as a consultant. Being a volunteer member of a Pharmacy and Therapeutics Committee in an institution may, for example, restrict your service as a consultant to a purveyor of products to that institution or its owners (such as the federal or state government).

These restraints may extend to presenting your own research work if expenses are reimbursed by a commercial source or in giving lectures sponsored in part by industry. Most of us give the same talk and answer questions the same way whether the meeting is unsponsored, sponsored by a manufacturer of products to be named, or sponsored by their competitors. But, candor in disclosing all financial relationships is always appropriate and now is often mandatory.

Financial Disclosures

Many institutions will ask you to disclose all financial relationships with other institutions. Carefully consider all direct and indirect support you receive or solicit. These relationships may be very complex. Your institutions may request disclosure of only major relationships, or they may wish a full disclosure of every conceivable relationship. You may receive or be promised donations of speakers, books, or products. Expenses of your continuing self-education may have been supported in part or you may have received gifts of goods or services.

You may be asked to disclose financial investments you have made, have been given, or are promised including collective instruments, such as mutual funds, the value of which may be influenced by the deliberations or actions of those with whom you consult. Be especially careful about standing orders to buy or sell stock at certain prices or times as these transactions may occur, automatically, at embarrassing moments. These disclosures usually extend to family members and all means by which you exercise control over investments (such as those held in "street names").

Ensure that you make a full and complete disclosure of all such relationships and be especially sensitive to the possibility that antagonists may, at a later time, apply different judgments to the thoroughness of your disclosures and any investment actions you take while in a position that you might have received insider information.

Are these rules necessary? Aren't honest physicians honest? Can't physicians sift opinions from facts, prejudice from evidence? Of course, and these rules do not guarantee truth and objectivity. But heightened sensitivity to real conflicts and to the possible appearance of prejudice, are valuable practices to make habits even when they may appear at first to be unnecessary for us.

Practitioners and Sales Representatives

Practitioners are experienced in the evaluation of scientific data. Sales representatives should be educators. They should present data from peer-reviewed journals. They should present valid scientific data from other sources with appropriate caveats. In all cases they should represent fair balance in the safety and efficacy of their products and those of competitors. As practitioners, and guardians of the health of her patients, the critical care practitioner should ask informed tough questions and evaluate critically the objectivity and fair balance of information presented by the representatives of a manufacturer, a scientist pursuing her own research program, or a famous opinion leader giving an "educational" lecture. No one is immune from bias and scientists are distinguished by their ability to avoid and detect bias and to challenge it whenever it appears.

Collaborative Research

Investigators often share their thoughts and research tools. The authorship of many publications illustrates the significance of such collaborations. In each such collective endeavor, it is important to define precisely what contributions are made by each party and what is expected in return. A gift of antibodies or cells may at first seem like an unencumbered donation, only to become the focus of litigious conflict over its commercial value which is later discovered.

Commercial enterprises often are asked to provide products, information, financial support, or other goods and services for research, education, or patient care. Most restrict such gifts and are required to do so if the product is for use in animals or patients.

Often the restriction is an agreement on the use of the materials, their disclosure to or use by other parties, and the intellectual property rights of the grantor and grantee. Protocols and reports may be required, and the grantee should not stray from the agreed uses. A critical care practitioner should carefully build a trusting relationship with those firms who can provide her with valued goods, services, and financial support.

Sometimes a firm cannot provide the materials requested. There may be an insufficient supply. The proposed use may not be proven safe, appropriate, or legal in the opinion of the manufacturer. Sometimes a new use of a compound may be patented by another party. In the US, this prohibits the manufacturer of the compound from researching the patented use. Such use patents may thereby restrict support of free academic investigation of a product by the manufacturer who holds the composition of matter patent.

Complication of Preapproval Research

A particular difficulty arises during the preapproval period of research of a product. Each research study must be documented fully with a plan, with validated auditable data, and with complete reports of results. This consumes resources of the manufacturer and complicates and prolongs regulatory review. Many manufacturers wish, therefore, to restrict the variety of research studies before regulatory approval of the first use of a product. They may be very interested in your innovative ideas, but wish to delay initiation of the investigation you propose until after regulatory approval.

Consider the special case in which a small dose of a product is to be used in a benign illness that is associated with few side effects. If you were to pursue studies of a much more aggressive treatment regimen in a serious disorder, there would be many adverse events that would complicate the regulatory review, approval, and labeling of the product for its benign application.

Compassionate Use of Investigational Materials

Compassionate use is the uncontrolled application of an investigational therapy in hopes of helping a sick patient. Compassionate use of an investigational drug may delay its approval for general use. Each such use must be well documented, all adverse effects must be analyzed and reported, and events different from those in controlled trials must be explained. These exercises consume resources, of the sponsor and regulators, which detract from the review of controlled trials.

Such decisions bring into ethical conflict the care of an individual patient today with the potential care of many future patients. Manufacturers and investigators should be careful to consider such requests carefully and to make consistent judgments. What decision would be made in the case of an executive employee of the manufacturer, a prominent shareholder, a powerful politician, or an evocative news reporter? Ethically, should that special patient be differentiated from the unknown patient of a concerned practitioner?

New Academe—Industry Relations

Health care institutions seek bargains and often are willing to restrict choice of their practitioners to discounted products that are good enough. Health care manufacturers need research investigators to show that their products are significantly better. This provides a win-win collaboration between institutions' practitioners performing, for a fee, quality scientific research, especially on health outcomes, and research-intensive manufacturers. The ethics of these relationships should be judged by the quality of the research, the payments for research, the separation of paid researchers from those who make purchasing decisions, and a focus on providing quality care to the ultimate customers—our patients.

Institutions may also agglomerate into buying groups to exert collective influence on the distribution channels. Such collaborations may foster quality research and careful selection of products with real value, but their members should ensure that these evaluations are made by qualified scientists who have the time to thoroughly investigate the products.

Recently, new products have been introduced after there have been scholarly studies of cost benefit. These studies, if well done, should stand as objective criteria in the selection of products and techniques for application in your critical care unit. Unfortunately, we have much to learn about these studies. Should costs only be direct health care costs or should they include indirect costs both medical and general. If a spouse has to miss work or hire a babysitter to provide care, should that be included? Should we measure just objective short-term outcomes for acute effectiveness? Should we measure total lifetime health benefits? Should we assess the patient preferences, utilities? Total lifetime costs and lifetime utilities are the best measures of therapies. If we accept short-term assessments, death is the best way to minimize direct health care costs.

Another serious problem is partitioning health care costs into budgets or benefits into systems rather than having a total view. Some studies have set out to minimize the pharmacy budget by limiting use of drugs, despite increased nursing, physician, and overall health care costs. That is shortsighted. Similarly, many studies take a restricted view of efficacy and report only supine diastolic arterial pressures rather than longevity, sexual function, or quality of life. We will have many opportunities to compare alternative treatments from objective studies and be sure they have measured the important variables in an appropriate manner.

Educational Collaboration

Manufacturers of complex goods and services depend on the knowledge, experience, and judgment of their customers. In health care, many devices and drugs require special expertise for their appropriate use. Manufacturers are especially willing to support initial and continuing education of health care practitioners.

The distinction between education and promotion of specific products is often the source of conflict between government, academe, and industry. If someone markets a safe and effective means of preventing AIDS, would not government, academe, and that firm share an interest in widespread education about its use? What would constitute promotion as distinct from education?

As opinion leaders and role models, critical care practitioners must be cautious in their participation in exercises sponsored by others. If asked to lecture, ensure that your lecture would be the same if it were hosted or supported by a competitor. If invited to attend a special exercise, examine carefully the educational and promotional aspects of it. Any good scientist is experienced in evaluating conflicting data, and in detecting bias, and should not be confused by its source. Remember always Caesar's wife. As a leader you should avoid the suspicion of bias or undue influence, even when you yourself are certain that you would not be unduly influenced by participation in an inappropriate event. Health care practitioners are the guardians of truth and the eschewers of bias—be always thus.

Conclusions

Collaborations between critical care practitioners and industry in education, research, and patient care can be most advantageous to them and patients worldwide. Collaborations are built on trust, mutual respect, clear definition of relationships, strict adherence to agreements, avoidance of suspicion, and an equal devotion to truth.

References

1. DiMasi JA, Bryant NR, Lasagna L: New drug development in the United States from 1963 to 1990. Clin Pharmacol Ther 1991;50:471–486.
2. Morningstar Inc. cited in Business Week 1991, Dec. 30, p. 133.
3. Grabowski H, Vernon J: A new look at the returns and risks of pharmaceutical R & D. Management Science 1990;36:804–882.

Chapter 8

Managing Information as a Resource

Edward D. Sivak, M.D.

Central to the issue of the "Business" of critical care is information that will facilitate definition of the scope of critical care services within a health care institution. The proper definition of services is essential for staffing, equipment purchases, utilization of ancillary support services such as laboratory and radiology, research, education, and budgetary processes within the intensive care unit (ICU). Such definition provides proper focus on external issues such as technology assessment, outcome measures, and health services research. Just as personnel, equipment, physical plant, and the knowledge and experience of the patient caregivers are considered essential resources for operation of an ICU, information is an equally valuable resource. It is the management of information derived from the delivery of patient care that will contribute to success of intensive care units in the 1990s.

When faced with the responsibility of managing information within the ICU, there seems to be little choice but to incorporate the use of

From: Sibbald WJ, Massaro T (eds.): The Business of Critical Care: A Textbook for Clinicians Who Manage Special Care Units. © Futura Publishing Co., Inc., Armonk, NY, 1996.

microprocessing technology into the tasks of patient care. Such effort must encompass both clinical as well as administrative tasks with the end result of a clinical information system (CIS) for the ICU. The final product should not stand alone, but rather mesh with the entire operation of a larger information environment, the hospital information system (HIS). Finally, because of requirements for the health care industry to meet needs of entire communities, data from external information systems should be incorporated into the clinical and administrative databases that originate from the care of the critically ill.

The purpose of this chapter is to acquaint the reader with an understanding of automation of data collection, device interfaces, report generation, and creation of a CIS for the ICU. The use of data modeling to facilitate report generation will be reviewed. This process allows the manager to speculate on the day to day operation of a unit if key information would be available. Finally, the use of large databases in assessing and evaluating health care delivery will be reviewed.

The Evolution of Requirements for CIS for the ICU

The evolution of ICUs represents a requirement to control pathophysiological processes that have either the potential to go awry or have already disrupted life's delicate balance to the point of the risk of death. In the 1960s, patients were placed in coronary care units (CCUs) to be monitored for lethal cardiac arrhythmias associated with myocardial infarction. In the 1970s, there was expansion into medical, surgical, and neurosurgical ICUs using newer technologies to improve clinical observation and physiological intervention. As expected, however, the length of stay, equipment requirements, numbers of caregivers, and physical resources to provide this care began to escalate. The 1980s gave way to an explosive growth in research in intervention, which furthered the science of physiological monitoring. The end result is massive amounts of data derived from the process of patient care.[1,2]

The process of physiological monitoring has exceeded early requirements to monitor cardiac rhythm, blood pressure, pulmonary capillary wedge pressure, and cardiac output. The vast amount of information required for decision-making in the delivery of patient care now reveals deficiencies of the written medical record in the following areas:

Table 1
Deficiencies of the Written Medical Record

Record Content
Missing, illegible, or inaccurate data
Excessive or redundant data
Failure to capture rationale of providers
Lack of standardization of terminology
Failure to describe patient experience
Lack of patient-based generic health outcome measures
Format
Not easily adapted to multiple problems
Data fragmented and not sorted for relevance
Data organized by source and chronologically
Access, Availability, and Retrieval
Patients records required simultaneously in two places
Excessive time required for retrieval of information
Records often difficult to locate
Linkages and Integration
Lack of integration of inpatient and outpatient records
Suboptimal use of available information
Records not easily transferrable

Adapted from reference 3.

1. Content
2. Format
3. Access, availability, retrieval
4. Linkages and integration.

Table 1 expands the natures of these deficiencies.[3]

These deficiencies will be magnified in the 1990s because economic and societal forces are placing increased demands upon critical care practitioners to account for the application of technology to the care of their patients. The phrase "technology assessment" as applied to the ICU, places demands upon the clinician to provide a quality of life beyond just survival of critical illness. Return to home, work, and society must be quantitated in terms of financial cost of years of life gained. For accurate cost accounting, descriptions of indications for services, documentation of services delivered, and resources required for the delivery of the services must be available and easily retrieved and summarized. The effectiveness, efficacy, and efficiency of the ICU must be assessed.[4]

There are requirements for the efficiency of the care to improve. The method for documentation of data derived from bedside monitors, ventilators, and other bedside devices must be improved. Time utilized for documentation of patient care services must be efficiently utilized. Abstraction of data derived from the medical record for reimbursement of services, hospital accreditation, and quality assurance must become less labor intensive. Time required to abstract clinical information from charts for research and education purposes must be reduced. If comparisons of patient populations are made, there must be adjustment for severity of illness.[5,6] In theory, such factors have even raised the interest of the Federal Government of the US to recommending computerization of the medical record with the perception that the quality of medical care will improve.[7]

Economy as a Driving Force for Computerization

Perhaps the most important event that suggested that computerization of the medical record was the wave of the future was a change in the method of reimbursement for medical services. In the US, the change took place in 1984 when reimbursement by Diagnostic Related Groups (DRGs) was mandated by law.[8] The basis for reimbursement became presumed cost rather than charge for service. This shift brought about the necessity to demonstrate quality of care. With this emphasis comes the requirement for documentation of severity of illness and adjustment in mortality figures.[5,6] Unless the data for these processes are computerized and become a by-product of patient care, the cost may exceed the benefit of the exercise.

Computerization of the medical record in Europe has a similar but perhaps more nationalistic focus. With the unification of the European community in 1992, requirements for more uniform health care will increase. By the same token, uniformity in information will follow. A greater exchange of medical information on individual patients is expected as citizens of various countries move freely across previously traditional borders. Since the European vision of health care dictates that the medical record should be . . . "patient centered and linked to allow continuous monitoring of quality of health care and its relevance", computerization is a necessity.[9,10]

Beyond national levels smaller scale projects of equal importance are under way. For example, the Cleveland Health Quality Choice (CHQC) Program has been organized to measure and improve the quality and efficiency of health care services community wide.[11] This common goal is shared by employers, hospitals, and physicians in Cleveland, Ohio and surrounding communities. With reference to the ICU, all hospitals belonging to the Cleveland Hospital Association must document the severity of illness of all ICU patients using the APACHE III scoring system.[6,11] Actual mortality from critical illness will be compared to predicted mortality by APACHE III methodology to define quality. The purpose of such an exercise is to provide information that payers can make available to their beneficiaries to allow them to seek health care from quality institutions. Additionally, hospitals will use the information to improve quality in appropriate areas. But, because of the intensity of data collection, labor costs, borne by individual hospitals remain high.

Along with the change in reimbursement, administrative officers within hospitals have placed increased pressures on caregivers to deliver patient services in an efficient manner and to demonstrate that this is indeed being done. Demands for data to demonstrate quality and efficiency have perpetuated the never ending saga of the "we" (caregivers) versus the "they" (administrators) conflict.

The demand for information to respond to the challenges of improving quality, reducing cost, and increasing access to medical care is so labor intensive that computerization will be the major utility for advancement. Although data to support the benefits of information management systems within ICUs remains anecdotal, East[12] has summarized the intuitive benefits of computerization of the ICU (Table 2). For the most part, however, the lack of proliferation of such systems within ICUs is testimony to the skepticism that exists on the part of executives who make decisions on installation of such systems.[13]

Administrative Versus Clinical Information Management

The incorporation of computer technology into the hospital practice of medicine has been from the financial office and materials handling departments into the more clinically relevant areas.[14] In the past, computing has focused on financial and administrative functions simply because of a matter of economics. The driving force in hospital operations was change capture. As expected, administrators also controlled expenditures, thus seeking technology that could facilitate their jobs.

As mentioned, clinical data is now driving the issue of reimburse-

Table 2
Cost-Justification of Commercial ICU Computer Systems

Category Data	Impact of Computer Systems	Documented Effects
Staffing Personnel retention	Reduced charting time Reduced documentation burden	Reduced FTEs* Increased nursing satisfaction Lower turnover Less training costs
Record management	Complete, detailed, and legible record that is easily searched	Less time spent on QA† Better risk management Better insurance audits (fewer lost charges) More complete billing information DRG management‡ Automated assignment of diagnosis
Supply and resource waste	Elimination of paper record and reduction in errors in medication calculations and duplication of laboratory test orders	Less cost for paper forms Less wasted medication Fewer duplicate lab tests
Improved quality of care	Better quality charts Automated data entry Automated calculations Extensive error checking	Impact on length of stay Questionable outcome Questionable morbidity Questionable quality of care

[a] FTE = full time equivalents (re, staff positions.
† QA = quality assurance.
‡ DRG = diagnosis-related groups.
Reproduced with permission from reference 12.

ment, thus administrative information is derived from the delivery of patient care. The medical record is the by-product of patient care, not the purpose of it. It is this latter point that has perhaps been one of the deterrents to the design and development of computerized clinical record systems. Administrators have not traditionally taken into account the flow of data and information from the point of delivery of patient care. In addition, physicians and other caregivers have not been traditionally involved in design of clinical systems.[14]

Friedman and Martin[14] have concisely outlined the distinction between administrative and clinical information management (CIS) by stating their view of the ideal HIS. Such systems would be composed of six distinct components summarized in Table 3. Medical documentation, medical support, and department management should be placed into the hands of a "Medical Computing Group".[14] This group would be deeply involved in the design and development of computerization of patient care areas. This separation of administrative and clinical computing is perhaps a reasonable outline that best suits a discussion on information management and computerization of the ICU.

Information and the technology required for its management are separate but interdependent entities. The information revolution has fueled the development of computerized information management systems. However, the application of this technology requires strict definition of the tasks that generate data and the processes that generate their derivatives (i.e., information). Regardless of which computer system is selected, users will be required to spend time defining their requirements for such a system. These requirements arise from the need to manage the data collected and to apply it to clinical and administrative situations. Therefore, when designing systems for clinical computing, needs for data should not be defined, but rather, development should begin with the tasks of patient care. Table 4 gives examples of data derived from the tasks of patient care. The definition of information derived from the data will be dependent upon the decisions to be made (clinical vs administrative). For the most part, decisions can be summarized as follows:

Table 3

Components of a Hospital Information System

Core
Registration-ADTR, order entry, results resporting
Business and Financial
Accounts receivable/payable, payroll, etc.
Medical Documentation
Medical record, quality assurance, utilization review, infection control, nursing, discharge planning
Department Management
Pathology, radiology, pharmacy, laboratory, anesthesia, etc.
Medical Support
Treatment protocols, pharmokinetic dosing
Communications/Networking
Connecting all of the above components

Adapted from Friedman and Martin.[14]

Table 4
Examples of Data Derived from the Tasks of Patient Care

Tasks	Data
Clinical Assessment	Provisional/final diagnoses
Physical Examination	Documented findings
Patient Orders	
Laboratory Studies	Hematology, chemistry, microbiology, arterial blood gases
Radiology	Confirmation of diagnosis; new diagnoses; therapeutic assessment
Monitoring	Hemodynamic, respiratory, mental status, therapeutic response, ventilator status
Fluid management	Fluid intake/output (balance)
Nutrition	Amount and type of caloric intake
Medications	Date, time, type, name, dosage
Respiratory	Ventilator settings, oxygen delivery systems, therapeutic intervention
Nutritional Assessment	Caloric intake/nutritional deficiency
Patient Care Plan	Goals of care/impediments to achievement of the goals
Calculations	Therapeutic response, clinical deterioration
Fluid balance	
Hemodynamic indices	
Respiratory indices	
Nutritional requirements	
Flow Sheet Generation	Trends in hemodynamic and respiratory status
	Trends in electrolytes, glucose, hemoglobin, etc.
	Trends in fluid balance, requirements for vasoactive drugs, etc.
	Changes in neurological status if Glasgow coma scale is used
Procedures	Indications, patient tolerance to procedure, technique, complications
Quality Assurance	Abstraction and documentaion of sentinel events

1. Selection of appropriate diagnosis
2. Therapeutic intervention
3. Assessment of efficacy of therapy
4. Implementation of improved patient care process.

Table 5 gives examples of information derived from the data derived from the tasks of patient care. Most important, with respect to clinical information systems is the requirement for caregivers to be involved in the development and implementation processes. Caution

Table 5
Examples of Information from Data Derived from the Tasks of Patient Care

Data	Information
Provisional diagnosis	DRG assignment, billing category, complexity, comorbid condition, complications
Final diagnosis	ICD-9-CM assignment
Procedures	Confirmation of diagnosis, therapeutic response, etiology of pathophysiological process, nutritional status, severity of illness
Flow sheet	Therapeutic response, clinical deterioration, severity of illness (APACHE II & III, SAPS, MPM when combined with laboratory data)*
	Requirements for fluids
Goals of care	Utilization of resources, quality of care, background for ethical decision making in limiting therapeutic intervention
Medication documentation	Medication errors, drug-drug interaction, utilization of resouces
Sentinel events	Deficiency in patient care process
	Identification of opportunities to improve patient care

* APACHE = Acute Physiology and Chronic Health Evaluation; SAPS = Simplified Acute Physiology Score; MPM = Mortality Prediction Model.[5,6,15,16]

should be given to executive decision to implement systems that are principally administrative in origin. Unless information systems have a clinical focus, there is no incentive for the caregiver to utilize them as there is no "pay-back" in the form of facilitated patient care.

Interdependency of Administration and Clinical Systems

As suggested above, there is an interdependency between administrative and clinical computing. Administrative officials of hospitals are in charge of providing adequate facilities for caregivers to deliver safe, effective, and efficient medical care. Caregivers are charged with the responsibility of utilizing appropriate resources to the advantage of their entire patient constituent. When resources are limited, efficiency and appropriateness of care become key issues.[1] In the long run both

Table 6
The Flow of Data Required for Admission to an ICU

Data Elements Authorize a Patient to Receive Care
- A patient has an assigned identity within a community
  - Name, social security #, date of birth, gender
  - Address, employer, health insurance policy #
  - Admitting physician
- The patient becomes a customer within the hospital upon admission
- Verification of identity required for delivery of care
  - Lab studies, x-ray, medication, administration, etc.

Verification Allows for New Data to be Created
- Information is created in multiple databases
  - Laboratory, x-ray, clinical narrative

The Patient Record Becomes a Depository for Information Required for Decision Making
- Decisions include medications, surgical procedures, patient care plans, monitoring frequency, patient orders
  - All decisions are authorized by the attending physician based upon the clinical needs of the patient

The Medical Record Becomes a Depository for Documentation of Outcome of Decisions, Therapy and Qualtiy of Outcome
- The medical record is abstracted for clinical as well as administrative documentation
  - ICD-9-CM coding, DRG classification, UHDA, billing, utilization, UCDS, QA, marketing, education, research

parties are responsible for the delivery and improvement of quality patient care. Administrators cannot exert too much control as clinicians will find other alternatives—other hospitals or other care systems. Clinicians cannot be irresponsible in the use of resources, otherwise hospitals will cease to exist. There is interdependency between both groups entrusted to provide patient care.

This interdependency extends down to the area of information management. Just as the management of critically ill patients requires a team effort by many practitioners within a hospital, an information management system for an ICU requires connections, communications, and data from disparate sources around the hospital. Table 6 represents the flow of information as a patient enters a hospital with subsequent admission to an ICU. Step one of the data flow essentially institutes the cascade of information on a patient. A patient is hospitalized, his identity is established within the hospital computer (usually through the admission/discharge/transfer-ADT-system), and all authorization for further care is based upon the established identity. This identity is administrative in nature but as patient care systems evolve within hospitals, the electronic transfer of the authorization within a hospital to various subsystems will direct the subsystems to accumulate new data. Basic demographics of a patient transferred to an ICU must be sent to the ICU patient care management system. Upon receipt of such data, a file is opened within the ICU system to electronically receive data from the bedside monitor, ventilator, and so forth. In essence the bedside devices and ICU information system require administrative authorization to receive new data on the patient.

A clinical information system should not require manual input of patient demographics that have already been entered into the hospital information system at the time of admission. By the same token, laboratory systems should automatically receive room location and essential demographics from ADT. Similar logic can be extended to the ICU system. The cascade of basic demographic information clearly defines the dependency of a clinical information system upon administrative information from the hospital information system.

Since no single system can stand alone within a hospital without high administrative overhead to enter basic patient demographics and other essential operational data, the conclusion is that information management within a hospital is done on an integrated basis through an extensive distributed network of databases or a large integrated central database. Figure 1 schematically illustrates the difference between the two methods. The patient care system for the ICU is no exception. It does not stand alone. The converse is also true, i.e., a hospital information system does not stand alone. If it is expected to facilitate patient care, it cannot function adequately without clinical orientation. Attempts to create stand alone systems will also result in high administrative costs required for data entry, abstraction, and retrieval.

Data Management Systems Versus Patient Care Systems

Computerized systems to manage data derived from the delivery of patient care have been described (patient data management systems—PDMS). Such systems automatically calculate indices, trend data, and perhaps store it for future review.[17,18] Other systems convert analog signals to digital signals for caregiver interpretation and documentation. The best examples of these later devices are bedside hemodynamic monitors, cardiac output computers, and microprocessor

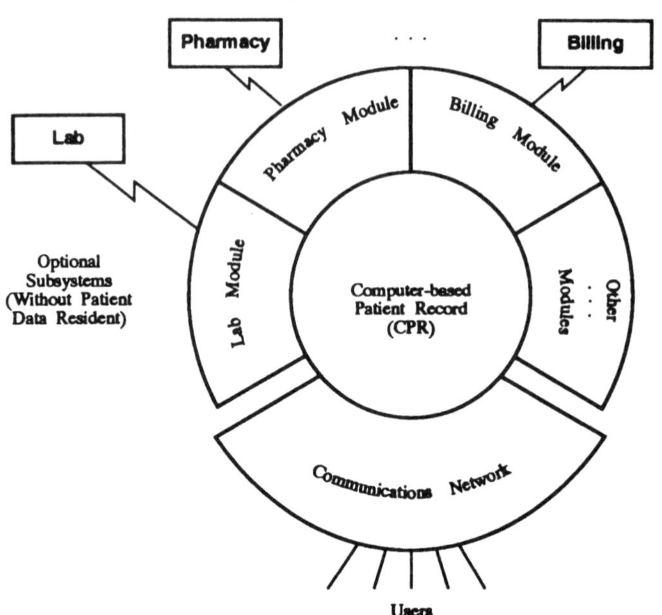
The Centralized CPR
Pharmacy
. . .
Billing
Lab
Pharmacy Module
Billing Module
Optional Subsystems (Without Patient Data Resident)
Lab Module
Computer-based Patient Record (CPR)
Other . . . Modules
Communications Network
Users

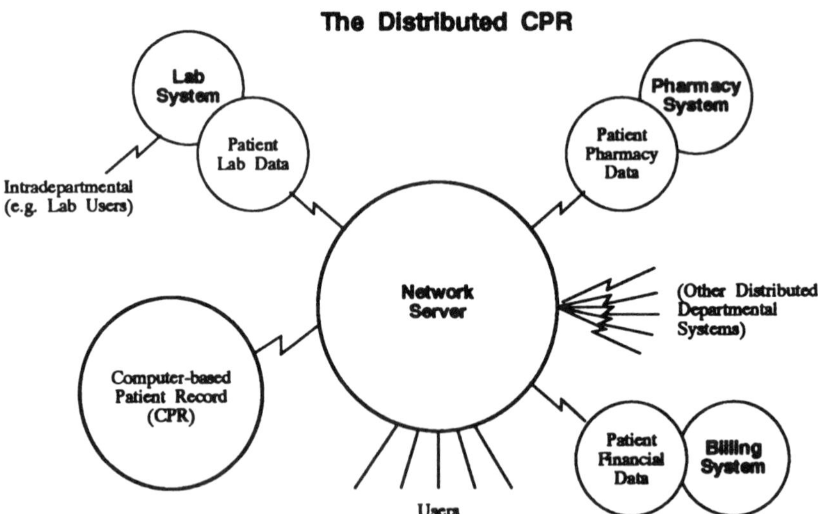
The Distributed CPR
Lab System
Patient Lab Data
Intradepartmental (e.g. Lab Users)
Pharmacy System
Patient Pharmacy Data
Network Server
(Other Distributed Departmental Systems)
Computer-based Patient Record (CPR)
Patient Financial Data
Billing System
Users

Figure 1.

based ventilators. Bedside oximeters, infusion pumps, and capnographs also serve as data management systems. On a larger scale, laboratory systems distribute results to various terminals within a hospital, x-ray systems report interpretations of images to the caregivers, and dietary systems facilitate the calculation of metabolic requirements for critically ill patients.

In contrast, a patient care management system facilitates the tasks of patient care. Such a system allows for automatic data capture and organization, displays the data in an easily interpretable fashion and allows for easy retrieval for retrospective review. If displays are done in an ergonomic fashion, decision-making can be facilitated. It is the patient care system that facilitates the collation of data from disparate sources to create information that is useful to the caregiver as well as the administrator. Properly designed systems also provide for creation of hard copy "flow sheets", medication records, fluid balance, clinical observations, and patient care plans, which can be generated to be placed into the patient's permanent medical record. These documents replace the handwritten medical record.[19]

Technical Components for Computerization

The principle component for computerization of the medical record within the ICU is the bedside terminal. Its location is logical, based upon the requirements for the caregiver to be close to the bedside. The configuration for the system is either to have the processing power located in a bedside microcomputer (decentralized), to have the bedside terminal with some processing power connected to a centrally located

←

Figure 1. In the Centralized Computerized Patient Record (CPR) (left), all patient data are stored in the central CPR, which is the core of the CPR system. The CPR system may be complete, supporting laboratory and nearly all other departmental functions, or it may receive data from remote distributed department subsystems for purposes of maintaining a complete central CPR. In the Distributed CPR (right), patient data are distributed in departmental systems or subsystems. Consequently, the complete CPR does not exist in any one place; rather, portions of the record are distributed among several computer systems. A node on the network might regularly gather data from the distributed computers to present a "view" of the patient's complete CPR.[3] (Reprinted with permission from The Computer-Based Patient Record: An Essential Technology for Health Care. Copyright 1991 by the National Academy of Sciences. Published by the National Acadamy Press, Washington, D.C.)

Table 7
Centralized vs Distributed Architecture

Centralized	Distributed
User outlines requirements	User performs definition
User controls source documents	User manages independent databases
User gets training from others	User is responsible for training
All data files are central	User has independent local files
Central report printing	User prints out reports
Priorities set by central unit	User sets priorities
User does not decide data access	User sets privileges for data access
User keys in data	User responsible for data integrity
User is not involved in evaluation	User evaluates system performance
Hardware is usually a large mainframe	Micro/mini computer
Operating system is complex	Operation and programming possible by user

Adapted from: Distributed information systems. In: Ahituv N, Neumann S. Principles of Information Systems for Management. Second edition. Wm. C. Brown Publishers, Dubuque. 1986, p. 328–329.

computer within the unit (distributed), or to have the terminal access the hospital mainframe computer (centralized). There are advantages and disadvantages to each of these configurations. These can be classified under developmental, operational, and control issues as summarized in Table 7. Since the ICU practitioner usually functions more independently, the distributed architecture with access to the HIS may be the best fit for the ICU.

Regardless of which architecture is selected for an ICU patient care management system, there will be requirements for software that can generically be classified as:

1. Operating systems
2. Database management system
3. Application software.

Operating System

The operating system is responsible for institution of instructions from either the user or other systems that enter or retrieve data from the system. Some operating systems are able to support only a single user (an example of such a system is DOS—disc operating system). More complex operating systems can support multiple users (OS 2 by IBM). While still others are able to support multiple users while performing multiple tasks (UNIX, UNIX Systems Laboratories, Summit, NJ, USA and QNX, Quantum Software Systems, Ottawa, Canada). For the ICU, the operating system should be analogous to the methods by which patient givers perform their daily tasks (i.e., caregivers are usually required to perform multiple tasks, while using multiple resources within the unit as well as the hospital).

Database Management System

The database management system is responsible for storage as well as rapid retrieval of data for clinical as well as administrative decision-making. The more logical the arrangement of this component of the system, the more rapid will be retrieval and display of data for review. It is on this point that one should begin to define the tasks of patient care so that computer programmers can understand the requirements to retrieve data from the database. Table 8 lists examples of patient care tasks that will have data as a by-product.

Application Software

Application software performs specific tasks that meet specific needs of the user. For example, a data input screen may allow for manual entry of hemodynamic data to facilitate the automatic retrieval of data from a monitor or a ventilator. In the background, the calculations of hemodynamic or respiratory indices will be performed and automatically displayed on the computer screen following calculation. A different screen may allow for the input of fluid intake and output while the total of each type of intake and output is accumulated. When the caregiver requests a 24-hour calculation, a numerical display or graphic display may be produced. The application software is responsible for calculation as well as formulation of specific displays. Tables 9 and 10 and Figure 2 illustrate these points.

To the bedside caregiver issues of operating system, database management system, and application software are perhaps "transparent". They represent a vast amount of complex technology below the surface of the bedside terminal. The patient caregiver interacts with a system through an interface. Such an interface is by keyboard, mouse, trackball, touch screen, voice, and so forth. Utilization of the system is through commands communicated via screen displays. Table 11 displays the menu approach and Figure 3 displays a graphical user interface (GUI)

Table 8
Data as a By-Product of Patient Care

- Vital Signs Assessment
  - Data—Temperature, pulse, respiration, blood pressure
  - Information—hemodynamic indices
  - Editorialized information—presentation of therapeutic response
- Ventilator Care Tasks
  - Data—FiO2, tidal volume, rate, peep, peak pressure, pressure support, arterial blood gases, oximeter, capnography
  - Information—oxygen delivery, ventilation/perfusion mismatch, compliance, etc.
  - Editorialized information—therapeutic response
- Fluid Balance
  - Intake by type and name
  - Output by type and name
  - Calculation of excess or deficit
- Medication Record
  - Orders given
  - Orders executed
- Dietary Orders
  - Calculated requirements
  - Administered (percent of requirements)
- Patient Care Plans
  - Patient orders
  - Administered orders
- Progress Notes
  - Physicians
  - Nurses
  - Therapists
- Review of Laboratory Data
  - Chemistry
  - Hematology
  - Microbiology
  - Specialized data

through the use of "windowing" techniques. Regardless of which method is used to allow the user to access the utilities within a bedside patient care management system, the interface must be accomplished in a fashion that is intelligible to patient caregiver.

Utilization of Information Derived From an ICU Patient Care Management System

The technical and administrative aspects of information management within the ICU have been discussed. Closely interwoven into these issues are the clinical elements that provide the thread responsible for cohesiveness of the operation of the entire ICU team. The fuel for the operation is derived from influx of information from outside of the ICU (laboratory, radiology, pharmacy, dietary, microbiology, etc.), from bedside devices (monitor, ventilator, oximeter, infusion pumps, etc.) and from caregiver observations. On these points, the purpose of the ICU patient care system begins to emerge. Although the logic necessary to justify the construction of ICU information management systems may seem obvious, the lack of proliferation of such systems raises the question: "How would one utilize such a system beyond facilitation of the delivery of patient care?" To answer the question, the critical care practitioner must examine his or her daily routine and data utilization, both clinical and administrative. For purposes of discussion, the data model for quality assurance proposed by Sivak and Perez[20] will be

Table 9

Example of Computerized Flow Sheet Illustrating Patient Data

	Vital Signs							
	08/24 13:00	08/24 14:00	08/24 15:00	08/24 16:00	08/24 17:00	08/24 18:00	08/24 19:00	08/24 20:00
Temp °F	99.2	99.5	99.4	98.7	99.4	99.6	99.3	99.2
Heart Rate	155	155	155	155	138	138	132	129
Resp Rate	22	2	22	22	21	22	21	22
Sys	72	73	73	75	75	66	84	66
Dia	46	47	47	46	46	43	55	42
MAP	54	55	55	55	55	50	64	50
PAS	30	30	31	31	30	31	30	30
PAD	16	17	17	17	14	13	15	14
PAM	23	24	24	24	21	19	19	21
CVP	7	7	7	7	7	7	7	7
PCWP	9	9	10	10	8	8	8	8
CO	3.20	3.20	3.20	3.20	3.20	3.20	3.20	3.20
CI	1.9	1.9	1.9	1.9	1.9	1.9	1.9	1.9
Heart Sound	click	wnl	click	click	wnl	wnl	wnl	rub
SVR	1174	1198	1198	1198	1198	1074	1423	1074
Skin Color	pink	pale	pink	pale	pink	pale	pink	pale
Bowel Sound	wnl	defer	wnl	absent	absent	absent	absent	absent
Left Rad	boundi	boundi	boundi	strong	wnl	strong	strong	strong
Rght Rad	wnl	wnl	wnl	strong	wnl	strong	strong	strong
Left Ped	wnl	wnl	wnl	faint	wnl	faint	faint	strong
Rgt Ped	wnl	wnl	wnl	faint	wnl	faint	faint	strong

An example of the use of application software illustrating data taken from various parts of the medical record. It is summarized in tabular form to facilitate caregiver analysis of patient status. This table is a facsimile of a computer screen.

utilized. Data elements are grouped according to structure, process, and outcome as shown in Table 12. The logic of the model is illustrated in Figure 4, which demonstrates that on first observation of an activity, the immediate information derived is that of an outcome. The process responsible for the outcome requires closer observation and finally, the structure or rules that regulate the process require the closest scrutinization for understanding. To derive information from data, proper grouping of the data is essential. Table 8 is a suggested model. When viewed in longitudinal fashion, temporal quantitation is possible. For example, if one wishes to quantitate the use of a technology such as mechanical ventilation used on a patient, it would be expressed in percent of patient

Table 10
Ventilator Rounds

ARGUS 2000 user: rai | Pt. Status: ADMITTED | Page: 1
Pt. Name: | Sex: F | Race: CAUC
Pt. ID #: | Unit/Bed: G62/07 | Admitted: 08-18-91 | Age: 59 yrs
Dr: | Diagnosis:

Date	08/19	08/19	08/19	08/19	08/19	08/19	08/19	08/19	08/19
Time	1055	1100	1320	1400	1425	1429	1433	1434	1439
vmode	SIMV	SIMV	SIMV	SIMV	SIMV	SIMV	SIMV	SIMV	SIMV
PEEPCPAP	0	0	0	0	0	0	0	0	0
presssupp	0	0	0	0	0	0	0	0	0
waveform	RA	RA	RA	RA	RA	RA	RA	RA	RA
sens	3.0	3.0	3.0	3.0	3.0	3.0	1.0	1.0	1.0
PkAirwayP	45.5	40.2	34.5	36.3	35.7	35.2	37.7	36.3	36.2
PlateauPress	.0	.0	.0	.0	.0	.0	.0	.0	.0
VTMech	800	800	800	800	800	800	800	800	800
VTPatient	877	885	854	877	862	862	834	831	862
TotalMV	11.40	11.50	11.10	11.40	11.20	11.20	10.90	10.80	11.20
SpontMV	.00	.00	.00	.00	.00	.00	.06	.00	.00
RRMech	13	13	13	13	13	13	13	13	13
RRPatient	13	13	13	13	13	13	13	13	13
pkiflow	80	80	80	80	80	80	80	80	80
IERatio	3.0	3.0	3.1	3.0	3.1	3.1	3.1	3.1	3.1
FiO_2	50	50	50	50	50	50	50	50	50
SighVol	1000	1000	1000	1000	1000	1000	1000	1000	1000
SighRate	1	1	1	1	1	1	1	1	1
SighHiPress	20	20	20	20	20	20	20	20	20
LoExhVT	100	100	100	100	100	100	100	100	100
LoExhMV	8.0	8.0	8.0	8.0	8.0	8.0	7.0	7.0	7.0
HiPressLt	68	68	68	55	55	55	55	55	55
LoPressLt	20	20	20	20	20	20	20	20	20
HiRR	35	35	35	35	35	35	40	40	40
CircTemp	.0	.0	.0	.0	.0	.0	.0	.0	.0
CircChg									
TubePos	0	0	0	0	0	0	0	0	0
CuffP	0	0	0	0	0	0	0	0	0

An example of automatic capture of ventilator parameters and settings at various times from a ventilator-dependent patient. This table is a computer printout of data.

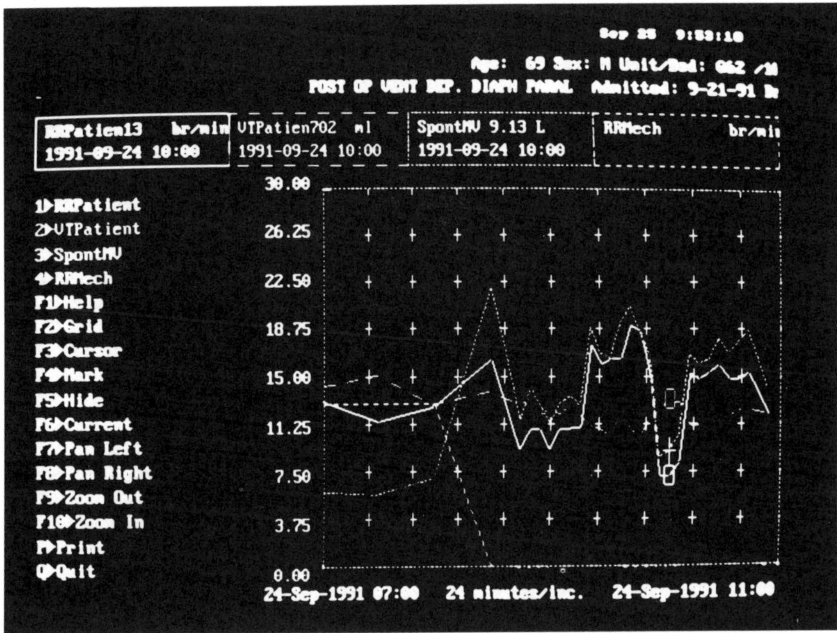

Figure 2. This screen illustrates spontaneous respiratory parameters of a patient being weaned from a ventilator. The patient's respiratory rate (RR patient), title volume (VT patient), and spontaneous minute ventilation (SPON MV) for the marked times (boxes on graft) are shown in rectangular boxes on the top of the graft.

days. If the patient required 10 days of ICU care and used the ventilator for 8 days, then the quantitation would be 8 of 10 days of ICU care. If the patient required 25 days of total hospitalization, then ICU utilization would be 10 of 25 days.

Outcome Analysis

Freedom of choice, financial pressure, and limited resources have driven the science of outcome prediction.[21] Although recent literature scientifically validates numerous probability estimates of outcome, classification of disease, per se, is not a recent development.[6,15,16,22] Table 13 lists some of the documented classifications in recent literature that can be applied to various components of a patient's illness. If one uses the ICU as a focal point in a patient's life cycle, the true panorama

Table 11

Meridia Huron Patient Care Physician's Patients Assigned to a Bed Processor

Mon Sep 28, 1992 01:41 pm

No	Name	Sex	BD	Room	Physician	SVC	Status	
00000–00000	DOE, JOHN	M	08/16/31	107-2	SIVAK, EDWARD	MED	INP	14
	Option No.	Option						

	Option No.	Option
Orders	1	Selected departments
	2	All active/pending
	3	Charge inquiry
	4	Pharmacy profile inquiry
	5	Consultation
Results	6	Laboratory orders
	7	Radiology orders
Information	8	Display patient care profile
	9	Patient information
	10	Patient appointment inquiry
Print	11	Attestation form
	12	Information cards
	13	Face sheets

Enter option number—

The above table is a printout of a computerized screen, displaying the menu approach of interfacing with application software.

is that of events that take place prior to, within, and after ICU admission and discharge. Classifications can be organized into databases both within the ICU environment and from without. The data elements contained in the classifications provide the basic background for outcome analysis. Each focuses on a different component of illness—the pre-ICU phase, the ICU phase, and the post-ICU phase of illness.

Within the ICU environment, databases of hemodynamic and respiratory variables can be collected electronically through device interface. Patient observation and disease classifications can be combined with the former to define physiological status, severity of illness, and outcome prediction. Fortunately, most classification systems lend themselves to computerization and database construction. Spreadsheet utilization provides an inexpensive method for sorting and analyzing data.[20,37] The APACHE III system (APACHE Medical Systems, Washington, DC, USA), can facilitate construction of databases based upon severity of illness and outcome prediction. The theme for such construction is:

1. Data collection (manual and automatic)
2. Data entry (manual and automatic)
3. Data editorialization (information creation)
4. Data reporting (for analysis and decision-making).

The ICD-9-CM (ICD-8 in Europe) and soon ICD-10 systems of disease classification are used to create a hospital discharge abstract—in the US, the Uniform Hospital Discharge Abstract (UHDA). This abstract available in any hospital certified by the Joint Commission on the Accreditation of Health Care Organizations (JCAHCO), consists of information as listed in Table 14. This information is frequently computerized and can be available for passage into a format for use in the microcomputer environment (PC). Information on length of stay, hospital discharge status, and co-morbid conditions are of particular use in outcome analysis and provide additional data according to the data model shown on Table 8. Table 15 illustrates a typical computerized printout of a

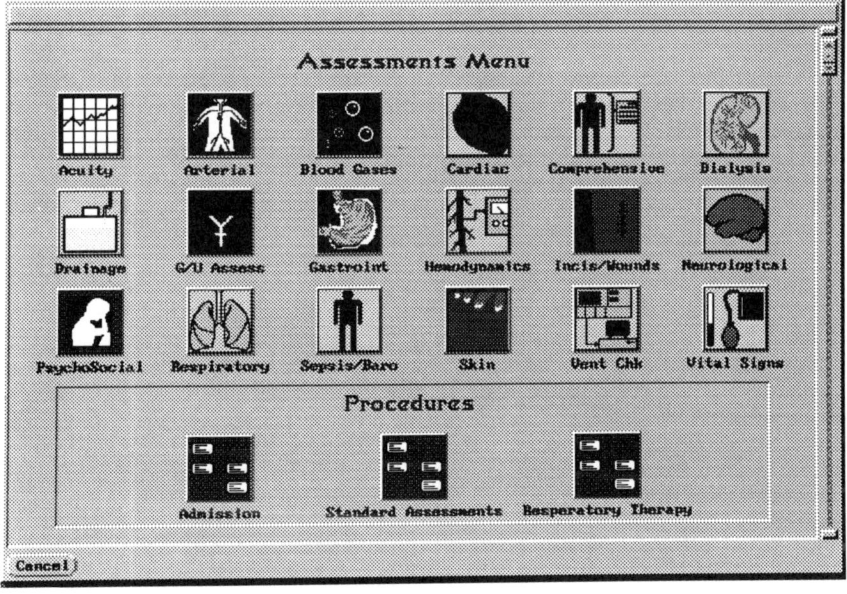

Figure 3. A computer screen from a commercial computer system for the ICU illustrates a completely different approach to the utilities within the system. Various icons are selected through the use of a "mouse" rather than by selection of written "menu" items. Although not reproduced, one can conceptualize how the user may rapidly access the various utilities by visual review of the icons. This particular screen is customized to access administrative utilities such as acquity as well as data from laboratory (blood gases), bedside devices (monitor and ventilator), and for the input of various clinical observations (gastrointestinal, neurological, psychosocial, and so forth). Certainly, more frequently performed assessments and procedures (Admission, Standard Assessments, and Respiratory Therapy) are set aside in the lower portion of the screen. (Photo courtesy of Mr. George Morrison, ACT/PC, Madison, Wisconsin.)

Table 12
Data Model for Quality Assessment in the ICU

Structure (pre-ICU phase)	Process (ICU phase)	Outcome (post ICU phase)
Name	ICU admission diagnosis	ICU discharge status
Identification number	Severity of illness on admission	Condition on discharge
Age	Technologies used in patient care (dates started and discontinued)	Custodial care
Sex	Mechanical ventilation	Rehabilitation care
Hospital admission date	Hemodynamic monitoring	Ventilator-dependent
Hospital admission service	Pressor agents	Hospital discharge date
Severity of illness on admission	Inotropic agents	* Post-ICU hospital days
Pre-ICU diagnoses	Vasodilator agents	Hospital discharge status
Pre-ICU procedures	Antibiotics	Home
* Pre-ICU days (number)	Parenteral nutrition	Nursing home
ICU admission day	Plasmapheresis	Ventilator-dependent
ICU admission diagnosis	Cardiopulmonary resuscitation	Hospital discharge status
	If appropriate, date DNR order written	Home
	ICU discharge date	Nursing home
	* ICU days (number)	Ventilator-dependent (home, nursing home)
	Discharge Status (died, survived, ventilator dependent)	Follow-up (1,3,6,12 months post-discharge); survived, died, quality of life

* Quantitation is obtained by dividing the number of days in each category by the total number of hospital days.

Reproduced by permission from reference 20.

UHDA derived from the HIS at Meridia Huron Hospital (Meridia Hospital System, Cleveland, OH, USA). This printout is readily available to a patient's attending and consulting physicians. This information combined with, for example, prediction of outcome, provides an adjusted mortality ratio.[6] The principle of information management applied is that data from two different databases can be combined electronically with properly designed information systems interfaces.

Outcome of illness beyond hospital discharge is becoming a major concern for all segments of society. Success can no longer be based upon survival alone. Quality of life is a more significant quantifier.

Numerous studies have documented long-term survival beyond ICU and hospital discharge. To such end, a prospective study is usually required for data acquisition. For long-term follow-up national databases may be useful. For example, in the US, the National Death Index (NDI) provides a suitable source of information for long-term survival. Table 16 illustrates a typical method of cross-indexing a database created within an ICU and the NDI. This information can be accessed electronically using a microprocessor environment (PC) or larger mainframe environment. The date of death, state of death, and death certificate number are within the public domain and are readily available on a yearly basis. Data is available from a previous year and is updated on a yearly basis. For example, data from 1992 would be available at the end of 1993. A researcher may also request a copy of a death certificate for cause of death but must design a formal research proposal and define methods of confidentiality if any further follow-back is desired.

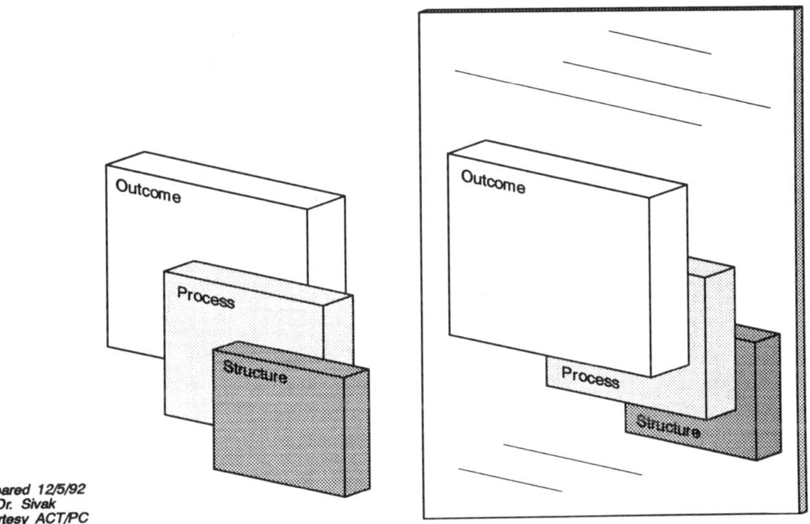

Figure 4. One problem with quality assessment has been the natural tendency to focus on the outcome, rather than on the structure and process that lead to the outcome. This figure, a "mirror image" model demonstrates the need to place structure and process in the forefront when assessing quality. For example, the outcome of a patient's ICU course may be death. If one examines the process, which involved judicious application of technology without unnecessarily prolonging life, one may show that the structure, or rules that governed the process, is responsible for the outcome. (Reproduced with permission from Sivak ED, Perez-Trepichio A: Quality assessment in the medical intensive care unit: Evolution of a data model. Cleve Clin J Med 1990;57:273–279.)

Table 13
Patient Classification Systems for Entire Patient Populations

Pre ICU-Entire Hospitalization	ICU Indices	Post-ICU Quality Evaluation
Diagnosis related groups[23]	APACHE and APACHE II[29]	Activities of daily living (ADL)
International classification of diseases (ICD-9-CM)[24]	Simplified acute physiology score (SAPS)[15]	Karnofsky performance status scale[31]
Physician's current procedural terminology (CPT)[25]	Mortality prediction model (MPM)[16]	Sickness impact profile[33]
Disease staging[26]	APACHE III[6]	Nottingham health profile[34]
Severity of illness index[27]	Therapeutic intervention scoring system (TISS)[30]	Functional status questionnaire[35]
Medical illness severity grouping system (MEDISGRPS)[28]		Quality adjusted life years[36]

Pre-ICU indices are often applied to patient populations throughout the entire course of hospitalization.

ICU indices are applied to specific portions of hospitalization.

Post-ICU indices are used to quantitate the long-term outcome of the patient care process.

For the future, as information systems facilitate the capture of data, clinicians will be able to utilize indices such as those listed in Table 13. The clinical record will quantitate quality of life in a more objective fashion rather than in terms of "feeling well" or "no complaints". Electronic files for the pre-ICU, ICU, and post-ICU phases of illness combined with outpatient records will provide better insight into quality of care, technology assessment, and utilization of resources quantitated in terms of life-years gained.[35]

Process of Care

Quantitation of the process of patient care is traditionally a financial matter. Cost accounting, however, has been difficult to validate because hospital financial charges have been average costs rather than patient specific. To circumvent the shortcomings of such systems, various scoring systems such as Therapeutic Intervention Scoring System (TISS) have been devised.[30] Such a system quantitates the process of patient care based upon the intensity of the tasks of patient care. Table 17 is an editorialized version of TISS, which demonstrates the quantitation of patient care. As one examines some of the data points listed in

Table 17, it becomes clear that each is documented somewhere in the patient's chart. Computerization of the patient record would facilitate abstraction of these data points thus making the quantitation of patient care, a by-product of the care itself as documented in the patient record.

The process of patient care can be analyzed by auditing sentinel events. Databases can be constructed utilizing a simple spread sheet or by utilizing commercial systems such as that marketed by APACHE Medical Systems. This latter system provides the user with a method of entering data on severity of illness, TISS events, and user defined sentinel events. Sentinel events may include pneumothorax, accident extubation, continuous patient agitation, medication orders, and so forth. If sentinel events are documented into the electronic medical record, data abstraction can be done automatically.

Additional administrative information about the process of patient care can be derived from other external databases within hospital information systems. Table 18 is an example of a computer screen that exists on the HIS within Meridia Huron Hospital. As can be seen, financial charges are summarized for review. Such information is useful in analyzing the financial impact of critical care, particularly long-term patients. Note that certain areas are designed as cost centers—pharmacy, surgery, laboratory, radiology, and respiratory therapy.

As one seeks to enlarge the information contained within an ICU information system, data on severity of illness can be accompanied with data that quantitates the process of patient care. Figure 5 illustrates the

Table 14
Uniform Hospital Discharge Data Sets

Patient name
Hospital number
Date of birth
Age
Gender
Admission date
Discharge date
Discharge status
Medical diagnostic category (MDC)
Diagnosis related group (DRG)
Principle diagnosis and description
Secondary diagnoses and description
Primary procedure and description (Date & surgeon)
Secondary procedures and descriptions (Date & surgeon)

Table 15

Uniform Hospital Discharge Abstract Derived From the Hospital Information System

MERIDIA HURON HOSPITAL
P.O. BOX 74299, CLEVELAND, OHIO 44112

Date	Name		Account #		Financial Class
09/13/92					
Sex	Birth Date	Age	Adm Date	Dsch Date	LOS
M					102

Attending Physician — Discharge Status

Coder: — 10 - Rehabilitation

MDC: 1 DISEASES/DISORDERS OF THE NERVOUS SYSTEM
DRG: 483 TRACH EXC MTH, LAR, PHAR DIS

		DIAGNOSIS	DESCRIPTION		DIAGNOSIS	DESCRIPTION
1.	(P)	952.10	*T1–T6 SPIN CORD INJ NOS	9.	510.0	*EMPYEMA WITH FISTULA
2.		512.8	*SPONT PNEUMOTHORAX NEC	10.	862.8	INTRATHORACIC INJ NOS-CL
3.		510.9	*EMPYEMA W/O FISTULA	11.	E965.4	ASSAULT-FIREARM NEC
4.		486	*PNEUMONIA ORGANISM NOS	12.	296.23	DEPRESS PSYCHOSIS-SEVERE
5.		263.9	*PROTEIN-CAL MALNUTR NOS	13.	518.81	RESPIRATORY FAILURE
6.		780.3	*SEIZURE DISORDER			

Table 15. (con't)

7.		038.9	*SEPTICEMIA NOS		
8.		518.5	*POST TRAUM PULM INSUFIC		
		PROCEDURE	DESCRIPTION	DATE	SURGEON NAME
1.	(P)	33.22	FIBEROPTIC BRONCHOSCOPY	06/04/92	
2.		96.56	BRONCH/TRACH LAVAGE NEC	06/04/92	
3.		34.04	INSERT INTERCOSTAL CATH	06/01/92	
4.		96.72	CONTIN MECH VENT>=96 HR	06/04/92	
5.		03.31	SPINAL TAP	06/14/92	
6.		33.23	OTHER BRONCHOSCOPY	06/09/92	
7.		31.1	TEMPORARY TRACHESTOMY	06/17/92	
8.		34.04	INSERT INTERCOSTAL CATH	06/17/92	
9.		33.23	OTHER BRONCHOSCOPY	06/17/92	
10.		43.11	PERCUT ENDO CASTROST/PEG	07/17/92	
11.		34.09	OTHER PLEURAL INCISION	07/21/92	
12.		97.23	REPLACE TRACH TUBE	07/21/92	
13.		45.13	SM BOWEL ENDOSCOPY NEC	09/03/92	
14.		97.51	REMOV GASTROSTOMY TUBE	09/03/92	

HOSPITAL NUMBER DIAGNOSES SUMMARY WORKSHEET
09/12/92

The table represents the summary of a hospitalization of a young gunshot victim. The items are self-explanatory. Note that each item—medical diagnostic category, diagnosis related group, and diagnosis and procedure code is followed by a text description. Diagnosis and procedure codes are ICD-9-CM codes. Procedures are listed chronologically and by the performing physician (the identities of patient and physicians have been erased). This information is readily available to the patient's attending and consulting physicians through any terminal within the hospital.

Table 16
National Death Index Data Set Items

Data Element	Tape Position	Descriptors
*Name		
Last	1–20	First and last names required
First	21–35	
Middle initial	36	
*Social Security #	37–45	All nine digits required
*Date of birth		
Month	46–47	May be sufficient with first and last names without social security #
Day	48–49	
Year	50–51	
*Father's surname	52–71	
Age at death	72–74	
*Sex	75	
Race	76	
Marital status	77	
State of residence	78–79	
State of birth	80–81	
Control #	82–91	Users identification (e.g., hospital record #)
Optional data	92–97	
Blank	98–100	

* Data sets for possible NDI record match.

Data output includes: State of death, death certificate #, first name, middle initial, last name, father's surname, social security #, date of birth, age, sex, race, marital status, state of residence, state of birth, user ID.

From: National Death Index User's Manual. U.S. Department of Health and Human Services. Public Health Service. Centers for Disease Control. National Center for Health Statistics. Hyattsville, Maryland. Sept. 1990. DHHS Publication No. (PHS) 90-1148.

concept of the comparison. Beyond this analysis, quantitation of patient days devoted to mechanical ventilation, utilization of Swan Ganz catheters, the care of the survivor and nonsurvivor provides better understanding about resource utilization. Table 19 is an example of how spread sheet formation could facilitate data analysis on resource utilization and process quantitating.

Decision Support Systems

The foregoing discussion implies that computerized patient care management systems for the ICU provide only administrative utilities.

Table 17
Examples of Therapeutic Intervention Scoring System Data Elements

4 Points
- Cardiac arrest and/or countershock within 48 hours
- Controlled ventilation with or without PEEP
- Balloon tamponade of varices
- Pulmonary artery line
- Atrial or ventricular pacing
- Platelet transfusions
- IABA (Intra-aortic balloon assist)

3 Points
- Hyperalimentation or renal failure fluid
- Chest tubes
- Nasotracheal or orotracheal intubation
- Complex metabolic balance (e.g., frequent I & O)
- Vasoactive drug infusion
- Peripheral arterial line
- Active diuresis or fluid overload or cerebral edema

2 Points
- Central venous pressure
- $>$ 2 IV lines
- Fresh tracheostomy
- Spontaneous respiration via E-T tube or tracheostomy

1 Point
- EKG monitoring
- Hourly V.S. or Neuro V.S.
- Decubitus treatment
- I.V. antibiotics
- Supplemental oxygen (nasal or mask)

Adapted from Keene, Reference 30.

Each data element is assigned a weight according to the above scale. Quantitation can be by shift by adding the total number of points for each data element recorded from the patient care process.

Perhaps far more reaching is the expectation that properly integrated databases will provide decision support systems for the patient caregiver. The number of data points that the practitioner must analyze during the delivery of patient care has multiplied to the point where it is unrealistic for the human mind to manage them without assistance.[37] The HELP systems at the LDS Hospital in Salt Lake City, Utah is perhaps the most extensively described decision support system in use, at least in the US. It contains decision support utilities for antibiotic therapy, nutritional management, and mechanical ventilation manage-

Table 18
Patient Care Charge Injury From the Hospital Information System

Meridia Huron Patient Care Charge Inquiry Processor

Mon Sep 28, 1992 01:32 pm

No	Name	Sex	BD	Room	Physician	SVC	Status
00000–00000	DOE, JOHN	M	08/16/31	107-2	SIVAK, EDWARD	MED	INP 14

Department	Today	All	Department	Today	All
CARDIOPULMONARY	0.00	103.00			
CENTRAL SUPPLY	0.00	620.00			
DIETARY	0.00	0.00			
LABORATORY	0.00	1215.00			
PHARMACY	12.46	583.73			
RADIOLOGY	0.00	507.00			
RESPIRATORY THERAPY	0.00	1782.00			
SURGERY	0.00	983.00			
OTHER	185.00	8736.80			
*** Total	197.46	14530.53			

The table represents a summary of charges for a patient with motor neuron disease admitted for placement of a feeding gastrostomy tube and treatment of associated respiratory insufficiency requiring noninvasive mechanical ventilation. This information is available to a patient's attending and consulting physicians on any terminal within the hospital.

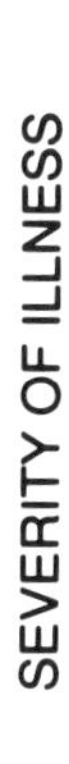

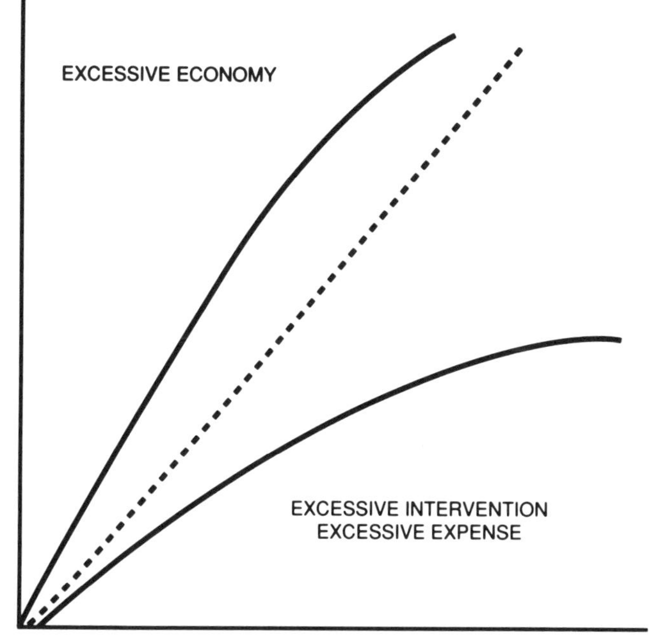

Figure 5. The dotted diagonal line represents a balance between severity of illness and the appropriate application of technology. The X axis could be calibrated with the Therapeutic Intervention Scoring System (TISS) and the Y axis with severity of illness (e.g., APACHE II or III). The balance between these two variables can be determined only over time and through comparison with other institutions. Excessive intervention (or higher TISS) with low or moderate severity of illness could be associated with excessive cost or with iatrogenic problems related to excessive intervention. Thus, quality is compromised. On the other hand, high severity of illness with a low TISS could result in high mortality, prolonged ICU stay, or compromised quality of life after discharge. (Reproduced with permission from Sivak ED, Perez-Trepichio A: Quality assessment in the medical intensive care unit: Evolution of a data model. Cleve Clin J Med 1990;57:273–279.)

ment including respiratory evaluation, ventilation, oxygenation, weaning, and extubation.[38–41] The generic goals of the use of decision support utilities can be summarized as follows:

1. Use of uniform logic in decision-making
2. Use of a uniform database for decision-making

Table 19

A Theoretical Resource Utilization and Process Quantitation Report

Patient #	Severity	Pre-ICU Days	ICU Days	Post-ICU Days	*Vent Days	Swan Days	Pharm	Rad	RT	LAB
1	22	1	3	7	2	1	$ 2000	$ 700	$ 1000	$ 1500
2	10	0	1	3	0	0	$ 800	$ 300	$ 200	$ 800
3	35	8	14	0	13	10	$ 9500	$ 1800	$ 7000	$ 9800
4	18	1	2	3	0	0	$ 2200	$ 1100	$ 750	$ 1500
5	42	14	22	21	18	5	$ 12500	$ 3800	$ 16000	$ 13000
100	38	6	15	12	12	3	$ 9900	$ 1650	$ 8500	$ 7500
TOTAL		400	800	1600	600	100	$350000	$180000	$480000	$150000
AVERAGE	28	2	8	12	9	5	3500	$ 1800	4800	$ 1500
MEDIAN	22	1	5	10	5	2	3200	$ 1900	$ 5400	$ 1400

* Vent Days = Ventilator days; Swan Days = Days of use of Swan Ganz catheter; Pharm = Pharmacy charges; Rad = Radiology charges; RT = Respiratory Therapy charges; LAB = laboratory charges.

The spread sheet can be sorted to derive median values, added to determine total values and averaged to figure average values. Additional values can be derived using the mathematical functions of the spread sheet. For example, Percentage of ventilator day to total days is 75%, percentage of Swan days to total 12.5%. The spread sheet can be significantly larger accommodating data in individual columns as suggested from Table 9.

3. Equal frequency of monitoring
4. Equal intensity of care for all patients[42,43].

Other decision support systems can be customized according to the requirements of the patient care team. Graphic and tabular displays of data are two generic methods of creating decision support systems. For example, a graphic display of pulse, tidal volume, and respiratory rate during the process of weaning from mechanical ventilation, which is favorable (e.g., respiratory rate < 30, tidal volume > 400 cc, and pulse < 100) will prompt the caregiver to continue the weaning process. An unfavorable trend (e.g., an increase of respiratory rate to 40, tidal volume of < 300 cc, and pulse > 130) over the second hour of weaning will signal that respiratory muscle fatigue may be happening by the second hour of weaning. A graphic display of worsening oxygenation, increasing respiratory rate, and declining urine output may indicate sepsis or congestive heart failure depending upon the clinical status of the patient. A tabular display of a patient's CBC during the course of treatment of severe pneumonia may reveal a declining white blood cell count signaling the time to stop antibiotic therapy when accompanied by a prolonged period of afebrility. Each of these utilities constitute decision support systems.

Structure of the Patient Care Process

This component of quality assessment and assurance is more difficult to grasp. It implies the resources necessary to deliver patient, the nature of patient illnesses treated in the ICU, the attending physician's expertise, and so forth. In short, structure could be defined as the rules or circumstances that dictate or control the process of patient care. Patients are admitted to an ICU by or upon the recommendations of physicians who admit patients to the hospital. The demographics of the attending physicians by service or specialty suggests the types of resources required for their patients. Large numbers of cardiology patients imply that arrhythmia monitoring may be much in demand. Large numbers of surgical patients with large swings in fluid balance may suggest that meticulous attention to fluid balance and weight may be in order. The point to be made that descriptions of patient and physician demographics as listed in Tables 20 and 21 may provide additional insight into the requirements for patient care within an ICU. Many times the construction of an electronic patient log within the ICU can facilitate defining requirements for services within the ICU.[20,44]

Table 20
Analysis of Utilization of Various Technologies Used in Patient Care (1988)

	Mechanical Ventilation	Flow Directed Catheter	Dialysis
Number of Admissions	281	79	38
Number of Patients	201	76	35
Number of Readmissions	17	3	3
Percent of Total Admissions	44%	16.0%	7.7%
Percent of Patient Days (MICU)	72%	13.2%	20.3%
Male (percent)	53%	51%	42%
Female (percent)	48%	49%	59%
Mean age (median)	59 (62)	61 (65)	66 (62)
Percent greater than 65 years	45.9%	54.4%	31.2%
Average pre-ICU Days (median)	17.4 (3)	9.6 (2)	12.2 (1)
Average ICU days (median)	11.4 (5)	11.7 (7)	16.9 (9)
Average days of ICU use (median)	10.5 (5)	5.3 (4)	
Average post ICU days (median)	15.0 (4)	15.6 (1)	10.0 (5)
Unit mortality	42.0%	53.6%	36.8%
Hospital mortality	56.0%	62.0%	55.0%
Unit mortality with ventilator		63.0%	39.5%
Hospital mortality with ventilator		74.0%	56.2%

Data from patients admitted to a medical intensive care unit in a large tertiary health care institution are listed. The population from which the data was derived from 501 MICU admissions which represented a subset of 31377 total hospital admissions for the year 1988. (Reproduced by permission from reference 44).

In the case of information management systems for the ICU, there will be requirements for integration into other databases within the hospital. In a sense, the ICU system will require the resources of the hospital's admission/discharge/transfer system. Other requirements include interfaces to laboratory, pharmacy, and radiology systems. These interfaces will provide structure to the ICU information management system as illustrated in Figure 6.

Access to Peripheral Databases

The themes of utilization of information within the ICU both for clinical and administrative decision-making have centered around access to data and integration of data from multiple sources to create useful information. Since economy is the foremost priority for the

Table 21
Utilization of Mechanical Ventilation by Key Services for 1988

Service	Age			Number of Admissions*	M	F	Median Stay Days			Percent Ventilator Days	Percent Patient Days	Unit Mortality	Hospital Mortality
	Avg	Med	Range				Pre-UCU	ICU	Post-ICU				
Cardiology	61	68	(24–77)	11	6	4	4.5	7.0	2.0	2.8%	2.0%	50%	88%
Gastroenterology	59	58	(36–84)	17	6	10	2.0	5.0	2.0	6.9%	5.0%	47%	62.5%
Hematology/ oncology	47	50	(23–73)	31	14	14	20.0	6.0	1.0	14.0%	10.2%	54.8%	62.5%
Pulmonary	61	65	(19–84)	60	38	22	0.0	4.5	5.5	16.2%	13.7%	36.7%	48.2%
Hypertension/ nephrology	59	60	(32–79)	13	4	9	0.0	5.0	1.0	6.0%	4.8%	53.8%	81.8%
Internal medicine	63	68	(33–80)	16	7	9	3.0	3.5	5.5	5.0%	3.9%	43.8%	53.3%
Neurology	63	67	(39–83)	11	4	7	1.0	3.5	15.0	13.2%	10.1%	27.3%	36.4%
Thoracic surgery	63	63	(29–83)	22	11	11	25.0	16.0	16.0	21.5%	14.5%	18.2%	31.2%

* Includes readmissions.

Data from the patient population described in Table 14 are shown for the utilization of mechanical ventilation by Key services which admitted patients to the same MICU are shown. (Reproduced by permission from reference 44).

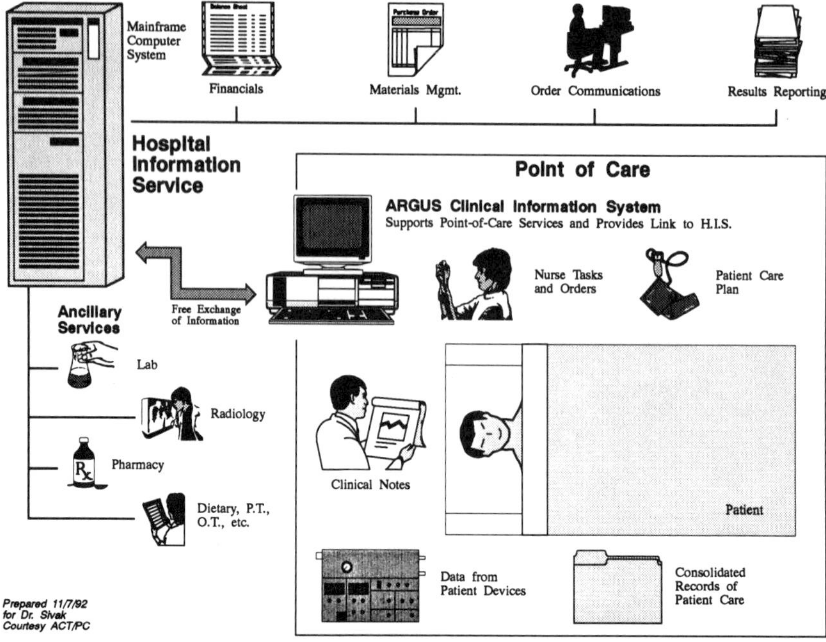

Figure 6. The concept of integration of information from the "Point of Care" in a commmercially produced patient care system is illustrated. Note free, bidirectional exchange of information between the Hospital Information System (Mainframe) and the Patient Care System closest to the point of patient care. The patient care system is clearly a component of the entire HIS and cannot exist in a freestanding environment. (Courtesy of Mr. George Morrison, ACT/PC, Madison, Wisconsin.)

1990s, efficient and economical methods for data access are mandatory. Daily utilization of data necessitates immediate, electronic access to data. For example, laboratory data, ordered on a daily routine basis, should be accessed via keyboard and CRT screen. If calculations are performed on such data to derive additional information, electronic transfer is necessary. For example, in calculation of nutritional intake and estimation of daily requirements, data from pharmacy and chemistry laboratory are necessary. The calculations would be done in the ICU system rather than either the pharmacy or laboratory system. As the requirements for information move into the administrative mode, the necessity for immediate access and extensive electronic interfaces begins to diminish. For example, length of stay reports, summaries of severity of illness, pharmacy, and laboratory utilization reports are usually not required for daily decision-making. However, there is frequently a requirement to analyze such data within one large customized database. Hence, the ability to draw data from the respective databases of the UHDA, severity of illness (e.g., APACHE III work station), pharmacy, and laboratory charge systems and to transfer it into a spread sheet such as Lotus (r) or Excel (r) allows the administrator to customize his summary reports without extensive and expensive programming of custom utilities. The only limitation of this latter method is the possibility that hospital information services departments may not have demographic and financial databases programmed to permit searching for data limited to ICU patients and to their individual ICU lengths of stays. At times, it may be necessary for the physician or administrator to construct his own internal database for creation of such reports as listed in Tables 20 and 21. These reports were derived from the data model listed in Table 12.

As information systems evolve, the quality of the information exchanged will allow for a better understanding of the utilization of intensive resources as they relate to the entire utilization of health care resources by individual patients. One particular example of this evolution is the approach that the Health Care Financing Administration (HCFA) is taking to improve the care for Medicare beneficiaries. The Health Care Quality Improvement Initiative (HCQII) has a three pronged approach to achieve this goal. First, peer review organizations will nationally uniform criteria to examine patterns of care and outcome. Second, peer review organizations will focus on the difference between observed and achievable outcomes. Third, peer review organizations will help providers identify problems of patient care and suggest solutions by monitoring patterns of care and outcomes. This will allow the providers to conduct more detailed reviews and to improve the process of patient care.[45]

To achieve these goals, two new data systems will evolve: the National Claims History (NCH) file; and the Uniform Clinical Data Set (UCDS). The NCH will contain bill payment records on Medicare claims to include physician, hospital, home health, and outpatient claims. This database will be all inclusive. The UCDS will provide for detailed clinical information describing patient demographics, history, physical findings, and treatments to allow for standardization in patient care monitoring and risk adjusted outcome analysis. This particular database will provide clinical information on a sample of discharged patients per year (about 1 million.[45] As clinical elements are defined, the UCDS could be incorporated into clinical information systems to allow caregivers to monitor the process of patient care in a proactive manner

Table 22
Uniform Clinical Data Sets (Medical and Surgical ICU)

Severity of Illness	
Clinical findings	Nervous system, cardiovascular, respiratory and renal systems
Vital signs	Temperature, pulse, blood pressure, respiration
Radiography/ultrasonography/ tomography	CNS, chest and abdomen
EKG	Ischemia, infarction, arrhythmias, pericarditis
Hematology	Hemoglobin/hematocrit, platelets, prothrombin time, partial thromboplastin time, serum lactate
Chemistry	Potassium, sodium, PaO2, PaCO2, pH, glucose, calcium, toxic levels of drugs/ chemicals
Intensity of Service	
Monitoring	Hourly, at least 3 of: blood pressure, neurovital signs, urine output, pulmonary artery pressure, intracranial pressure, arterial line, CVP, blood gases, pulse oximetry, capnography
Treatment/therapy	Fluid replacement (greater than 6 liters/24 hours), ventilator, balloon pump
Medication	At least daily: vasoactive agents, diuretic, antiarrhythmics, insulin phentoins, steroids, antimicrobials, beta blockers, anticoagulation (All agents must be given Intravenously)
Protective isolation	
Discharge Screens	
Clinical/functional	Blood pressure, absence of arrhythmias, respiratory status, neurovital signs stable, absence of invasive lines, absence of chest pain, DNR order
Options	Care safely rendered in alternate setting

before government and peer review organization analysis. Table 22 represents the data that are addressed in the UCDS with respect to ICU admission. At the present time UCDS are used only for application to the Patient Care Algorithm System (PACS) to . . . "select cases for physician review in a more uniform and reliable way."[45] In the future, the UCDS will be asked for risk adjustment of outcome and monitoring patient care. Such adjustments may not be as sophisticated as those offered by ICU severity of illness classifications, but, nevertheless, they can be expected to be incorporated into larger government databases, at least in the US.[45]

The essence of the NCH and the UCDS, when combined, will be similar to the logic illustrated in Figure 5. Outcome, adjusted to severity (UCDS) will be linked to process (some subsets of the UCDS and cost—NCH).

The population of patients within the ICU environment is aging. Such circumstances make the application of Medicare claims data to the analysis of patients receiving ICU services, a reasonable exercise to compare charges and reimbursement to outcome, severity, and process of care. To this end, the Medicare Automated Data Retrieval System (MADRS) provides a linked Medicare Part A and Part B utilization file. The file, available from the Health Care Financing Administration (HCFA) to researchers, contains institutional, physician, and supplier bills for all Medicare utilization by date of service. The data are person based and retrievable using beneficiary Health Insurance Claim (HIC) numbers. The availability of dates of service makes this data file ideal for examining expenditures associated with hospitalization requiring ICU admission.[46] This file is restricted and all efforts to protect patient confidentiality must be demonstrated before accessing the file.

Summary

The care of critically ill patients represents a point of service, located along the time line of an individual's health care history. Recognizing that the 1990s must be associated with efficiency and cost reduction, the application of ICU services must be analyzed from the point of outcome and process of care. The analysis is data intensive and can only be facilitated by proper management of information derived from the data that is derived from patient care. The entire management process will require the use of computer technology placed at the bedside with linkages throughout the entire hospital information system and beyond to the large databases maintained by third party payers and federal governments. Figure 7 illustrates these concepts.

The management of the information is the responsibility of the entire patient care team. On the clinical side, caregivers must actively seek ways to enhance the delivery of patient care through the use of microprocessors placed at the bedside. Automatic retrieval of data from bedside devices will facilitate charting. Automatic organization of pa-

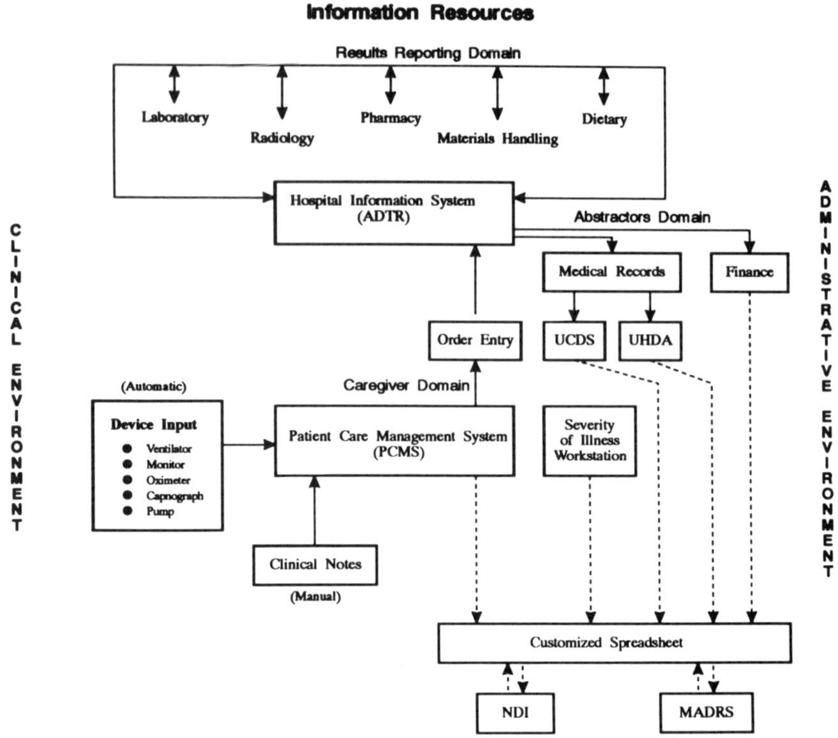

Information Resources

Results Reporting Domain
Laboratory
Radiology
Pharmacy
Materials Handling
Dietary
Hospital Information System (ADTR)
Abstractors Domain
Medical Records
Finance
Order Entry
UCDS
UHDA
Caregiver Domain
(Automatic)
Device Input
Ventilator
Monitor
Oximeter
Capnograph
Pump
Patient Care Management System (PCMS)
Severity of Illness Workstation
Clinical Notes
(Manual)
Customized Spreadsheet
NDI
MADRS
CLINICAL ENVIRONMENT
ADMINISTRATIVE ENVIRONMENT

Figure 7. The information domain of this chapter is illustrated. Authorization for collection of data is provided by the HIS through ADTR (Admission/Discharge/Transfer module). Patient data are collected through the PCMS (Patients Care Management System) located at the point of patient care. Data input into the PCMS is both automatic and manual. Peripheral to the PCMS is an administrative work station for calculation of severity of illness (e.g., APACHE III). Information for the Clinical environment is listed to the left of the figure and information from the Administrative environment is listed to the right. The solid lines represent real time flow of information and the dashed lines represent the exchange of information through medium such as magnetic disc (floppy) or tape. The latter information is used for administrative purposes, such as quality assessment, utilization review, technology assessment, and research. There is usually no requirement for real time capture of this data as its analysis does not contribute directly to patient care. Customization of data retrieval for creation of files for accessing the National Death Index (NDI) and Medicare Automated Data Retrieval System (MADRS) will facilitate creation of information that can be fed back into a stand alone spread sheet to allow the ICU practitioner to perform independent analysis. Information exchange by disc or tape is considerably less expensive than retrieval electronically. The dashed lines in the figure represent this indirect derivation of data. (UCDS = uniform clinical data sets; UMDA = uniform hospital discharge abstract.)

tient data will facilitate flow-sheet generation and the creation of decision support systems ranging from graphic displays to computerized patient care algorithms. On the administrative side, vital linkages become even more important. The transfer of clinical information from bedside patient care management systems (PCMS) and HIS will facilitate automatic collection of data for on line calculation of severity of illness and quantitation of the utilization of resources. The same PCMS will facilitate abstraction of data for medical records (UCDS and UHDA) and for financial records. Thus administrative data becomes a by-product of the delivery of patient care.

Selective abstraction of files through such media as a floppy disk will permit inexpensive data retrieval for analysis of the operation of the ICU. Severity of illness, resource utilization, and long-term outcome can be analyzed in the microprocessor environment with spread sheets used as application generators.

The entire process of information management will require caregiver commitment and executive sponsorship. The creation of HISs, which authorize data collection down to the caregiver level, will strategically place the ICU for assessment of the efficiency, efficacy, and effectiveness of its care in the 1990s.

References

1. Reiser SJ: The intensive care unit. The unfolding and ambiguities of survival therapy. Int J Technol Assess Health Care 1992;8(3):382–394.
2. Dragsted L, Qvist J: Epidemiology of intensive care. Int J Technol Assess Health Care 1992;8(3):395–407.
3. Dick RS, Steen EB, eds: The Computer-Based Patient Record. An Essential Technology for Health Care. Washington, DC, National Academy Press, 1991, p. 58.
4. Sibbald WJ, Inman KJ: Problems in assessing the technology of critical care medicine. Int J Technol Assess Health Care 1992;8(3):419–443.
5. Knaus WA, Draper EA, Wagner DP, et al: An evaluation of outcome from intensive care in major medical centers. Ann Intern Med 1986;104: 410–418.
6. Knaus WA, Wagner DP, Draper EA, et al: The APACHE III prognostic system. Risk prediction of hospitalized mortality for critically ill hospitalized adults. Chest 1991;100:1619–1636.
7. GAO 1991: Medical ADP systems. Automated medical records hold promise to improve patient care. GAO?IMTEC-91–5. January 22.
8. Vladeck BC: Medicare hospital payment by diagnosis-related groups. Ann Intern Med 1984;100:576–591.
9. Commission of the European Communities. AIM. Requirements board report on requirements and options in the field of research and development in health care and biomedical informatics. Ref: A10459. 10 October 1989.

10. Castren A, Grimmes S, Kari A, et al: User requirements for data systems in anaesthesia and intensive care. Int J Clin Monit Comput 1988;5:137–146.
11. Shaller DV, McAuliffe PS, Pinzone SM: Greater Cleveland Health Quality Choice Coalition. Incentive Benefits Committee. 1990 Workshop Series Compendium. April 1991.
12. East TD: Computers in the ICU: Panacea or Plague? Res Care 1992;37: 170–180.
13. Kaplan B: The medical computing "lag": Perceptions of barriers to application of computers to medicine. Int J Technol Assess Health Care 1987;3: 123–136.
14. Friedman BA, Martin JB: Hospital Information Systems. The physician's role. JAMA 1987;257(13):1792.
15. LeGall JR, Loriat P, Alperovich A, et al: A simplified acute physiology score for ICU patients. Crit Care Med 1984;12(11):975–977.
16. Lemeshow S, Teres D, Pastides H, et al: A method for predicting survival and mortality of ICU patients using objectively derived weights. Crit Care Med 1985;13(7):519–525.
17. Gardner RM: Computerized management of intensive care patients. MD Computing 1986;3:36–51.
18. Gardner RM, Shabot MM: Computerized ICU data management: Pitfalls and promises. Int J Clin Monit Comput 1990;7:99–105.
19. Kuperman GJ, Gardner RM, Pryor TA: HELP: A Dynamic Hospital Information System. New York, Springer Verlag, Inc., 1991.
20. Sivak ED, Perez-Trepichio A: Quality assessment in the medical intensive care unit: Evolution of a data model. Cleve Clin J Med 1990;57:273–279.
21. Knaus WA, Wagner DP, Lynn J: Short term mortality predictions for critically ill hospitalized adults: Science and ethics. Science 1991;254:389–394.
22. Higgins TL, Estafanous FG, Loop FD, et al: Stratification of morbidity and mortality outcome by preoperative risk factors in coronary artery bypass patients. A clinical severity score. JAMA 1992;267(17):2344–2438.
23. St. Anthony's DRG Working Guidebook, 1992. Alexandria, VA, St. Anthony's Publishing, Inc., 1991.
24. The International Classification of Diseases, 9th revision, Clinical Modification. ICD-9-CM. DHHS Pub # (PHS) 80–1260. US Department of Health and Human Services, Public Health Service—HCFA. Vol. 1, 2nd ed, 1980.
25. CPT-1992. Physicians' Current Procedural Terminology. American Medical Association, Chicago, 1991.
26. Gonella JS, Hornbrook MC, Louis DZ: Staging of disease. A case-mix measurement. JAMA 1984;251:637–644.
27. Horn SD, Horn RA, Sharkey PD: The severity of illness index as a severity adjustment to diagnosis-related groups. Health Care Fin Rev 1984;6(Suppl): 34–45.
28. Brewster AC, Karlin BG, Hyde LA, et al: MEDISGRPS(r): A clinically based approach to classifying hospital patients at admission. Inquiry 1985;22: 377–387.
29. Knaus WA, Draper EA, Wagner DP, et al: APACHE III: A severity of disease classification system. Crit Care Med 1985;13(10):818–829.
30. Keene AR, Cullen DJ: Therapeutic intervention scoring system: Update 1983. Crit Care Med 1983;11(1):213–216.
31. Katz S, Ford AB, Moskowitz RW, et al: Studies of illness in the aged. The

index of ADL: A standardized measure of biological and psychosocial function. JAMA 1963;185(12):914–919.
32. Karnofsky DA, Ableman WH, Carver LF, et al: The use of nitrogen-mustards in the palliative treatment of carcinoma. Cancer 1948;1:634–656.
33. Berger J, Bobbitt RA, Pollard WE, et al: The sickness impact profile: Validation of a health status measure. Med Care 1976;14(1):57–67.
34. O'Brien BJ, Banner NR, Gibson S, et al: The Nottingham health profile as a measure of quality of life following combined heart and lung transplantation. J Epidemiol Community Healthcare 1988;42(3):232–234.
35. Jett AM, Davies AR, Cleary PD, et al: The functional status questionnaire: Reliability and validity when used in primary care. J Gen Intern Med 1986; 1:143–149.
36. Torrence GW, Feeny D: Utilities and quality-adjusted life years. Int J Tech Assess Health Care 1989;5:559–575.
37. Eddy DM: Clinical decision-making. JAMA 1990;263:1265–1275.
38. Pestotnik SL, Evans RS, Burke JP, et al: Therapeutic antibiotic monitoring: Surveillance using a computerized expert system. Am J Med 1990;88: 43–48.
39. Bradshaw KE, Sittig DF, Gardner RM, et al: Computer-based data entry for nurses in the ICU. MD Computing 1989;6(5):274–280.
40. East TD, Yank W, Tariq H, et al: The IEEE medical information bus of respiratory care. Crit Care Med 1989;17:580.
41. Sittig DF, Gardner RM, Morris AH, et al: Clinical evaluation of computer-based respiratory care algorithms. Int J Clin Monit Comput 1990;7:177–185.
42. East TD, Bohm SH, Wallace CJ, et al: A successful computerized protocol for clinical management of pressure control inverse ratio ventilation in ARDS patients. Chest 1992;101:697–710.
43. Morris AH, Menlove RL, Rollins RJ, et al: A controlled clinical trial of a new 3-step therapy that includes extracorporeal CO2 removal for ARDS. Trans Am Soc Artif Int Organs 1988;11(1):48–53.
44. Sivak ED, Perez-Trepichio A: Quality assurance in the medical intensive care unit. Continued evolution of a data model. Qual Assur Util Rev 1992; 7(2):42–49.
45. Jencks SF, Wilensky GR: The health care quality improvement intensive. A new approach to quality assurance in medicare. JAMA 1992;268(7): 900–906.
46. Sneen M, Linked A/B Files—Medicare Automated Data Retrieval System (MADRS), in Conference Proceedings—1989 Data Users Conference. NCFA, US Department of Health and Human Services, Baltimore, MD, 1989, pp. 79–83.

Chapter 9

Developing a Quality Improvement Program

Albert A. Driedger, M.D., Ph.D.

"The argument in our previous Reports has been somewhat as follows:

That the Trustees of our Charitable Hospitals do not consider it their duty to see that good results are obtained in the treatment of their patients. They see to it that their financial accounts are audited, but they take no inventory of the Product for which their money is expended. Since the Product is given away, they do not bother to standardize and to see whether it is good enough to be sold."

EA Codman 1916[1]

In one sense, professionals devoted to providing health care have always understood that all human processes are capable of indefinite improvement: that understanding of essential improvability is intrinsic

From: Sibbald WJ, Massaro T (eds.): The Business of Critical Care: A Textbook for Clinicians Who Manage Special Care Units. © Futura Publishing Co., Inc., Armonk, NY, 1996.

to the scientific method through which the current abilities to provide effective health care have become possible. In another sense, these same professionals have lived within the value systems of their contemporary societies and, with the exception of visionaries such as Dr. Codman, have tended to express those values in their practices. On the one hand, it is true that hospitals and health care professionals have largely come late to formally consider the application of continuous quality improvement (CQI) to their activities: after all, the industrial sector in North America recognized the potential value of these strategies a decade ago. On the other hand, the concepts of CQI are little more than systematic articulation of values and principles that are nominally espoused by professionals and managers in any resource limited enterprise.

Change is difficult for both people and organizations and tends not to occur without an adequate stimulus. Complex pressures for change in relation to societal, economic, technological, and professional issues currently have convinced most players in the health care scene of the need to change the system through which health care is delivered. The outstanding questions are—how is change to be accomplished? Who will set the parameters and direction of change? How will it be done? How will we know if there is improvement as a result and by whose definition is it to be an improvement?

CQI is an approach to change that is capable of modifying organizational cultures through a systematic approach to specific concrete issues that occur at any level in the workplace. It depends critically on involvement of the workforce in conceptualizing and solving all issues. The methodology for the involvement of key workers and their managers and for focusing them on their issues is key to the application of the approach. The success of CQI depends critically on the understanding that it is customers who define and judge quality and that it is the customer's level of satisfaction with the quality of the product or service that is the primal value. Customers are the recipients of every value-added activity that occurs within the organization. Hence, opportunities for quality improvement will be best recognized through dialogue between customers and suppliers. Suppliers are those workers, not only their management, whose activities actually add value to the relevant goods or services. The culture that fosters CQI, values workers and supports their efforts to excel. The role of management in the culture of CQI is ever more to teach, coach, and strategize than it is to supervise or discipline the workers. The operational impact of CQI is that with adequate education about the nature and purpose of the job, workers tend increasingly to take responsibility for their performance and to supervise themselves.

Organizations that choose to espouse CQI must accept living with a lot of unresolved, and possibly unresolvable, tensions. The replacement of hierarchical organization structures with their seemingly clear lines of command and accountability by more fluid and horizontally structured teams may be unacceptable to some senior managers. The necessary reduction of supervisory functions may threaten some middle level managers. The perceived potential for job losses through realization of efficiencies may be difficult for union members. However, many will recognize that they too can benefit in an organization in which they as customers can define the quality inputs that they need to perform at their assignments.

What alternatives are there, if any? The experiences of industry outside of health care have been that there really aren't any. The fault finding mentality of the quality assurance paradigm infantalized workers and increased costs of production through the development of supervisory hierarchies that were required to recognize and reject substandard products. In the present day competitive environments of health care and in other industries, no one can afford to neglect the power that customer opinion represents.

Prerequisites

The successful implementation of CQI has several prerequisites.

1. Foremost among these is the *leadership* issue: CQI implementation is a process of education and re-education of management and the workforce that will require 5–10 years to mature if the workforce is of any size. The process will periodically encounter resistance from one level or another within the organization and it will require diversion of resources to achieve the quality targets. Without the unqualified support of the Board, the CEO, and senior management the effort will fail.
2. Although the operative principles of CQI are *scientifically based*, they are not intuitively obvious and education on an ongoing basis and in some depth is required at all levels of the organization. The end product of CQI is not only improved product but a changing, dynamically structured organization in which the nature of power is forever altered.
3. The *implementation* of a CQI program in most organizations requires significant change in the organizational structure in response to the values that drive the program: it is not possible

to have staff function as equals in the "quality" part of their jobs while the remainder of the organization retains traditional hierarchies.

4. The cornerstone of CQI is the recognition of the primary importance of the CUSTOMER, as defined earlier. Every step of every necessary process that occurs within the organization has a customer who will be distressed by failures in that process. Customers are found both inside and outside the organization and their inputs have equal validity. Successful CQI programs characteristically have clearly identified their customer(s) and failed programs can often be shown to have lost this critical focus.
5. The efforts in CQI must be consciously linked to the mission and goals of the organization. This requires focusing on the improvement of activities that are strategically important. CQI takes time and time is always a limited resource. CQI is not a panacea, but only a methodology: application of CQI in an uncritical fashion is more likely to create than to solve significant issues. It remains for the organization to provide relevant content. Organizations that have simply trusted the process without assessing the content have characteristically been hurt rather than helped by CQI.
6. Perhaps most importantly, in the CQI way it is necessary to learn to think differently about the provision of health care in the distinction of medical care processes from the "Product" of health care, to use Dr. Codman's term. It may be because of the historical relation of procedures to fees that physicians tend to think of the procedures as the products of medical practice. However, to the patient the only desirable product is the recovery of some measure of well being. The distinction of processes from the product lead logically to the new definition of quality as the achievement of wellness through the process of care from the quality assurance view of quality as mere excellent workmanship.

Principles of CQI

Berwick, Godfrey, and Roessner[2] have identified ten principles that underlie CQI; namely, that:

1. Productive work is accomplished through processes.
2. Sound customer-supplier relationships are absolutely necessary for sound quality management.

3. The main source of quality defects is problems in the process.
4. Poor quality is costly.
5. Understanding variability is a key to improving quality.
6. Quality activities should focus on the most vital processes.
7. CQI is grounded in scientifically based statistical thinking.
8. Total employee involvement is critical.
9. New organizational structures can help achieve quality improvement.
10. CQI activities encompass planning, control, and improvement.

Framework for CQI

An organization seeking renewal through application of CQI must ensure that there is clear understanding within all levels of what is the entity's business. An update of the strategic planning process with definition of the internal and external forces that impact the organization is necessary because the consensus for change arises from the recognition of those same forces. Understanding the nature of the business is not a trivial matter and requires visionary reflection: what is the business of a hospital in an increasingly "wellness minded" community? What is the business of a hospital in ambulatory care if that is known to be competitive with the private practices of its own medical staff? Is it the business of the hospital only to provide services that are remunerative? What unfilled niches exist in the market? These and many other provocative questions need to be addressed at the outset.

Linked to the question of the organization's business is that of the identity of its customer(s). Who will be delighted by excellence in the products and distressed by defects? In health care, the customer may be a patient, but may equally also be a family, a physician, an insurance company, an HMO, or the office of a regulatory agency to name but a few of the external variety. Internally, the staff alternately are suppliers and customers of each other and the understanding of this interdependency is critical to the success of a CQI program. Each customer has a right to be heard about his/her experience of quality at the hands of the supplier. Loss of the customer focus is a recognized cause of failure of some CQI programs.

Health care institutions need also to address the question of who is(are) the community(ies) that they serve. In the current cost conscious, competitive environment, the traditional provider-based paradigm is being questioned and the option of a community needs based model is touted. The expectations of the community will drive the definition of the business and identification of the primary customer. CQI will not likely be able to revive an institution that is rooted in the wrong paradigm.

Against the background of the foregoing it becomes possible to ask questions that have a higher likelihood of being answerable through the methodology of CQI. Input from external and internal customers and reference to the mission of the organization will define the products or services whose improvement will be noticed.

The CQI process does not happen merely through goodwill and public announcement of intent. The CEO should ideally mandate and lead the effort and organize a senior management support structure, usually known as the Quality Council, whose function it is to strategize around the key quality issues and to mandate and empower each individual quality process team. The empowerment must include the ability of the team to call on staff from relevant tasks or units and the provision of necessary resources together with the assurance of process through which the recommended solutions will be adopted, implemented, and their performance monitored.

The CQI process is critically dependent on the interpersonal dynamics of the team. There are rules of conduct and association that need to be agreed to and there are processes to be followed that allow all team members to participate as equals: these rules and processes are not intuitively obvious to all and must be explicitly agreed to. Professional credentials tend to inhibit support staff and upset the credo of equality of all team members. It is important to provide education on the process to team members at such times as they recognize the need. The provision of such education and of necessary technical support to teams requires that the organization provide appropriate infrastructural support; in short, a "Quality Office" whose members are able to operationalize the CQI program, to educate staff, and to facilitate the team processes. The infrastructure should be proportionate to the size and complexity of the organization. In some organizations it has been felt preferable to engage consultants to act in the support role rather than to develop the expertise in house.

The optimal strategy of CQI usually is to select opportunities for improvement in areas where difficulties are recognized but where the solution is not within the power of any one manager or managerial unit to implement. A cross-functional team with representation from all involved disciplines and managerial units should be struck to deal with each quality issue. The team should set an appropriate timeline to complete its task. On completion of the task and submission of the report to Quality Council, the team should be dissolved except that follow-up on the results of the implementation may be assigned to the committee by the Council.

The foregoing has described some of the structural and staffing issues relative to CQI. In the remainder of this chapter we will now concentrate on the major process issues that bear on the functioning of the program.

Stages and Steps

The CQI process is best conceptualized as a continuous cycle whose stages progress through the elements of project definition, diagnosing the causes of quality limitation, formulation of a remedy and, finally, maintenance of the improvement. The cycle can go on indefinitely. The stages in the cycle have a close analogy with the clinical process in which consultation progresses to diagnostic testing and the formulation of a diagnosis, then on to a plan of treatment and ultimately to follow-up. Within these stages, it is possible to define a number of discrete steps that require specific activities and skills of the team as seen in Table 1. These steps are reviewed in greater detail below.

1. List Problems and Priorities: Any process may be the subject for quality improvement irrespective of whether it is a planning, a management, or production issue. The list may be developed in

Table 1
Stages and Steps of Continuous Quality Improvement

Stages	Steps[3]
Project Definition	1. List problems and priorities
	2. Define project and enlist team
Diagnostic Stage	3. Analyze symptoms
	4. Formulate theories of cause
	5. Test theories
	6. Identify most likely causes
Remedial Stage	7. Consider possible solutions
	8. Design an optimal solution and controls
	9. Address resistance to change
	10. Implement solution and controls
Holding the Gains	11. Check performance (indicators)
	12. Monitor control system

a number of ways including suggestion boxes, brainstorming, customer complaints, etc. Items may come from patients or other internal or external customers, internal reports, quality assurance audits, liability issues, financial considerations, human resource issues, or regulatory requirements. The ideas may come from any level of the organization.

It will not be possible to address more than a few of the items on the problem list on account of the limitations of time and resources. The selection of the problems that will be studied should be made through open discussion with reference to the organization's mission and needs. Further, in CQI, decisions must be made wherever possible through reference to data; the opinions of senior medical staff or managers must be muted to allow all input to be heard. Quality Council may need to determine the order and priority in which problems are supported.

2. Define Project and Enlist Team: CQI is not an idle game. Once a problem has been deemed worthy of study it must be resolved if the program is to retain credibility. Definition of the problem must be based on data. The potential consequences of improving or failing to improve the process in question must be assessed; that is, the strategic significance of the process must be known. The mission of a proposed CQI team should be written and presented to the Quality Council in order to receive a mandate.

   The membership of the team should be selected from among those workers who own the process in question. All disciplines involved must be represented while maintaining an effective team size. Some disciplines may have an interest in only limited aspects of the problem and it may be appropriate to involve them only at those times when their concerns are on the agenda. The team should be led by a chairperson who understands but does not own the process. In addition, it is essential to have a facilitator who understands the CQI process and the group dynamics. That the facilitator may not know very much about the technology or other specifics about the subject of the team's mission is irrelevant. The facilitator is the link to the quality office infrastructure and the source of the necessary education for the team.
3. Analyze Symptoms: The analysis of symptoms in the CQI process is analogous to the clinical process. The symptoms themselves are identified through a methodical analysis of the prob-

lem in a manner that avoids attribution of blame. The symptom is an indicator of a problem (e.g., late starts in the operating room) and requires to be understood before it is responded to. As in medicine, so also in CQI, a premature response to symptoms may preclude achievement of a correct diagnosis. Symptoms are pointers toward cause and not the causes in themselves. The purpose of analyzing symptoms is to arrive at an understanding of underlying causes.

The process for the analysis of symptoms might best begin with a brainstorming session and the organization of all possible causes in a "herringbone diagram" (Figure 1). The diagram serves the purpose of classifying causes into major types while concentrating on system issues without highlighting the shortcomings of people. In a typical analysis symptoms may be classified under the "PM4" schema; i.e., people, machines, materials, measurements, and methods.

4. Formulate Theories of Cause: This step follows logically from the preceding analysis of symptoms. It is of crucial importance in that successful treatment of a problem requires that the remedy be targeted on the cause, and not merely on the obliteration of a symptom. The formulation of theories proceeds directly along the lines through which scientific theories are developed in which care is taken to ensure that all relevant observations are accounted for in accordance with the basic principle of parsimony.
5. Test Theories: CQI proceeds on the basis of facts, not unsubstantiated opinions. Therefore, it is essential that data be collected and analyzed as the basis on which the preferred theory is to be selected. It should not usually be necessary to collect a lot of new data for the purpose of validating a theory. Often it is sufficient to use a routinely collected dataset with which the organization is familiar and that is deemed able to act as a proxy of the events under scrutiny: e.g., lengths of stays of patients awaiting placement in chronic care may support a provisional hypothesis that there is a shortage of available chronic care places in the community, without the expense of a direct study of the number of places available. It is essential to remain aware of the assumptions that are being made and sometimes it is necessary to go to the expense of collecting a new dataset. The point being made is that it is necessary for the CQI team to maintain a sense of perspective and to ensure that the data are adequate to the scope of the problem and serve to evaluate

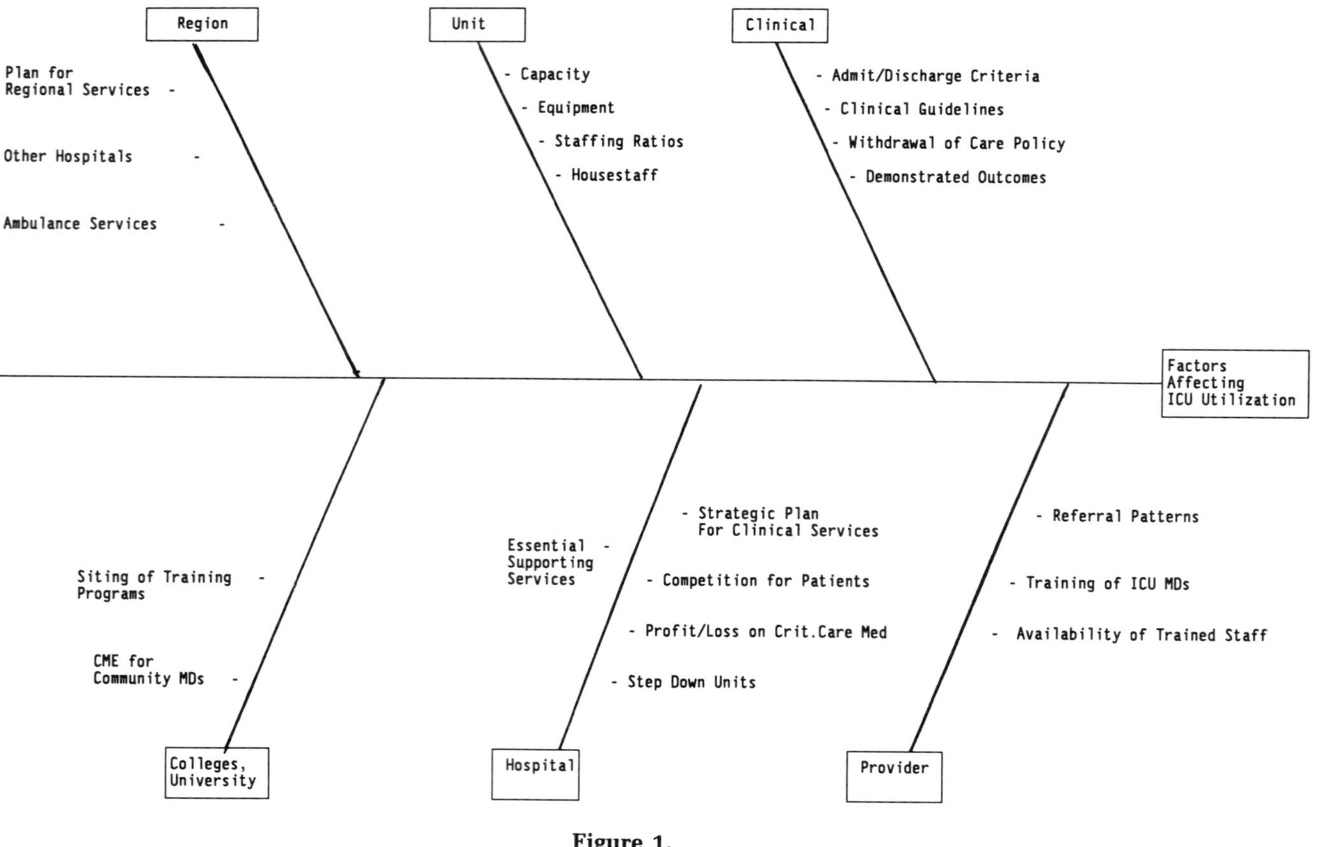
Region
Plan for Regional Services -
Other Hospitals -
Ambulance Services -
Unit
- Capacity
- Equipment
- Staffing Ratios
- Housestaff
Clinical
- Admit/Discharge Criteria
- Clinical Guidelines
- Withdrawal of Care Policy
- Demonstrated Outcomes
Factors Affecting ICU Utilization
Siting of Training Programs -
CME for Community MDs -
Colleges, University
Essential Supporting Services -
- Strategic Plan For Clinical Services
- Competition for Patients
- Profit/Loss on Crit.Care Med
- Step Down Units
Hospital
- Referral Patterns
- Training of ICU MDs
- Availability of Trained Staff
Provider

Figure 1.

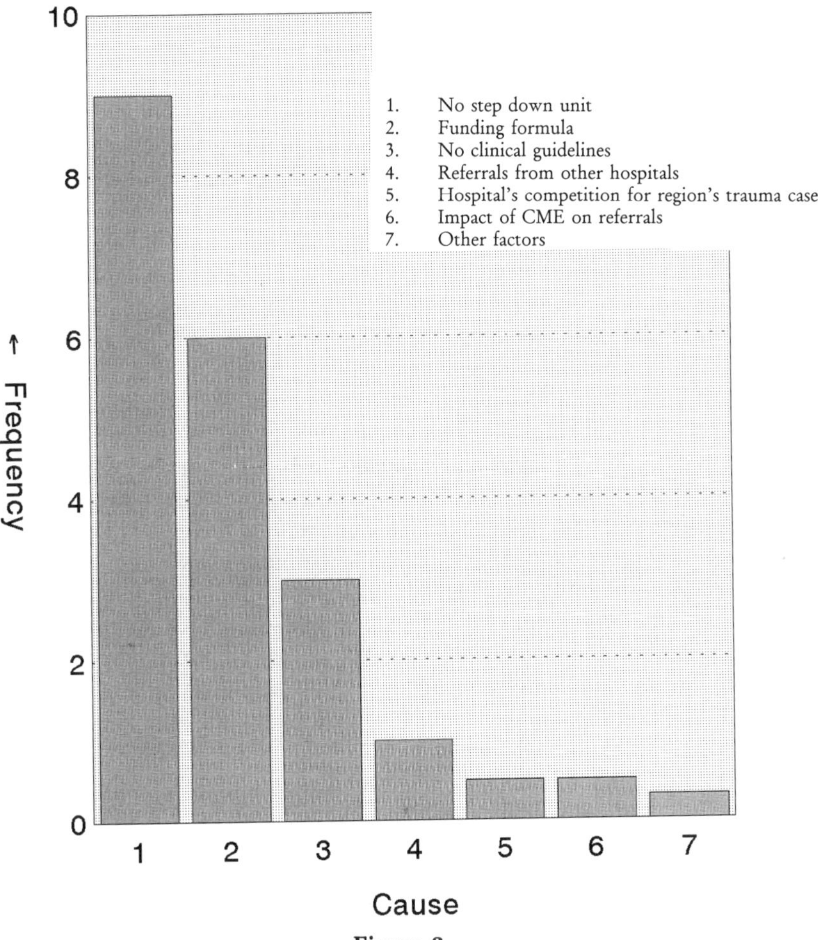

Figure 2.

the theories in a manner that is consistent with scientific principles while the costs remain proportionate to the strategic importance of the problem.

6. Identify Underlying Causes: After the most favored theory has been established, it is possible to determine a list of the root causes of variability in the process under examination. Usually, only one or a few causes will serve to explain the majority of the variation. The relative importance of the root causes can be visually demonstrated in a "Pareto" diagram (Figure 2). The significance of this process is that it is not possible to

attack all causes of variability at once and that it is necessary to secure the agreement of the team as to the relative importance of each prior to the development of solutions.

7. Consider Solutions: It is important that all members of the team participate in the consideration of potential solutions. The group dynamics by this time should allow discussions of each team member's insights: the best solution may come from the most junior or the least educated member and no proposed solution should be rejected out of hand. For example, the best solution to an infection control problem may elude the medical staff but be obvious to the housekeeping staff who are sensitive to the implications of a traffic pattern in the area of concern.
8. Design Optimal Solution/Controls: The design of an optimal solution must take into consideration the organizational setting in which it will operate. In addition to the narrowly defined problem undergoing resolution, the environment in which the solution will operate must be understood. Issues of the strategic importance of the solution to the organization as well as its potential impact on people and resources must be clarified. The implementation of a solution must include the training required to acquaint workers with it. Training must clarify the objectives, the customer-supplier relationship visualized in the solution, the expected behaviors of the staff, and the anticipated outcome of the change.

   Finally, the solution is incomplete unless *indicators* are built in that will allow monitoring of its performance. Only in this way will it ultimately be possible to determine whether the mooted solution has delivered the expected results.
9. Resistance to Change: Even perfect solutions encounter resistance in application (because it is in the nature of people to resist change). The resistance may come from within the team or from within the organization. The factors that contribute to resistance may variously be rooted in lack of understanding of the reasons change is needed, in genuine belief that the old way is the best way, in fear of the new way or in some form of self-interest. The cost of overcoming resistance to change must be factored into the cost of making change. It falls within the role of managers to understand on what basis change is to be resisted. It also falls to managers to work with the CQI team to anticipate resistance and to craft strategies through which to overcome it. Solutions that are technically correct are likely to be rejected if their social impact is not addressed.

It is important to ensure that the affected workers know in advance of the existence of the CQI task team and are aware of their objectives and management's view of the need. Openness is a sine qua non of the CQI process: it may be helpful to leave the team's charts hanging in the staff room where they meet for others to see. It will be essential that staff meetings include briefings on the status of the team and of the processes that exist for securing of input from those who are not team members. Concerns should be openly addressed. Recommendations and proposed solutions should not without reason be held in confidence within the organization. Issues that lie behind resistance should be addressed head on when detected: commonly, there is fear about the ability to function in a post-solution environment or fear about job security.

When the team along with management has done whatever seems necessary to overcome resistance in prospect, then the solution should be implemented. In some cases the reality of the solution may of itself be convincing. For a few workers in almost every organization the CQI environment is too difficult and too full of tensions and these workers may require assistance to be relocated within or outside the organization. If the CQI process is to grow in credibility it is incumbent upon management to work with the team so that it will be able to support the team's recommendations and accept the proposed solutions.

10. Implement Solutions and Controls: At this stage it is time to implement the proposed solution. In the technical sense the implementation is the job of management and not of the team. The team has essentially done its work and the members might now be reassigned to their former duties. However, it is helpful to the credibility of the process if the team members are given some role along with management in the implementation in order that they may report back to their colleagues on the integrity of management in its dealings through the CQI process. Perhaps the team should meet at infrequent but regular, intervals to maintain an overview of the implementation until its completion.
11. Check the Performance of the Solution: Upon the implementation of the solution, the indicator data required to track the performance of the solution should begin to be collected. The solution may require periodic adjustment in order to achieve the projected outcome. Performance tends not to be maintained

unless there is ongoing review. Unmonitored implementation of a solution may result in only a temporary improvement through the so-called Hawthorne Effect (i.e., that workers' performance tends to improve if they believe that attention is being paid to them) rather than through operation of a genuine solution.

12. Recognize and Reward Success: An essential part of the CQI process is the recognition of employees for the additional effort that quality improvement requires and for the achievement of goals. Recognition may take the form of an announcement in the house newsletter, a letter to the employee signed by the CEO or the Chairman of the Board, an annual invitation to dinner with the President, or in other ways. Rewards may take the form of a bonus or of an educational opportunity for individuals or of a capital opportunity for the unit or department. Organizations differ in the nature of actions that are open to them depending on their culture, labor relationships, whether they are publicly or privately funded, and in other ways. In an academically orientated organization such as a teaching hospital it may be reward enough for the professional staff to be supported in their CQI involvements at a level that permits of career advancement through peer-reviewed publication.

Applications of CQI to Intensive Care

The CQI approach to management of an intensive care unit (ICU) is applicable across the entire spectrum of activity ranging from policy setting to alteration of operational and patient care issues.

A commonly recognized issue is that of the operational cost of ICUs which approximates 1% of the gross national product of the USA whereas their overall clinical effectiveness remains uncertain.[4] Many hospitals in the US regularly lose money on reimbursement received for admissions to the ICU.[5] It has been documented that during times of reduced ICU bed availability with admission triage of some patients to standard wards who would otherwise have been admitted to the unit, mortality did not rise.[6] The factors that contribute to the decision to admit a patient to an ICU bed are not only related to the clinical status but also to considerations of psychosocial and economic reasons; i.e., patient/family pressures, physician's perception of liability related to not admitting to the unit, economic benefits to providers of providing care inside versus outside the ICU, etc. How then might a hospital respond to pressure from the community or its medical staff to provide more ICU beds?

The CQI based approach would, by way of example, require review of data on community need with reference to other demographically similar communities as benchmarks, factors affecting the outcomes of ICU care,[4,5,7] admission policies including actual practices and variations, categories of illness (DRGs or CMGs) being admitted to the unit, discharge policies, and outcomes data. The process improvement process would utilize these data to allow systematic evaluation of issues related to effective use of the ICU by its users and staff. The evaluation of processes is capable of extension to any level down to such specific operational issues as nursing time required to care for angioplasty patients,[8] development of critical pathways for the care of trauma patients,[9] protocols for management of respiratory care,[10] guidelines for the management of chest pain,[11] or of acute myocardial infarction,[12] etc.

Education of all staff in the objectives of the activity is crucial to the possibility of success. Activities whose objectives are not understood are likely to be resented. For instance, physicians may wonder whether review of the variances in their outcomes among cases reflects on their competence or nurses may believe that high patient staffing ratios reflect excellent care in and of themselves and, hence, resent monitoring and documentation of their care. Hidden agendas and professional turf issues must give way to openness, commonly agreed upon objectives, and functionality.

In hospitals, the format of continuous quality improvement may need to be modified so as to fit the standards of the JCAHO (USA) or CCHFA (Canada), but that can be done without substantively altering the values and principles described and exemplified above. The more traditional quality assurance activities of the medical and nursing staffs are not rendered redundant by CQI but, remain a useful tool for selective use within the overall quality program. Stevens[13] has described a model of quality assurance in the ICU in the context of JCAHO standards. The CCHFA standards for quality are currently in revision, but it is clear that they will require multidisciplinary, unit-level implementation.

The cost of a CQI program in an institution or in an ICU are not inconsiderable. It is not helpful to break out the ICU portion of the costs separate from the rest of the hospital because the orientation of CQI is to stress the outcomes of care. It is not unusual for a hospital to devote 1%–2% of its annual budget to bootstrapping a CQI initiative. The major predictable elements of cost are in relation to education of staff, establishing functional teams, collection of data and their analysis, securing of consensus for models of change, and implementation of the change itself. A failure may be very costly. On the other hand, a success may, and often does, result in significant improvements of care or service and reduction of cost as exemplified by the Brigham and Women's Hospital study on drug delivery schedules.[14] The gains tend not to come about through dramatic major shifts in the way that care is delivered but in a series of modest quantifiable achievements. In this respect the ICU is not different from the hospital in general and the health care sector is not different from other industries.

Conclusion

There is nothing about CQI that is startlingly new except perhaps its appearance of naivety in its commitment to place optimization of patient care and outcome and a high value on the opinions and abilities of workers ahead of all other issues.

The CQI effort is unending. As soon as the current opportunity for improvement has been resolved, it is time to look again at the process and to envisage what further potential there may be for improvement. Always be aware of what the best of your peers and competitors have been able to accomplish and build on that. No improvement is too small to implement if it will be noticed by a potential customer. The breakthroughs will come about through attempting to improve on what is already the best and every worker who has any involvement whatever in the production process has potential to contribute to that.

References

1. Codman EA. A Study in Hospital Efficiency. Privately published, 1916, p. 5. Reprinted by the Classics of Medicine Library 1992.
2. Berwick DM, Godfrey AB, Roessner J, eds: Curing Health Care. San Francisco, CA, Jossey-Bass Publishers, 1991, pp. 32–43.
3. Principles and Processes in "Methods and Tools of Quality Improvement". National Demonstration Project on Quality Improvement in Health Care. 1991, pp. I-11.
4. Knaus WA, Wagner DP, Zimmerman JE, et al: Variations in mortality and length of stay in intensive care units. Ann Intern Med 1993;118:753–761.
5. Shortell SM, Zimmerman JE, Gillies RR, et al: Continuously improving patient care: Practical lessons and an assessment tool from the National ICU Study. Qual Rev Bull 1992;18:150–155.

6. Singer DE, Carr PL, Mulley AG, et al: Rationing intensive care—Physician responses to a resource shortage. N Engl J Med 1983;309:1155–1169.
7. Luce JM: Improving the quality and utilization of critical care. Qual Rev Bull 1991;17:42–47.
8. Laughon D, Ax S, Boyington C: From unit-based quality assurance to multidisciplinary continuous quality improvement in the coronary care unit. J Nurs Care Qual 1993;7:19–27.
9. Latini EE, Foote W: Obtaining consistent quality patient care for the trauma patient by using a critical pathway. Crit Care Nurs Q 1992;15:51–55.
10. Elliott G: Computer-assisted quality assurance: Development and performance of a respiratory care program. Qual Rev Bull 1991;17:85–90.
11. Weingarten S, Agocs L, Tankel N, et al: Reducing lengths of stay for patients hospitalized with chest pain using medical practice guidelines and opinion leaders. Am J Cardiol 1993;71:259–262.
12. Gunnar RM, Bourdillon PDV, Dixon DW, et al: Guidelines for the early management of patients with acute myocardial infarction. J Am Coll Cardiol 1990;16:249–292.
13. Stevens B: Implementing a quality assurance program at the unit level in intensive care: Essential elements for successful implementation. AACN Clin Issues Crit Care Nurs 1991;2:69–76.
14. Laffel G: "A Hospital Pharmacy Applies the Quality Improvement Process" in Improving Health Care Quality; sponsored by the National Demonstration Project Unit XI, 1991.

Chapter 10

Managing the Internal Evaluation Process

Jack E. Zimmerman, M.D.

An aging population and a growing demand for sophisticated medical and surgical procedures are likely to increase the complexity and demand for intensive care unit (ICU) services throughout the 1990s. At the same time, health care regulatory agencies and both private and governmental payers are likely to place even greater emphasis on programs aimed at controlling costs while maintaining quality. To meet these challenges, ICU managers will need to better describe their unit's patients, the resources used in their care, and assume accountability for the effectiveness and efficiency of its operations and processes. The goals of this chapter are to provide ICU physician and nurse managers with the tools for characterizing their unit's patients, measuring its resource utilization, and for assessing and improving the quality and productivity of care.

From: Sibbald WJ, Massaro T (eds.): The Business of Critical Care: A Textbook for Clinicians Who Manage Special Care Units. © Futura Publishing Co., Inc., Armonk, NY, 1996.

ICU Patient Input

Few physicians or nurses would treat a pneumonia patient without first obtaining information about the patient's acute illness, past history, physical findings, laboratory studies, and prior therapy. But as ICU managers the same individuals often make management decisions with little information about the characteristics of the unit's patients or the type and amount of services it provides. Under such circumstances decisions are often made using perception and impulse rather than facts. But if management decisions require the same kinds of information used in treating critically ill patients, what data is needed and how should it be collected?

I believe we should concentrate on data that has the greatest proven impact on resource use and patient outcome. Information about demographic features such as age, comorbidity, and diagnosis is vital, but knowing that a patient is elderly, in poor health, and has congestive heart failure provides little information about the need for intensive care. Severity of physiologic abnormalities is what best explains a patient's need for ICU admission and is the most important single determinant of outcome and resource use. During the last decade the principles used in developing severity and prognostic scoring systems have made it possible to identify, organize, and collect data that predicts both outcome and resource use.

Ideally, this data would be entered into a computerized management system, much of it via electronic interfaces with the hospital's clinical information system, laboratory, and bedside monitoring system. Because this new technology is available in only a few ICUs, however, data collection is usually performed manually and either maintained in a log book or entered into a personal computer. Despite the value of input data and the availability of computers, few ICU managers have adequate data. The reasons include: a substantial data collection burden; poor institutional support; lack of a standardized format; and the absence of major incentives to analyze utilization and outcomes. In the future, however, increasing demands for ICU care, shrinking resources, and regulatory or requirements are likely to increase the need for patient input data as an essential first step in analyzing resource use and quality of care.

This section will provide guidelines for measuring patient input. Its major emphasis will be on severity systems, particularly those with demonstrated applications in providing management information. This will be followed by a more detailed description of the APACHE III system, which receives particular emphasis because of its application for ICU utilization review, and quality improvement.

Demographic Data

Studies of ICU admissions in the US and other countries have demonstrated marked differences in patient characteristics.[1–4] In aggregate, these studies encompass the universe of potentially valuable demographic data. But what data should your ICU collect; and how should the data be recorded?

Table 1 summarizes the patient input data, which is most useful for supplementing ICU management decisions. Variables such as diagnosis, age, comorbidity, operative status, admission source, and severity of illness are important determinants of outcome from ICU care.[5,6] But this same information is also essential in assessing how your ICU is utilized and in performing quality review. Additional information such as the date and time of admission and discharge can also be used for evaluating bed utilization, e.g., total patient days, occupancy rate, and length of stay.

Severity and Prognostic Scoring Systems

Table 2 lists the scoring systems that are most useful for defining ICU patient input, resource use, and evaluating quality of care. These severity systems can be categorized as disease specific or general. The Burn Index,[7] Trauma Score,[8] Injury Severity Scoring system,[9] and Glasgow Coma Score,[10] are examples of disease or injury specific systems. General severity scoring systems include: Acute Physiology and Chronic Health Evaluation (APACHE II and APACHE III), the Simplified Acute Physiology Score (SAPS), the Mortality Prediction Model (MPM), and the Therapeutic Intervention Scoring System (TISS) for adult ICU admissions; and the Physiology Stability index (PSI) and Pediatric Risk of Mortality Score (PRISM) for children.

Severity measurement is a confusing concept because no uniform scientific definition exists. In some instances severity implies extent of injury. The burn index, which uses percent body surface area burned, is an example.[7] Some severity systems examine the impact of disease or injury on function, as in the Glasgow Coma Scale[10]; others monitor the amount of therapy received, using the premise that the sicker the

Table 1
Patient Data Used for Supporting ICU Management Decisions

Patient Name: ______________ Bed Number: ______________

Admission date/time: ______________ Discharge date/time: ______________

Chronologic Age* ______________

Comorbidity*: ______________ ______________

______________ ______________

Operative Status*: _____ Elective surgery _____ Emergency surgery

_____ Nonoperative

Admission Source*:

ER _____ OR _____ RR _____ Ward _____ Other _____

Another ICU _____ Another Hospital _____

Diagnosis*: ______________

Severity of Illness*: ______________

Admitting Service: ______________

Admitting Physician: ______________

Services during first ICU day:

Active treatment _____ Monitoring only _____

Discharged from ICU to:
Floor _____ Step-down unit _____ Another ICU _____

Another ICU _____ Another hospital _____

Discharge status: Alive / Dead

* Data are part of and can be recorded using the APACHE III Prognostic system.[50]

Table 2
Severity Scoring Systems for Describing ICU Patient Input

Burns and Trauma	
Burn Index	Injury Severity Score
Glasgow Coma Scale	TRISS method
Trauma Score	Pediatric Trauma Score
Abbreviated Injury Scale	
Adult ICU Populations	
Acute Physiology and Chronic Health Evaluation APACHE II* and APACHE III*	
Mortality Prediction Model * (MPM)	
Simplified Acute Physiology Score (SAPS)	
Rapid Acute Physiology Score	
Pediatric ICU Populations	
Physiologic Stability Index (PSI)	
Pediatric Risk of Mortality* (PRISM)	

* System also provides prognostic estimates

patient, the more treatment required. The Therapeutic Intervention Scoring System (TISS) is the best example. APACHE, SAPS, MPM, and PRISM measure severity using physiological measurements; increasing severity is reflected by the extent of derangement from normal physiology, which is closely associated with hospital mortality.[11]

Some general systems can measure severity and estimate prognosis as well as, and in some cases, more precisely than systems developed for specific diseases. Because these general systems are applicable to many diseases, they are the preferred measure for most ICUs. An in-depth review of the many general and disease specific methods for measuring disease severity and predicting clinical outcome is beyond the scope of this chapter. For further details, readers are referred elsewhere.[5,6,12,13]

Severity Scoring for Injury and Trauma

Several systems have been developed for comparing input, outcomes, and quality of care for trauma patients. These systems are also an important element in the certification of trauma units. In general, an increasing score is associated with higher mortality, but these estimates are not used for individual patient predictions or as an aid in clinical decision-making. The following briefly describes the most useful trauma scoring systems.

The Trauma Score[8] uses points for respiratory rate and effort, systolic blood pressure, capillary refill, and Glasgow Coma scale. The Abbreviated Injury Scale (AIS)[14] grades the severity of blunt trauma by assigning 1 (minor) to 6 (fatal) points to the extent of injury in six anatomic regions. The Injury Severity Score[9] is the sum of squares of the highest AIS points for the three most severely injured anatomical regions. Triss[15] represents a combination of the Trauma Score with the Injury Severity Score and can be applied for both blunt and penetrating trauma. The Pediatric Trauma score[16] grades injury severity among infants and children by assigning three point categories for six different patient variables.

Acute Physiology and Chronic Health Evaluation (APACHE)

The original APACHE system was completed in 1981[17] and consisted of two parts: (1) an Acute Physiology Score (APS) reflecting the degree of physiological derangement; and (2) a Chronic Health Evaluation reflecting status before the acute illness. The system used 34 potential physiological measurements, with the relative weight for each variable determined by expert opinion and review of clinical literature. APACHE provided a reliable and valid method for risk stratification and severity measurement, but was too complex and required multi-institutional testing.

The APACHE II system was introduced in 1985, and incorporated many important changes in APACHE.[18] APACHE II consists of a numerical score that varies from 0 to 71. The score consists of three parts: (1) points for the extent of abnormality of 12 physiological measures; (2) points for increasing age; and (3) points for chronic health abnormalities (Figure 1). An increasing APACHE II score reflects an increased severity of illness and risk of hospital death.

First day APACHE II scores and diagnosis can be used in an equation to estimate group probability of hospital mortality. This prognostic capability has been used by researchers to stratify patients into clear, well defined groups with discretely different risks of hospital death.[19–21] The success and acceptance of APACHE II as a case-mix control and means for group risk stratification is attributable to the system's statistical and clinical validity.

Although some investigators have attempted to use APACHE II scoring over time to assess prognosis for individual patients,[22,23] the

THE APACHE II SEVERITY OF DISEASE CLASSIFICATION SYSTEM

PHYSIOLOGIC VARIABLE	HIGH ABNORMAL RANGE						LOW ABNORMAL RANGE		
	+4	+3	+2	+1	0	+1	+2	+3	+4
TEMPERATURE — rectal (°C)	≥ 41°	39°-40.9°		38.5°-38.9°	36°-38.4°	34°-35.9°	32°-33.9°	30°-31.9°	≤ 29.9°
MEAN ARTERIAL PRESSURE — mm Hg	≥ 160	130-159	110-129		70-109		50-69		≤ 49
HEART RATE (ventricular response)	≥ 180	140-179	110-139		70-109		55-69	40-54	≤ 39
RESPIRATORY RATE — (non-ventilated or ventilated)	≥ 50	35-49		25-34	12-24	10-11	6-9		≤ 5
OXYGENATION: A-aDO$_2$ or PaO$_2$ (mm Hg) a. FiO$_2$ ≥ 0.5 record A-aDO$_2$	≥ 500	350-499	200-349		< 200				
b. FiO$_2$ < 0.5 record only PaO$_2$					PO$_2$ > 70	PO$_2$ 61-70		PO$_2$ 55-60	PO$_2$ < 55
ARTERIAL pH	≥ 7.7	7.6-7.69		7.5-7.59	7.33-7.49		7.25-7.32	7.15-7.24	< 7.15
SERUM SODIUM (mMol/L)	≥ 180	160-179	155-159	150-154	130-149		120-129	111-119	≤ 110
SERUM POTASSIUM (mMol/L)	≥ 7	6-6.9		5.5-5.9	3.5-5.4	3-3.4	2.5-2.9		< 2.5
SERUM CREATININE (mg/100 ml) (Double point score for **acute** renal failure)	≥ 3.5	2-3.4	1.5-1.9		0.6-1.4		< 0.6		
HEMATOCRIT (%)	≥ 60		50-59.9	46-49.9	30-45.9		20-29.9		< 20
WHITE BLOOD COUNT (total/mm3) (in 1,000s)	≥ 40		20-39.9	15-19.9	3-14.9		1-2.9		< 1
GLASGOW COMA SCORE (GCS): Score = 15 minus actual GCS									
[A] Total ACUTE PHYSIOLOGY SCORE (APS): Sum of the 12 individual variable points									
Serum HCO$_3$ (venous-mMol/L) [Not preferred, use if no ABGs]	≥ 52	41-51.9		32-40.9	22-31.9		18-21.9	15-17.9	< 15

[B] AGE POINTS:
Assign points to age as follows:

AGE(yrs)	Points
≤ 44	0
45-54	2
55-64	3
65-74	5
≥ 75	6

[C] CHRONIC HEALTH POINTS
If the patient has a history of severe organ system insufficiency or is immuno-compromised assign points as follows:

a. for nonoperative or emergency postoperative patients — 5 points
or
b. for elective postoperative patients — 2 points

DEFINITIONS
Organ Insufficiency or immuno-compromised state must have been evident **prior** to this hospital admission and conform to the following criteria:

LIVER: Biopsy proven cirrhosis and documented portal hypertension; episodes of past upper GI bleeding attributed to portal hypertension; or prior episodes of hepatic failure/encephalopathy/coma.

CARDIOVASCULAR: New York Heart Association Class IV.

RESPIRATORY: Chronic restrictive, obstructive, or vascular disease resulting in severe exercise restriction, i.e., unable to climb stairs or perform household duties; or documented chronic hypoxia, hypercapnia, secondary polycythemia, severe pulmonary hypertension (>40mmHg), or respirator dependency.

RENAL: Receiving chronic dialysis.

IMMUNO-COMPROMISED: The patient has received therapy that suppresses resistance to infection, e.g., immuno-suppression, chemotherapy, radiation, long term or recent high dose steroids, or has a disease that is sufficiently advanced to suppress resistance to infection, e.g., leukemia, lymphoma, AIDS.

APACHE II SCORE
Sum of [A] + [B] + [C]

[A] APS points ____
[B] Age points ____
[C] Chronic Health points ____
Total APACHE II ____

Figure 1.

system was neither designed nor intended for use in individual patient decisions. What has been possible, however, is the use of APACHE II as a tool to examine outcomes from ICU care. In a series of articles, risk factors for disease combined with the APACHE II score were used to predict group death rates, which were then compared to the actual number of deaths as a measure of performance. This method has been used to compare outcomes among US ICUs,[24] and for comparing their performance with units in France,[1] New Zealand,[2] and Japan.[25]

Because of its ability to risk stratify groups of ICU patients, APACHE II has been used in studies aimed at improving ICU utilization. The same principles used to identify patients at low and high-risk of death during the first ICU day can also identify levels of risk in regard to need for life-support.[26,27] These studies demonstrated that ICU admissions who did not receive life-support during the first ICU day and had a low APS were at low (< 10%) risk of subsequently receiving these treatments.

The Simplified Acute Physiology Score (SAPS)

The SAPS[28] is a general severity of illness score based on APACHE. SAPS was developed in France and is primarily used in European ICUs. SAPS uses age and 13 of the 34 physiologic variables from the original APACHE system. The weights, i.e., scoring for abnormalities among these 13 physiologic variables are identical to those used in APACHE.

SAPS has three major uses: (1) risk stratifying ICU patients by prognosis[29]; (2) describing acuity and categorizing treatment services[30,31]; and (3) explaining cost differences among patients with similar diagnoses.[32] SAPS cannot be used for assessing individual prognosis.

Mortality Probability Model (MPM)

The MPM was designed to predict the probability of hospital mortality at the time of ICU admission, and after 24 and 48 hours in the ICU.[33,34] The admission model contains 11 patient specific variables that are independent of treatment received in the ICU. The 24- and 48-hour models reflect both patient condition and treatments. MPM has been used to estimate probability of hospital mortality for ICU patients,[34] and for ICU quality assessment.[35] Refinement of MPM is continuing with the aim of making it clinically useful.

Physiology Stability Index (PSI) and Pediatric Risk of Mortality (PRISM)

The PSI was developed to measure severity of illness in pediatric ICUs. Like the original APACHE system, PSI assigned points to each of 34 physiological variables depending on the degree of abnormality.[36] When scoring for physiological abnormalities is combined with scoring for age, a higher total score is associated with increasing severity of illness and risk for hospital mortality.

The PRISM score (Table 3) reduced the original 34 PSI variables to 14, but maintained the same 1–5 point scoring system used in PSI.[37] A logistic regression equation incorporating PRISM score, age (in months), and operative status can be used to estimate hospital mortality. The principles used to develop, streamline, and validate PRISM are similar to those used for APACHE II. PSI and PRISM have been used to compare pediatric ICU outcomes,[38] for utilization review,[39] and quality assessment.[40] PRISM was not designed to assess prognosis for individual patients, but the implications of daily changes in PRISM over time for individual survival have been examined.[41]

Therapeutic Intervention Scoring System (TISS)

The TISS is based on the premise that the more therapy a patient receives, the greater the severity of illness. The system was developed by Cullen and associates[42] in 1974 and expanded and updated in 1983.[43] TISS assigns from 1 to 4 points to various diagnostic, monitoring, and therapeutic tasks. The points assigned for each intervention reflect an increasing level of nursing time, skill, and effort. For example, the skill and effort required for intra-aortic balloon assistance is assigned a higher score (4 TISS points), than tracheotomy care (2 TISS points), or 10 hourly vital sign monitoring (1 TISS point). Table 4 presents a modified version of TISS, which was updated in 1988 for use in the APACHE III study. Variables have been added to reflect recent changes in ICU therapy and organized to characterize the type of services: active treatment; ICU monitoring; and standard floor care.

An increasing number of TISS points is associated with an increasing hospital death rate and has been used to measure severity of illness.[44,45] Because therapy varies greatly among institutions, however, TISS should not be used as a primary measure of severity of illness or outcome predictor. TISS has also been used to categorize ICU services

Table 3
Pediatric Risk of Mortality (PRISM) Score*

Variable	Age Restrictions and Ranges		Score
Systolic BP	Infants	Children	
(mmHg)	130–160	150–200	2
	55–65	65–75	
	>160	>200	6
	40–54	50–64	7
Diastolic BP	All ages		
(mmHg)	>110		6
Heart Rate	Infants	Children	
(beats/min)	>160	>150	4
	<90	<80	
Respiratory rate	Infants	Children	
(breaths/min)	61–90	51–70	1
	>90	>70	5
	Apnea	Apnea	
PaO2/FIO2[a]	All ages		
	200–300		2
	<200		3
PaCO2 (torr)[b]	All ages		
	51–65		1
	>65		5
Glasgow Coma Score[c]	All ages		
	<8		6
Pupillary reactions	unequal or dilated		4
	fixed and dilated		10
PT/PTT	All ages		
	1.5 × control		2
Total bilirubin	<1 month		
(mg/dL)	<3.5		6
Potassium	All ages		
(mEq/L)	3.0–3.5		
	6.5–7.5		1
	<3.0		
	>7.5		5
	All ages		
Calcium	7.0–8.0		
(mg/dL)	12.0–15.0		2
	<7.0		
	>15.0		6
	All ages		
Glucose	40–60		
(mg/dL)	250–400		4
	<40		
	>400		8
Bicarbonate[d]	All ages		
(mEq/L)	<16		
	>32		3

[a] Cannot be assessed in patients with intracardiac shunts of chronic respiratory insufficiency; requires arterial blood sampling.

[b] May be assessed with capillary blood gases.

[c] Assessed only if there is known or suspected CNS dysfunction; cannot be assessed in patients during iatrogenic sedation, paralysis, anesthesia, etc. Scores <8 correspond to coma or deep stupor.

[d] Use measured values.

* From Pollack et al.[37]

Table 4
Therapeutic Intervention Scoring System Modified According to Type of ICU Services

Active Treatment Tasks	
Respiratory	Renal
1. Controlled ventilation	19. Stable hemodialysis
2. Controlled ventilation with muscle relaxant	20. Unstable hemodialysis
	Gastrointestinal
3. IMV or Assisted ventilation	21. IV Pitressin infusion
4. Spontaneous PEEP or CPAP	22. Continuous arterial drug infusion
5. Nasal/oral intubation	23. Balloon tamponade for esophageal varices
6. Fresh tracheostomy (48 hours)	
7. Emergency bronchoscopy	24. Continuous NG Lavage
Cardiovascular	25. Emergency endoscopy
	Neurologic
8. Atrial/ventricular pacing	
9. Intraaortic balloon	26. Mannitol infusion
10. Vasoactive drug infusion (one)	27. Ventriculostomy*
11. Vasoactive drugs (>one)	28. Treatment of seizures
12. IV Antiarrhythmic infusion	29. Induced hypothermia <32C
13. >6 L/day IV fluids	30. Barbiturate anesthesia*
14. Rapid blood transfusion	Miscellaneous
15. Post arrest (>48 hours)	31. Treatment of metabolic acidosis/alkalosis
16. Trauma suit	
17. Cardioversion	32. Emergency operation
18. Pericardiocentesis	

(continued)

for both adult[46] and pediatric patients,[47] measure ICU costs and resource use,[48] and assess nurse staffing requirements.[49] Unfortunately, the complexity and burden of collecting TISS data have represented a major barrier to its more widespread use and acceptance as a tool for assessing ICU resource use.

The APACHE III Prognostic System

The APACHE III prognostic system was developed in 1991 to expand and improve the prognostic estimates provided by APACHE.[50] APACHE III consists of two options: (1) An APACHE III score; and (2) a series of predictive equations linked to the APACHE III database.

Table 4 *(continued)*

Active Treatment Tasks	
ICU Monitoring Tasks	
1. Hourly vital signs	5. Pulmonary artery/left atrial catheter
2. Hourly Neurologic checks	6. Cardiac output measurement
3. ECG monitoring (continuous)	7. Pacemaker (standby)
4. Peripheral arterial cannula	8. Intracranial pressure monitor
Standard Floor Care Tasks	
1. Intake and Output	26. Peripheral IV (>one)
2. Pump regulated IV	27. Central line
3. Urinary catheter	28. Urine for fractionation
4. Ostomy drainage	29. Drainage tube(s)/hemovac(s)
5. Extensive wound care	30. Standard orthopedic traction
6. Routine dressing changes	31. Complex orthopedic traction
7. Multiple dressing changes	32. Hyper/hypothermia blanket
8. Decubitus care	33. Parenteral chemotherapy
9. 1–2 IV antibiotics	34. Acute digitalization
10. >2 IV antibiotics	35. Active diuresis/overload
11. Bolus IV Med. (unscheduled)	36. Anticoagulation (acute)
12. Intermittent IV Med. (sched)	37. Anticoagulation (chronic)
13. Conc. K via central line	38. Chest physical therapy
14. Platelet infusion(s)	39. Incentive spirometry/IPPB
15. Central IV nutrition	40. Inhalation therapy
16. Peripheral IV nutrition	41. Tracheal suction (non-intub)
17. Enteral tube feedings	42. Oxygen via mask/cannula
18. Oral/NG fluid replacement	43. Spontaneous respiration via endotracheal tube
19. Chest tube(s)	
20. Thoracentesis/paracentesis	44. Endotracheal/trach. care
21. Diagnostic procedure (not in ICU)	45. Oximetry*
22. Peritoneal dialysis	46. Patient isolation*
23. Kayexalate/colonic enema*	47. Patient restraints*
24. Thrombolytic therapy*	48. Frequent blood tests
25. Peripheral IV (one)	49. Frequent blood product infusion

* Not included in TISS–1983 update.[43]

The APACHE III Score

The APACHE III score[50] can be hand calculated and consists of: (1) points for physiological abnormalities; (2) points for age; and (3) points for chronic health status (Table 5). Physiological scoring is based on the extent of abnormality for 17 variables reflecting vital signs, laboratory tests, and neurological evaluation. In addition, points are added

Table 5
Components of the APACHE III Score

Physiological Variables (APS)	0–252 Points
Mean blood pressure	PaO2 or A-aDO2
Respiratory rate	PaCO2
Temperature	Serum sodium
Pulse	Serum albumin
Urine output/24 hours	Serum bilirubin
Hematocrit	Serum glucose
White blood cell count	Serum creatinine
Blood pH	Blood urea nitrogen
Glasgow coma score (modified)	
Chronological Age	**0–24 points**
Chronic Health Evaluation	**0–23 points**
AIDS	Immunosuppression
Hepatic failure	Metastatic cancer
Lymphoma	Cirrhosis
Leukemia/multiple myeloma	

based on increasing age and seven comorbid conditions shown to have a significant impact on short-term mortality. The sum of points for APACHE IIIs components yields a numerical score that theoretically ranges from 0–299; physiological scoring contributes the majority (0–252) of the score compared to age (score 0–24), and chronic health evaluation (score 0–23).

The APACHE III score can be used to measure severity of disease and to risk stratify patients within a single diagnostic category or independently defined patient group. This is because an increasing score is associated with an increased risk of hospital death. APACHE III scores can also be used to compare patient survival, but can only be used for ICU admissions meeting the same diagnostic and selection criteria used in the APACHE III study.

APACHE III Predictive Equations

An automated version of APACHE III[51] provides prognostic estimates that are generated by a series of predictive equations. These equations link the APACHE III score to a 17,440 admission reference database and also uses additional variables to reflect disease classification and patient selection for intensive care. The database includes 212 potential diagnoses and there are weights for 66 specific reasons for ICU admission and 7 nonoperative and 5 operative organ system categories. Patient selection is accounted for by variables reflecting the hospital length of stay and location prior to ICU admission. These variables are included to control for differences in patient selection and response (or lack of) to prior therapy.

In addition to hospital mortality, a series of equations using similar, but not identical predictor variables, can predict outcomes such as ICU length of stay, resource use, nursing intensity, and risk for receiving active life supporting therapy. Each outcome is predicted on the basis of individual patient and institutional characteristics with reference to the APACHE III database. The ratio of actual to predicted outcome aggregated at the unit level provides a means for assessing and comparing ICU efficacy and efficiency.

Utilization Review

The resources used to care for ICU patients encompasses a unit's entire physical plant, equipment, supplies, professional staff, and all of its support services and personnel. This view of resource utilization is that of the hospital administrator, a perspective that is necessarily complex and involves a multitude of items and millions of dollars. But from a clinical perspective, ICU resource use is primarily related to the kinds of patients admitted, the type and amount of services they receive, and their length of stay.

There are three major reasons why resource utilization is a vital topic for ICU managers: first, resource shortages, mainly of beds and nurses, are common in ICU; second, managers are responsible for making "front line" utilization decisions; and third, measuring resource use is an essential step in assessing ICU costs. This section will suggest methods for categorizing ICU services and then discuss how this information can be used to assess and improve resource allocation and utilization.

Categorizing ICU Services

The services provided by ICUs are comparable to those provided by fire departments; they fight fires, but also work to prevent them.

Fighting fires is what happens when patients are admitted for life supporting therapy; and prevention when patients are admitted for monitoring because they are perceived at increased risk for needing life-support. The type and amount of patient services provided by ICUs are best measured using the TISS. As shown in Table 4, ICUs provide three major types of services: (1) *Active treatment*, which includes life supporting therapies or techniques best limited to an ICU; (2) *ICU monitoring*, nursing and technologic services that are observational rather than therapeutic; and (3) *Standard floor care*, services that are commonly provided in ICU but are neither unique nor limited to ICUs.[46]

Classifying ICU admissions according to type of services received during the first ICU day provides an excellent method for utilization review. ICU monitor admissions, are those who receive only monitoring and standard floor care services; and active treatment admissions, those receiving one or more active life supporting treatments in addition to monitoring and floor care services.[46,53] Active treatment admissions have the greatest need for ICU care, but among monitoring admissions priority is largely determined by their risk for subsequent active life supporting therapy.[52,53]

Low-risk monitoring admissions are patients who are at less than a 10% risk for receiving active treatment after their first ICU day.[26,27,52] These patients typically have such a low severity of illness and probability of death that their characteristics are often similar to ward patients. Low-risk monitor admissions typically receive minimal amounts of concentrated nursing care and observation, although some also receive technologic monitoring (e.g., an arterial catheter). Examples of low-risk monitoring admissions include many, but not all surgical patients who have undergone carotid endarterectomy or other peripheral vascular procedures, and elective craniotomy, thoracotomy, or laparotomy for a neoplasm. Low-risk medical admissions include many patients admitted for monitoring after episodes of chest pain, syncope, self-inflicted drug overdose, and diabetic ketoacidosis.

High-risk monitoring admissions are patients at greater than 10% risk for receiving active life supporting treatment after their first ICU day.[27] These patients usually have moderate severity of illness; a higher probability of death; and receive greater amounts of monitoring and concentrated nursing care. Examples of high-risk monitoring admissions include medical patients admitted for GI bleeding or pneumonia, and surgical patients admitted after intracranial aneurysm clipping, or laparotomy for intestinal obstruction.

Active treatment admissions, are patients who receive one or more of the life supporting therapies listed in Table 4 during their first ICU day.[27] These patients can be further classified according to whether their probability of hospital mortality is low, intermediate, or high.[54,55] Each of these probability ranges has an important impact on ICU resource use.[53,56] Patients who require life-support but have a relatively low (< 40%) probability of hospital death (e.g., drug overdose, asthma), not only need, but are also most likely to benefit from ICU care.

At the high (> 80%) probability end of the spectrum are patients who are so severely ill (e.g., respiratory failure due to neoplasm, cardiac arrest) that there is a reduced likelihood of benefiting from ICU admission because therapy will probably be ineffective.[56–59] Many of these patients use few resources because they die after a brief trial of therapy, but for others care is prolonged and often resource intensive.[60,61] Although unlikely to recover, these patients are rarely denied admission to US ICUs for reasons that range from prognostic uncertainty, to death-denying patients and families, or overzealous physicians.

Of greatest importance, is the active treatment patient admitted with an intermediate (40%–80%) probability of death. Many of these patients (e.g., septic shock, pneumonia) respond to aggressive therapy, but others deteriorate or fail to respond to therapy. The prognostic uncertainty and continuing life-support for such patients often results in the highest cost and poorest outcomes.[53,62,63] Identifying patients who are likely to die despite state-of-the-art support is a high priority for outcomes research.[64,65]

International comparisons have shown marked differences in the types of patients admitted to ICU. In general, monitoring admissions are less common outside the US.[1,2] But in the US, ICU admissions in teaching hospitals more often receive active treatment than in community nonteaching hospitals.[66,67]

Measuring ICU Resource Utilization

Most of the patient input data listed in Table 1 can be used to measure ICU resource utilization, but in the absence of automation, the volume of data to collect and analyze would be overwhelming. It is, therefore, critical to focus on a few issues that reflect both efficient resource use and important challenges in your unit. Some of the more important measures of resource use are listed in Table 6.

All ICU managers need basic volume measures (e.g., census, patient days, occupancy) for staffing and budgetary projections. Most patient level measurements, however, should focus on current challenges. For

Table 6
Measures for Evaluating ICU Resource Use

Volume Measures
Average census
Analysis by service, diagnosis, physician
Patient days and occupancy rate
Types of Patients
Referral sources
Analysis by service, diagnosis, physician
Active treatment admissions
Monitoring admissions—high risk vs low risk
Medicare admissions
ICU Length of Stay (LOS)
Analysis by service, diagnosis, physician
Analysis of process e.g., admission and discharge delays
Case-mix adjusted ICU LOS performance
Staff Utilization
Nursing care hours
Medicus
Case-mix adjusted nursing intensity
Type and Amount of Treatment
Analysis of process e.g., laboratory studies
Case-mix adjusted ICU therapy (TISS)
Ventilator days
Swan-Ganz Catheterization

some units, analysis might focus on utilization by high-risk patients (e.g., admissions with AIDS or far advanced cancer) or high-risk procedures (e.g., ventilator support). Units in referral hospitals might concentrate on admissions transferred from another ICU or hospital.[68] Units experiencing delays in patient admission or discharge may wish to monitor the time required to transfer patients from emergency, recovery, and operating rooms or in discharging patients to wards or intermediate care units.

The principle of focusing on efficiency and important challenges also applies to measures such as ICU length of stay, proportion of low-risk monitor admissions, nursing care hours, and the use of diagnostic services (e.g., laboratory testing) or treatment modalities (e.g., ventilator days). An ICU that frequently faces admission requests that exceed bed capacity, for example, should review its patient input, particularly the proportion of low-risk monitoring admissions. Since these patients seldom require unique services, units with a substantial proportion of such admissions may have the ability to reduce ICU use without jeopardizing quality of care.[27,39,69] This can be accomplished by exploring care alternatives such as floor care[70,71] or establishing intermediate care units.[72–74]

Many ICU managers would like to know—How does our unit's efficiency compare to others?—Unfortunately, simple comparison of measures such as ICU length of stay that are not adjusted for patient differences are unlikely to accurately reflect performance. The APACHE III prognostic system can now generate predicted utilization rates based on both institutional and patient characteristics using performance within a representative sample of US hospitals with 200 or more beds as a standard. Resource use (e.g., ICU length of stay) is predicted based on individual patient characteristics aggregated at the unit level and then analyzed over time. The difference between mean actual and predicted ICU length of stay provides not only a direct measure of efficiency, but also provide regarding methods for improving performance.

In a recent evaluation of differences in efficiency among 42 ICUs, mean ICU length of stay ranged from 3.3 to 7.3 days and 78% of the variation was explained by case-mix adjusted mean predicted length of stay.[75] The ratio of mean actual to predicted ICU length of stay ranged from 0.88 to 1.21. For six units, efficiency was significantly better ($P < 0.05$) than average and for five significantly worse ($P < 0.05$). There was no association between performance ranking by ICU length of stay and risk adjusted hospital mortality, but superior efficiency was associated with better ICU organization and management.[76] The ability to reliably adjust for variations in patient characteristics across these ICUs provided not only an objective evaluation of efficiency in resource use, but also permitted examination of the factors associated with superior performance.

Using scientific methods for monitoring performance and defining upper and lower control limits is the basis for modern quality improvement techniques.[77–80] By entering patient input data and applying a series of predictive equations, ICU can use the APACHE III system to monitor resource use and compare their efficiency with other units. In addition to ICU length of stay, a series of equations permit similar case-mix adjusted efficiency comparisons for measures such as unit level treatment intensity, nurse staffing, ventilator days, and use of Swan-Ganz catheters.

These techniques can permit ICU clinicians to increasingly "manage by facts".[81] For example, the leadership of an ICU might discover that their unit's length of stay exceeds that of similar units. Using this information as a focus for problem diagnosis, potential causes can be identified, solutions designed, and then implemented. Continued mon-

Table 7
Indicators of ICU Quality Related to Structure Process or Outcome

Process	
Cardiac arrest	Nosocomial sinusitis
Upper GI bleeding	Nosocomial pneumonia
Airway emergency	Medication error
Reintubation (within 24 hours)	Use of salt poor albumin
Self-extubation	Use of blood products
ICU readmission (within 24 hours)	Blood transfusion
Pneumothorax	Iatrogenic hyperkalemia
Bleeding from anticoagulation	Complication of transport
Ventilator complication	PA catheter complication
Catheter related bacteremia	Fall from bed
Postoperative wound infection	Right mainstem intubation
Structure	
Appropriateness of admission and discharge practices	
Equipment malfunction	
Appropriateness of ICU length of stay	
Proportion of low risk monitor admissions	
Delays in patient admission or discharge	
Management of patient overflow	
Outcome	
Review of ICU deaths	Review of low risk deaths
Patient satisfaction	Family satisfaction
Comparison of actual and predicted death rate	

itoring provides a means for confirming and maintaining improved performance (Table 7).

Managing ICU Resources

With knowledge of patient input and services, ICU leaders who wish to assess and improve resource use might concentrate on improving selection of patients for ICU admission and discharge, streamlining patient throughput, identifying more efficient patient care protocols, or more efficient use of laboratory services. The following examples illustrate how improved management can lead to more efficient resource use.

Civetta et al.[82] demonstrated how improving the process of ordering laboratory tests can effect cost savings. They found that some patients spent 15% of their total hospitalization in ICU, but generated 61%

of their total laboratory charges during this period. After a series of interventions, total laboratory tests per patient declined by 42% (from 134 to 78 tests) and laboratory charges by 53%. What were the interventions? They included: (1) The introduction of arterial and venous oximetry; (2) staff education; (3) elimination of standing orders, routines, and parochialism; and (4) the substitution of structured decision trees to help select appropriate tests in common situations such as "fever work-ups" and nutritional support monitoring.

Achieving better selection of patients for ICU admission and discharge is another major challenge for ICU. Rationing of critical care beds is an everyday occurrence in many hospitals and there is substantial evidence that current practices are often subjective and even based on political power, provincialism, and economic incentives.[83,84] Kalb and Miller[69] have suggested that hospitals should either adopt formal rationing guidelines or take clear steps to increase critical care resources by expanding ICU or intermediate care capacity. They believe the overriding determinant for allocating scarce ICU resources is medical suitability defined as a benefits/burdens test with priorities based on each patient's expected functional status and duration of survival.

Readers will find SCCM recommendations for ICU admission and discharge criteria[85] particularly useful in establishing policies and priorities that emphasize need and anticipated benefit. For most ICUs, patient autonomy and lack of alternative care sites make it almost impossible to refuse patients who seem "too sick" to benefit. At present a trial of therapy, ongoing dialogue with family and primary physician and, if needed, input from the hospital ethics committee are the best methods for avoiding prolonged futile care. When triage of low-risk monitoring admissions is a frequent issue, ICU managers need to document the problem and then explore floor or intermediate care alternatives with hospital administrators.[70–74]

The APACHE III system has considerable potential for assisting these allocation decisions. A series of predictive equations can assist admission decision-making by accurately predicting risk of hospital mortality and identifying low-risk monitor patients. Discharge decisions can also be supplemented by daily APACHE III predictions of risk for life-support in the subsequent 24 hours. Although estimates of probability of mortality and risk for requiring life supporting therapy are not the only considerations in making ICU admission and discharge decisions, risk prediction can provide objective criteria for establishing relative priorities.[86,87]

It is widely recognized that 90%–95% of low-risk monitor admissions never receive active intervention, but many physicians are unwilling to recommend routine ward admission. When all ICU beds are occupied, however, low-risk patients are frequently refused ICU admission or the ICU length of stay shortened.[70,72] By providing an objective method to identify risk for life-support, particularly among monitoring patients, APACHE III predictions should be helpful in supporting clinical judgments about ICU admission and in establishing priorities for ICU discharge during periods of limited bed availability. Thus, objective estimates of risk for life-support can now be used, not only to assess overall ICU resource use, but also to supplement clinical judgments regarding admission, discharge, and triage decisions.

Quality Assessment and Improvement

How do you define quality? To most of us quality is like beauty, it has a positive connotation but isn't measurable. But if quality can't be measured, how can it be assessed or improved? How, for example, can I determine which is the best quality car to buy? To communicate what I mean, "best quality" must be defined in terms of specific attributes, and then each attribute must be defined using quantitative measurements. Before buying a car I can review data on performance, fuel economy, and trouble spots for each make and model. Assessing and improving the quality of ICU care requires a similar approach; quality must be defined using specific attributes, and each attribute must be measured.

Delivering high-quality patient care has long been a core value of medical and nursing professionals. So why perform quality assurance studies? A frequent answer is, "The Joint Commission (JCAHO) says we have too!" Unfortunately, past efforts at quality assessment have been viewed as an ineffective forced bureaucratic chore rather than an attempt to improve quality of care.[88] Programs that tended to concentrate on negative events, were viewed as restrictive or punitive, and largely emphasized looking for "bad apples", passing inspections, and meeting subjectively developed minimal standards.[78]

The 1988–1990 APACHE III study demonstrated some of the shortcomings of recent approaches to quality assurance. Among the 42 ICUs studied, 95% had a nursing quality assurance (QA) program, but physicians participated in evaluating care processes in only 50%–60% of the units. During detailed on-site organizational analyses at nine of these ICUs, we found that physicians and nurses readily identified quality problems related to triage, emergency responses, etc. But their QA activities rarely addressed these problems. In some units there was minimal staff participation; and in others no internal QA program. When specific patient care issues were addressed, there was little feedback, or such a delay that nobody could remember the case. For most units, QA was perceived as a necessary evil to keep "JCAH0 off their backs".

Why should ICU approach JCAHOs agenda for change and its focus on continuous quality improvement (CQI) differently? The answer should be to deliver better care! Although CQI is of uncertain value medically, it has resulted in remarkable quality improvements among both manufacturing and service industries.[89–92] But the real driving force behind CQI is the pressure to contain health care costs and simultaneously improve quality. CQI (also called total quality management or TQM) enlists an entire organization to work toward a goal of continuous improvement in quality as defined by attributes needed or wanted by the customer.

The Monitoring and Evaluation Process

For most readers, adopting continuous quality improvement is not an option; it's implicit in meeting JCAHO standards. Thus, for ICU managers, the Joint Commission's perspectives and the ten step monitoring and evaluation process are required reading.[93,94] I will, therefore, only briefly summarize their content.

ICUs must have a planned, systematic process for monitoring and evaluating patient care and for resolving problems. JCAHO emphasizes that professionals in each unit should design these activities; that they be carried out in an ongoing, planned, and systematic fashion; and function as part of an organizationwide written plan. To do this, ICUs must use or adapt the ten-step process summarized below:

1. *Assign Responsibility.* The ICU medical director is responsible for monitoring and evaluating care, but may assign specific duties to others.
2. *Delineate Scope of Care.* Take an "inventory" of what the unit does (diseases treated, therapies provided) to provide a basis for identifying important aspects of care.
3. *Identify Important Aspect of Care.* Important aspects of care are defined as those that are high-risk, high-volume, or problem prone, and thus have the greatest impact on quality of care.
4. *Identify Indicators.* Indicators of quality, i.e., variables related to structure, process, or outcomes, must be identified and defined for each important aspect of care.

5. *Establish Thresholds for Evaluation.* Define a level or point at which intensive quality evaluation is triggered.
6. *Collect and Organize Data.* Data pertaining to each indicator should be collected and organized.
7. *Evaluate Care.* When there is sufficient data related to each indicator care should be evaluated to determine whether a problem exists and identify causes and methods for improvement.
8. *Take Action to Solve Problems.* Develop and enact plans to solve problems or improve care.
9. *Assess Actions and Document Improvement.* Assess and document the effectiveness of actions taken and identify if any further actions are needed.
10. *Communicate Relevant Information.* Document findings and conclusions of monitoring, evaluation, and actions and report them through hospital channels.

ICUs have excellent potential for implementing CQI. Their scope of practice (what they do) can be characterized using diagnosis, severity of illness, admitting service, etc. (Table 1). The scope of care (services provided) can be measured with regard to type (active treatment, monitoring) and amount of services (TISS) provided (Table 4). Many of these services represent important aspects of care, can be defined using indicators, and are well suited to explicitly defined standards or protocols. Systems involving human beings, however, combine both explicit and implicit elements into a "usual way of doing things". Thus an ICU, no matter how outstanding its written rules, standards, or protocols, will have a certain percentage of bad outcomes. This is because no system can account for all the ways by which bad outcomes might occur.

Implementing a Quality Improvement Program

The anesthesiologist sighed as he secured the endotracheal tube and ordered ventilator settings. Intubation hadn't been difficult, but the patient's acute pulmonary edema, newly clipped cerebral aneurysm, and recent vasospasm hardly represented a routine case. He had used thiopental because the patient was hypertensive, but the fall in blood pressure had been greater than expected. Since there was already hemiparesis due to vasospasm, the neurosurgery resident was worried about cerebral infarction. The blood pressure rose as the nurse increased the dopamine infusion.

The pulmonary edema cleared, there was no cerebral infarction, and outcome at ICU and hospital discharge was excellent. Although this instance of pulmonary edema complicating hypervolemic-hypertensive therapy was extreme, our ICU staff had been concerned about the frequency of this complication. The problem had been discussed among the ICU and neurosurgical staff; and complications of hypervolemic therapy recorded as a quality indicator for the past year. The incidence of complications seemed high, but was the same or lower than reported in several case series. Prior discussions had had little impact on the problem.

Although there were some differences about monitoring and use of vasopressors, the ICU and neurosurgery staff agreed that their approach reflected published recommendations. We were concerned, however, that the actual process was inconsistent. Using the literature as a foundation, we developed a protocol that provided a standard treatment approach. Following implementation and a period of education and adjustment the process improved and the complication rate fell. By the third and last year of monitoring the incidence of pulmonary edema had been cut in half; and when present, most instances represented only radiographic findings of pulmonary congestion.

The approach used in the above example follows the spirit if not the letter of the CQI process. In my opinion, the book "Curing Health Care" by Berwick et al.[95] provides the best description of how ICU managers can apply CQI in the health care setting. The authors describe quality improvement as "a process consisting of defining the problem, making the diagnosis, administering the remedy, and holding the gains". Your unit may not be ready to select projects through criterion matrices, use cause and effect or flow diagrams, or collect data using Pareto diagrams or control charts, but you can identify problems, collect data, and orchestrate a team approach to their definition analysis and correction.

ICUs will rarely identify a unique quality problem; most will have been described in the literature dealing with the complications of intensive care. Although rarely published for purposes of quality improvement, the literature dealing with complications of specific technologies, procedures, or adverse events are valuable sources for defining and solving quality problems.[96–99] Table 6 is a list of high-risk, high-volume, or problem prone aspects of ICU care. Classified according to their relationship to structure process and outcome, they can be used as indicators in collecting quality data.

Many of the problems or complications listed in Table 6 are infrequent and relevant data will require collection over prolonged periods.

In our unit we use a simple worksheet to record data concerning each indicator. More importantly, we emphasize concurrent review, i.e., we record, evaluate, and discuss each event daily as a part of our morning rounds. For each quarter our data is updated, summarized, and reported to the hospital quality improvement department via the critical care committee. For most indicators we simply display quarterly data, but when data is sufficient it is summarized, analyzed, and our findings reported. We also report what actions have been taken and then continue monitoring to provide evidence of problem resolution.

Our program, as outlined above, has worked. We've reduced the incidence of pulmonary edema during hypervolemic therapy, iatrogenic pneumothorax, self-extubation, and also improved our resource utilization. But as reported by others, we often fail to identify adverse events,[100,101] make reliable quality assessments,[102,103] and fail to focus on outcomes.[104]

It has been predicted that the quality assessment tools of the future will be more reliable, valid, based on meaningful guidelines, and performance measures.[105] Currently, the use of ICU outcomes, e.g., mortality or complication rates, as quality indicators is extremely inaccurate when data is not adjusted for pretreatment risk.[77,101] A prognostic scoring system that establishes a predicted mortality risk for each ICU based on individual patient characteristics, however provides a valid comparison of predicted and observed outcome. The difference between actual and predicted death rates is not only a measure of quality of care, but can also provide insight regarding means for improving performance.

The usefulness of this approach was demonstrated by an evaluation of outcome from intensive care in 13 major US medical centers.[24] When the predicted mortality rate for each unit was compared to its observed rate, 11 of the 13 units performed within two standard deviations. However, one ICU had 40% fewer deaths than predicted; another 58% more deaths than expected. The most striking difference between these two ICUs was related to how well the units were organized and managed. These findings have been prospectively examined as part of the APACHE III study.[75] Observed hospital mortality rates varied from 6% to 40% among the 42 units and 90% of the inter-hospital variation in death rate was accounted for by patient physiological and demographic characteristics on admission. The ratio of actual to predicted mortality varied from 0.67 to 1.25. Compared to average performance at all 42 units, risk adjusted mortality rate was significantly better at 5 and worse at 5 ICUs.

The automated version of APACHE III (51) can now provide hospitals with the capability of monitoring and comparing ICU outcomes.

By entering the clinical and physiologic data required for prognostic estimates ICUs can compare actual and predicted outcomes. The system allows ICU to compare their outcomes to units in hospitals with similar structural characteristics or to a nationally representative standard. For quality improvement activities, the system provides continuous monitoring and evaluation of group outcomes by service, diagnosis, and severity of disease. This type of information can, therefore, focus quality review by diagnosis, service, and facilitate detecting the underlying mechanisms causing mortality.[77–81]

We have recently explored using APACHE III in our unit to select charts for quality review. Case selection was based on results of a RAND corporation study,[106] which demonstrated that the majority of preventable deaths occur among patients at a low-risk of death on admission. We, therefore, reviewed the charts of patients who died and were at low (< 40%) risk of death on ICU admission. Using implicit (based on personal knowledge and our experience) judgment alone, we looked for and found preventable deaths and opportunities for improving care process. This preliminary experience suggests that risk prediction at ICU admission can be helpful in improving case selection for quality review by focusing the review process on cases that provide more meaningful insights for quality improvement.

Risk Management

Risk management has many of the same goals as CQI, i.e., the identification, analysis, and prevention of errors and mishaps.[107,108] Risk management's primary focus, however, is on: (1) preventing financial loss; and (2) controlling the frequency and severity of malpractice claims. Measures aimed at preventing financial loss include: staff orientation and training (e.g., standards for documentation and patient care); patient injury prevention; and fire safety programs. But the greatest challenge for loss prevention is maintaining effective incident reporting. Critical care is fraught with hazards and human error is the most important cause of mishaps and complications.[98,99,109] Obstacles to reporting these errors include defensiveness, denial, and an inquisitional style of investigation. To insure effectiveness, ICU managers should promote incident reports as important risk management and quality tools and avoid finger-pointing and a punitive atmosphere.

Liability control includes legal affairs, claims management, insurance programs, and the hospital's quality improvement program. ICU physician and nurse managers, however, are in the "front lines" of risk control; they are directly in contact with the patient or caregivers and can ensure a consistent approach to family relations and communication. The risk of litigation can be reduced by following four general rules[108,110]: (1) use common sense and avoid defensiveness and denial regarding errors and mishaps; (2) avoid elements of negligence. Legally, negligence has occurred if a nurse or physician owed a duty (determined by standards of care) to a patient, but failed to meet that duty resulting in damages that were directly caused by failure to meet accepted'standards; (3) maintain proper documentation. Write precise descriptions so events can be reconstructed; deficiencies imply sloppy practice; don't alter or add contrived facts. Avoid completing a chart in response to a potential suit and ablating entries, however, supplemental entries can be written immediately or within days, but should be accurately dated and labeled; and (4) use the unit's CQI program to avoid and correct problems.

An ICU manager's most important role in risk management occurs when there is a major disaster. The following is a suggested step-by-step approach. First, acknowledge the problem and avoid denial or cover-up. Second, review the medical record to define the problem and assess the extent of injury, care process, and adequacy of documentation. Third, discuss the situation with involved staff members. Get the facts, but be supportive and avoid finger-pointing. Fourth, notify the risk management department and wait their recommendations in regard to risk, documentation, and patient/family notification. Finally, evaluate causes, and opportunities for improvement and preventing recurrences.

References

1. Knaus WA, Legall JR, Wagner DP, et al: A comparison of intensive care in the USA and France. Lancet 1982$_\infty$:642.
2. Zimmerman JE, Knaus WA, Judson JA, et al: Patient selection for intensive care: A comparison of New Zealand and United States hospitals. Crit Care Med 1988;16:318.
3. Draper EA, Wagner DP, Knaus WA: The use of intensive care: A comparison of a university and community hospital. Health Care Financ Rev 1982; 3:49.
4. McClish DK, Russo A, Franklin C, et al: Profile of medical ICU vs. ward patients in an acute care hospital. Crit Care Med 1985;13:381.
5. Seneff M, Knaus WA: Predicting patient outcome from intensive care: A guide to APACHE, MPM, SAPS, PRISM, and other prognostic scoring systems. J Intensive Care Med 1990;5:33.
6. Knaus WA, Zimmerman JE: Prediction of outcome from critical illness.

In Ledingham I McA (ed): Recent Advances in Critical Care Medicine. Edinburgh, Churchill Livingstone, 1988, p. 1.

7. Feller I, Tholen D, Cornell RG: Improvements in burn care 1965 to 1979. JAMA 1980;244:2074–2078.
8. Champion HR, Succo WJ, Carnazzo AJ, et al: Trauma score. Crit Care Med 1981;9:672.
9. Baker SP, O'Neil B, Haddun W, et al: The injury severity score: A method for describing patients with multiple injuries and evaluating emergency care. J Trauma 1974;14:187.
10. Teasdale G, Jennett B: Assessment of coma and improved consciousness: A practical scale. Lancet 1974$_{\infty}$:81.
11. Wagner DP, Knaus WA, Draper EA: Physiologic abnormalities and outcome from acute disease. Arch Intern Med 1986;146:1389.
12. Teres D, Avrunin JS, Lemeshow S: Severity of illness modeling. In Rippe JM (ed): Intensive Care Medicine. Second Edition. Boston, MA, Little Brown, 1991.
13. Farmer JC, Kirby RR, Taylor RW (eds): Problems in Critical Care Medicine. Volume 3, Number 4. Philadelphia, PA, JB Lippincott, 1989.
14. Civil ID, Schwab CW: The injury severity score, 1985 revision: A condensed chart for clinical use. J Trauma 1988;28:87.
15. Boyd CR, Tolson MA, Copes WS: Evaluating trauma care: The TRISS method. J Trauma 1987;27:370.
16. University of South Alabama College of Medicine, Division of Pediatric surgery: Pediatric trauma score: A rapid assessment and triage tool for the injured child, 1986.
17. Knaus WA, Zimmerman JE, Wagner DP, et al: APACHE—acute physiology and chronic health evaluation: A physiologically based classification system. Crit Care Med 1981;9:591.
18. Knaus WA, Draper EA, Wagner DP, et al: APACHE II: A severity of disease classification system. Crit Care Med 1985;13:818.
19. Zeigler EJ, Fisher CJ, Sprung CL, et al: Treatment of gram-negative bacteremia and septic shock with HA-1A human monoclonal antibody against endotoxin. N Engl J Med 1991;324:429.
20. Durocher A, Saulnier F, Seuscart R, et al: A comparison of three severity score indices in an evaluation of serious bacterial pneumonia. Int Care Med 1988;14:39.
21. Teskey RJ, Calvin JE, McPhail I: Disease severity in the coronary care unit. Chest 1991;100:1637.
22. Chang RWS, Jacobs S, Lee B: Predicting outcome among intensive care unit patients using computerized trend analysis of daily APACHE II scores corrected for organ system failure. Int Care Med 1988;14:588.
23. Chang RWS: Individual outcome prediction models for intensive care units. Lancet 1989$_{\infty}$:201.
24. Knaus WA, Draper EA, Wagner DP, et al: Evaluation of outcome from intensive care. Ann Intern Med 1986;104:110.
25. Sirio CA, Tajimi K, Tase C, et al: An initial comparison in intensive care in Japan and the United States. Crit Care Med 1992;20:1207.
26. Wagner DP, Knaus WA, Draper EA, et al: Identification of low-risk monitor admissions within a medical-surgical intensive care unit. Med Care 1983; 21:425.

27. Wagner DP, Knaus WA, Draper EA: Identification of low-risk monitor admissions to medical-surgical ICUs. Chest 1987;92:423.
28. Le Gall JR, Loirat P, Alperovitch A, et al: A simplified acute physiology score for ICU patients. Crit Care Med 1984;12:975.
29. French Multicenter Group of ICU Research and the INSERM Unit 169 of Statistical and Epidemiological Studies: Factors related to outcome in intensive care: French multicenter study. Crit Care Med 1989;17:305.
30. Durocher A, Saulnier F, Beuscart R, et al: A comparison of three severity scores indexes in an evaluation of serious bacterial pneumonia. Int Care Med 1988;14:39.
31. French Multicenter Group of ICU Research and the INSERM Unit 169 of Statistical and Epidemiological Studies: Description of various types of intensive and intermediate care units in France. Int Care Med 1989;15:260.
32. Eisenber G: Diagnosis related groups, severity of illness and equitable reimbursement under Medicare. JAMA 1984;251:645.
33. Lemeshow S, Teres D, Pastides H, et al: A method for predicting survival and mortality of ICU patients using objectively derived weights. Crit Care Med 1985;13:519.
34. Lemeshow S, Teres D, Avrunin SJ, et al: Refining intensive care unit outcome prediction by using changing probabilities of mortality. Crit Care Med 1989;16:470.
35. Teres D, Lemeshow S, Harris D, et al: Mortality prediction models (MPM) for ICU patients. In Farmer JC, Kirby RR, Taylor RW (eds): Problems in Critical Care Medicine. Philadelphia, PA, JB Lippincott, Philadelphia, PA, 1989, p. 585.
36. Pollack MM, Yeh TS, Ruttimann UE, et al: Evaluation of pediatric intensive care. Crit Care Med 1984;12:376.
37. Pollack MM, Ruttimann UE, Getson PR, et al: Pediatric risk of mortality (PRISM) score. Crit Care Med 1988;16:1110.
38. Pollack MM, Ruttimann UE, Gaston PR, et al: Accurate prediction of the outcome of pediatric intensive care: A new quantitative method. N Engl J Med 1987;316:134.
39. Pollack MM, Getson PR, Ruttimann UE, et al: Efficiency of intensive care. A comparative analysis of eight pediatric intensive care units. JAMA 1987;258:1481.
40. Pollack MM, Alexander SR, Clarke N, et al: Improved outcomes from tertiary care center pediatric intensive care: A statewide comparison of tertiary and nontertiary care facilities. Crit Care Med 1991;19:150.
41. Ruttimann UE, Pollack MM: Objective assessment of changing mortality risks in pediatric intensive care unit patients. Crit Care Med 1991;19:474.
42. Cullen DJ, Civetta JM, Briggs BA, et al: Therapeutic intervention scoring system: A method for quantitative comparison of patient care. Crit Care Med 1974;2:57.
43. Keene AR, Cullen DJ: Therapeutic intervention scoring system; update 1983. Crit Care Med 1983;11:1.
44. Wagner DP, Knaus WA, Draper EA: Severity of illness and the relationship between intensive care and survival. Am J Public Health 1982;72:449.
45. Cullen DJ: Results and costs of intensive care. Anesthesiology 1977;47:203.

46. Knaus WA, Wagner DP, Draper EA, et al: The range of intensive care services today. JAMA 1981;246:2711.
47. Yeh TS, Pollack MM, Holbrook PR, et al: Assessment of pediatric intensive care—application of the therapeutic intervention scoring system. Crit Care Med 1982;10:497.
48. Wagner DP, Wineland TD, Knaus WA: The hidden costs of treating severely ill patients: A case study of charges and resource consumption in an intensive care unit. Health Care Financ Rev 1983;5:81.
49. Greenberg AG, McClure DK, Janus CA, et al: Nursing intervention scoring system: A concept for management, research and communication. In Lindberg DAB, Reichertz PL (eds): Lecture Notes in Medical Informatics. New York, NY, Springer Verlag, 1978, p. 729.
50. Knaus WA, Wagner DP, Draper EA, et al: The APACHE III prognostic system: Risk prediction of hospital mortality for critically ill hospitalized adults. Chest 1991;100:1619.
51. Knaus WA, Draper EA, Wagner DP: Utilization of findings from APACHE III research to develop an operating information system in the ICU: The APACHE III management system. In Symposium for Computer Applications for Medical Care. New York, NY, McGraw Hill, 1992, p. 987.
52. Henning RJ, McClish D, Daly B, et al: Clinical characteristics and resource utilization of ICU patients: Implications for organization of intensive care. Crit Care Med 1987;15:264.
53. Oye RK, Bellamy PE: Patterns of resource consumption in medical intensive care. Chest 1991;99:685.
54. Knaus WA, Draper EA, Wagner DP: Evaluating medical-surgical intensive care units. In Parrillo JE, Ayers SM (eds): Major Issues in Critical Care Medicine. Baltimore, MD, Williams Wilkins, 1984, p. 35.
55. French Multicenter Group of ICU research: Factors related to outcome in intensive care: French multicenter study. Crit Care Med 1989;17:305.
56. Knaus WA, Rauss A, Alperovitch A, et al: Do objective estimates of chances for survival influence decisions to withhold or withdraw treatment? Med Decis Making 1990;10:163.
57. Knaus WA, Draper EA, Wagner DP, et al: Prognosis in acute organ system failure. Ann Surg 1985;202:685.
58. Denardo SJ, Oye RK, Bellamy PE: Efficacy of intensive care for bone marrow transplant patients with respiratory failure. Crit Care Med 1989;17:4.
59. Murphy DJ, Murray AM, Robinson BE, et al: Outcomes of resuscitation in the elderly. Ann Intern Med 1989;111:199.
60. Jacobs S, Chang RWS, Lee B, et al: An analysis of the utilization of an intensive care unit. Int Care Med 1989;15:511.
61. Rapoport J, Teres D, Lemeshow S, et al: Explaining variability of cost using a severity of illness measure for ICU patients. Med Care 1990;28:338.
62. Murphy DJ, Knaus WA: Outcome prediction in critical care medicine: The role of probability estimates in clinical decision-making and resource allocation. In Lumb PD, Shoemaker WC (eds): Critical Care State of the Art. Eleventh Edition. Fullerton, CA, Society of Critical Care Medicine, 1990, p. 347.
63. Civetta JM, Kirby RR: Prediction and definition of outcome. Adv Anesthesia 1992;9:137.

64. Knaus WA, Wagner DP, Lynn J: Short-term mortality predictions for critically ill hospitalized adults: Science and ethics. Science 1991;254:389.
65. Murphy DJ, Matchar DB: Life-sustaining therapy: A model for appropriate use. JAMA 1990;264:2103.
66. Nelson JB: The role of an intensive care unit in a community hospital. Arch Surg 1985;120:1233.
67. McClish DK, Russo A, Franklin C, et al: Profile of medical ICU vs. ward patients in an acute care hospital. Crit Care Med 1985;13:381.
68. Borlase BC, Baxter JT, Benotti PN, et al: Surgical intensive care resource use in a specialty referral hospital: I. Predictors of early death and cost implications. Surgery 1990;109:687.
69. Kalb PE, Miller DH: Utilization strategies for intensive care units. JAMA 1989;261:2389.
70. Singer DE, Carr PL, Mulley AG, et al: Rationing intensive care—physician responses to a resource shortage. N Engl J Med 1983;309:1155.
71. Strauss MJ, LoGerfo JP, Yeltatzie JA, et al: Rationing of intensive care unit services. JAMA 1986;255:1143.
72. Popovich J: Intermediate care units graded care options. Chest 1991;99: 4.
73. Krieger BP, Ershowsky P, Spivack D: One year's experience with a noninvasively monitored intermediate care unit for pulmonary patients. JAMA 1990;264:1143.
74. Elpern EH, Silver MR, Rosen RL, et al: The noninvasive respiratory care unit: Patterns of use and financial implications. Chest 1991;99:205.
75. Knaus WA, Wagner DP, Zimmerman JE, et al: Variations in mortality and length of stay in intensive care units: Findings from the APACHE III study. Ann Intern Med 1993;118:753–761.
76. Zimmerman JE, Shortell SM, Rousseau DM, et al: Structural and organizational factors associated with variations in intensive care unit performance: Findings from the APACHE III study. Crit Care Med (submitted for publication).
77. Ellwood PM: Outcomes management—a technology of patient experience. N Engl J Med 1988;318:1549.
78. Berwick DM: Continuous improvement as an ideal in health care. N Engl J Med 1989;320:53.
79. Laffel G, Blumenthal D: The case for using industrial quality management science in health care organizations. JAMA 1988;162:809.
80. Kritchevsky SB, Simmons BP: Continuous quality improvement: Concepts and applications for physician care. JAMA 1991;266:1817.
81. Berwick DM, Godfrey AB, Roessner J: Curing Health Care: New Strategies for Quality Improvement. San Francisco, CA, Josey-Bass, 1991.
82. Civetta JM, Hudson-Civetta JA: Maintaining quality of care while reducing the charges in the ICU: 10 ways. Ann Surg 1985;202:254.
83. Marshall MF, Schwenzer KJ, Orsina M, et al: Influence of political power, medical provincialism, and economic incentives on the rationing of surgical intensive care unit beds. Crit Care Med 1992;20:387.
84. Perkins HS, Jonsen AR, Epstein WV: Providers as predictors: Using outcome predictions in intensive care. Crit Care Med 1986;14:105.
85. Task Force on Guidelines Society of Critical Care Medicine: Recommendations for intensive care unit admission and discharge criteria. Crit Care Med 1988;16:807.

86. Truog RD: Triage in the ICU. Hastings Center Report 1992;22:13.
87. Strosberg MA: Intensive care units in the triage mode: An organizational perspective. Hosp Health Services Admin 1991;36:95.
88. Duncan PG: Quality assurance and anesthetic outcome. Adv Anesthesia 1992:121.
89. Albrecht K, Zemke R: Service America. Homewood, IL, Time Warner, 1985.
90. Zemke R, Schaaf D: The Service Edge. New York, NY, NAL Penguin, 1989.
91. Walton M: The Deming Management Method. New York, NY, Putnam, 1986.
92. Crosby PB: Quality is Free: The Art of Hassle-Free Management, New York, NY, NAL Penguin, 1984.
93. Joint Commission for Accreditation of Health Care Organizations: Accreditation Manual for Hospitals. Chicago, IL, 1992.
94. Joint Commission for Accreditation of Health Care Organizations: Accreditation Manual for Hospitals. Chicago, Il, 1993.
95. Berwick DM, Godfrey AB, Roessner J: Curing Health Care New Strategies for Quality Improvement. San Francisco, CA, Josey-Bass, 1991.
96. Lumb PD, Bryan-Brown CW: Complications in Critical Care Medicine. Chicago, IL, Year Book, 1988.
97. Wollschlager CM, Conrad AR, Kahn FA: Common Complications in Critically ill Patients. Disease-a-Month 1988;34:225.
98. Abramson NS, Wald KS, Grenvik ANA, et al: Adverse occurrences in intensive care units. JAMA 1980;244:1582.
99. Wright D, Mackenzie SJ, Buchan I, et al: Critical incidents in the intensive therapy unit. Lancet 1991;338:676.
100. Brennan TA, Localio R, Leape LL, et al: Identification of adverse events occurring during hospitalization. Ann Intern Med 1990;112:221.
101. Sanazaro PJ, Mills DH: A critique of the use of generic screening in quality assessment. JAMA 1992;265:1977.
102. Caplan RA, Posner KL, Cheney FW: Effect of outcome on physician judgements on appropriateness of care. JAMA 1991;265:1957.
103. Goldman RL: The reliability of peer assessments of quality of care. JAMA 1992;267:958.
104. Dubois RW, Rogers WH, Moxley JH, et al: Hospital in-patient mortality: Is it a predictor of quality? N Engl J Med 1987;317:1674.
105. O'Leary DS: Beyond generic occurrence screening. JAMA 1991;265:1993.
106. Dubois RW, Brook RH: Preventable deaths: Who, how often, and why? Ann Intern Med 1988;109:582.
107. Knaus GP: Health Care Risk Management. Los Angeles, CA, National Health publishing, Rand Communications, 1986.
108. Dawson JA, McL Booth FV: Quality Assurance and Risk Management. In Rippe JM, Irwin RS, Alpert JS, et al. (eds): Intensive Care Medicine. Second Edition. Boston, MA, Little-Brown, 1991, p. 1962.
109. Shulman D, Yoel D, Shlomit D, et al: Human errors in an intensive care unit: A pilot study. Crit Care Med 1987;15:371.
110. American Society of Anesthesiologists: Professional Liability and the Anesthesiologist. Park Ridge, IL, American Society of Anesthesiologists, 1987.

Chapter 11

Managing the External Evaluation Process

David R. Massel, B.Sc., M.D.

Caring for patients in an intensive care unit (ICU) is expensive.[1] A disproportionate percentage (perhaps as much as 20%) of total hospital expenditures are consumed by ICU patients.[2] It is estimated that the provision of care in an ICU is approximately 3.8 times more expensive than in a general ward.[3] With the advent of newer and generally expensive technologies, it is anticipated that the cost of providing intensive care will continue to rise.[4]

In our society, life itself is valued above all else and in some instances above quality. Consequently, the prolongation of life (or the postponement of death) has been used as justification for the use of care that is expensive, unproved, or perhaps only marginally, if at all, effective. Moreover, the evidence that intensive care clearly decreases morbidity and mortality is lacking.[5] Therefore, from a societal viewpoint the overall value, *inter alia*, of the ICU remains unclear.

With the costs of health care escalating, pressure is increasingly

From: Sibbald WJ, Massaro T (eds.): The Business of Critical Care: A Textbook for Clinicians Who Manage Special Care Units. © Futura Publishing Co., Inc., Armonk, NY, 1996.

being applied to practitioners by hospital administrators, third party payers, government, and society to provide efficient and quality health care. The consumption of a large percentage of health care resources with unknown, if any, marginal returns in terms of health status begs to question whether intensive care is "shallow slope" or "flat of the curve" medicine.[6] Indeed, in some situations more is not necessarily better and intensive care may do more harm than good.[7] Therefore, it is incumbent among ICU practitioners and researchers to demonstrate, *ceterus paribus*, the added value of intensive care and to rationalize the various components.

The demonstration of efficient care would satisfy this goal. Efficiency has two components: technical and allocative. Technical efficiency is defined as the use of the least health care resources to obtain the desired outcomes. Allocative efficiency would exist if reallocation of health care resources from one type of activity (e.g., the ICU) to another (not necessarily involving the health care sector) could not be undertaken without making one person better off and someone else worse off. This chapter will focus on means of evaluating the technical component of efficiency through the formal assessment of technologies. Allocative efficiency requires a discussion of ethical, moral, philosophical, and political issues beyond the scope of the chapter but discussed elsewhere in this monograph.

This subject area constitutes a massive volume of literature that continues to expand. It would be impossible to be all-inclusive and address each of the individual topic areas in detail. Therefore, this chapter will attempt to serve as an overview and an introduction to the general concepts. An example will be provided so as to enhance the clinical relevance of the discussion.

Clinical Scenario

You are called by the nurses in your large community hospital late one evening and told that a 62-year-old man had been transferred back to the ICU 6 days following an inferior acute myocardial infarction (AMI). Up to that point he had been treated medically with aspirin and thrombolytic therapy without complications. You have difficulty assessing him, especially his central venous pressure, as he is quite a large man and tachypneic. His blood pressure is 80/50 with no obvious pulsus paradoxus. There is evidence of peripheral hypoperfusion and pulmonary crackles to 15 cm above the lung bases. You start initial resuscitative efforts and get things set up to insert a pulmonary artery (PA) catheter.

Just then, two of your colleagues enter the ICU accompanied by the ICU nurse manager. One of the colleagues, the local cynic, recalls an editorial calling for a moratorium on pulmonary catheters as they are associated with, and may cause, an increase in mortality.[8] *The other recalls a subsequent editorial contradicting this point of view.*[9] *The nurse manager is astounded as she has just reviewed the budget and is aware of the cost of this procedure to your unit. She questions how they could be used when there is no consensus as to whether they do more harm than good.*

What is a Technology Assessment?

Technologies can be defined as the techniques, drugs, devices, and procedures used for the prevention, diagnosis, treatment, and rehabilitation of health problems together with the systems through which they are supplied.[10] Assessment is the process that involves problem formulation, study design and methodology, data acquisition, data analysis, and interpretation concerning the properties of these technologies. Optimally, the assessment is comparative but this is not always the case.

In this context, technology assessment encompasses a broad perspective and includes most things in the delivery of health care and not just the "big ticket", highly visible or expensive items. Not all agree with such a broad definition. Donabedian[11] feels that technology assessment should be restricted to passing judgment on the technology itself and that quality assessment should judge the degree to which it is appropriately applied to the provision of health care: "Technology assessment establishes the criteria and standards of efficacious, effective, and efficient care; quality assessment determines the extent to which the criteria and standards have been observed."

In practice, the two forms of assessment are complimentary and at times the distinction between the two becomes blurred.

Technology assessments occur in a stepwise fashion (Table 1).[12,13] First, it will have to be shown that the technology is feasible, that it is producing the desired result in a safe fashion. Second, efficacy will have to be demonstrated (Table 2). Efficacy is related to the economist *ceterus paribus* assumption and refers to the impact of an intervention under ideal circumstances. Technology assessments have progressed beyond the mere examination of technical characteristics such as safety

Table 1
Sequential Steps in the Assessment of Technology

1. Feasibility—is it acceptable and safe?
2. Efficacy—does it work under ideal circumstances?
3. Effectiveness—can it work when applied more widely?
4. Economic evaluation—what are the costs and consequences?

Adapted from Jennet B.[12]

and efficacy. Presently, there is a greater awareness of clinical, societal, and economic outcomes of interest such as effectiveness, appropriateness, quality of life issues, and patient preferences.[13] Therefore, the next step is to test effectiveness, that is whether the intervention does more good than harm to those to whom it is offered. Finally, the economic impact of the technology is addressed, although this stage may be performed concomitantly with assessment of effectiveness.

McKinlay[14] has outlined the seven stages in the career of a medical innovation (Table 3) that is germane to the topic of technology assessment. In his scheme, a true assessment is frequently not undertaken until the technology is "established" as "standard" in terms of a procedure or care. Indeed, at this stage it is no longer an innovation but part of the norm.[14] Moreover, the more advanced the care, the greater the acceptance, the more difficult it will be to undertake a trial to critically assess the technology. In the future, demonstration of effectiveness should be a requisite prior to acceptance and diffusion.

Acceptance of the results of a technology assessment requires a consideration of scientific validity, generalizability, as well as the costs and consequences. Methodological principles as to the quality of medical evidence and economic evaluations are discussed in the following sections. Moreover, acceptance and implementation of technology assessments is only possible if the results are effectively communicated

Table 2
Study Objectives: Efficacy versus Effectiveness

Type of Trial	Synonym	Conditions	Goal	Question
Efficacy	Explanatory	Ideal	Understanding	Can it work?
Effectiveness	Management Pragmatic	Usual	Decision making	Does it work?

Table 3
Seven Stages of a Medical Technology

1. The promising report
2. Professional and organizational adoption
3. Public acceptance and third-party endorsement
4. "Standard procedure" and observational reports
5. The randomized controlled trial
6. Professional denunciation
7. Erosion and discreditation

Adapted from McKinlay JB.[14]

and disseminated to practitioners.[15] Last, the "diffusion" or "creep" of the technology must be continually monitored to ensure appropriate application.[16,17]

Technology assessments themselves have the potential for both good and harm (Table 4).[13,15,18] Nevertheless, as it is clear that it is impossible to do all things for all people, choices on the use of technologies will have to be made. With an increasing awareness of evidence based medicine and the scientific method, it is hoped that the barriers to technology assessment (Table 5) will be broken down and that increasingly efficient and quality care will ensue.[19,20]

Table 4
Potential Benefits and Concerns

Benefits
The provision of quality care
The abandonment of technologies that are of no clinical value
Possibly, the conservation of scarce resources
The priorization of expenditures for health care
The priorization of the distribution and development of technologies
Concerns
Lead to rationing of health care
Potential for inappropriate policy decisions
Formulation of restrictive practice guidelines with erosion of physician autonomy
Limiting reimbursement by third-party payers as a means of cost containment
Stifling research in certain areas

Adapted from Fuchs VR,[13] Winkler JD,[15] and Fineberg HV.[18]

Table 5
Barriers to Technology Assessment

1. The proponent is often given more weight than the scientific evidence
2. Physicians are prone to accepting new technology without critical appraisal
3. Physicians are generally resistant to change
4. Lack of scientific approach in medical education
5. Anecdote-based medicine versus evidence-based medicine

Adapted from Grimes DA.[20]

Quality of the Evidence

"The day is rapidly receding when ex cathedra judgments dominate therapeutics."[21]
Marvin Zelen

There are numerous different methods that can be used to assess technology (Table 6).[22–24] These have been segregated into primary and secondary research designs.[11] The primary designs include the traditional epidemiologic methodologies. The secondary designs have been less frequently applied to the critical care setting.

Table 6
Methods of Assessing Technology

Method	
Primary	
True Experiment	
Randomized controlled trial	√
Subexperimental Methods	
Cohort study with contemporaneous or historical controls	√
Case-control study	√
Case series	√
Secondary	
Meta-analysis	√
Consensus development	√
Decision analysis	√
Cross-sectional surveys and surveillance systems	√
N of 1 trials	
Outcomes research—Observational and administrative database	√
Before-after trials	√
Anecdote	

√ denotes that this method has applications to the critical care setting.

Primary Evidence

The strongest evidence in support of a technology comes from the randomized controlled trial (RCT). Less trust should be placed in the results of studies using subexperimental methodology. This is not only based on the numerous limitations (mostly biases) inherent in these latter studies but also that the results have been shown time and time again to be unreliable when compared to the randomized trial.[22] The biases present in analytical research and strategies to overcome them are discussed in two excellent publications.[25,26]

Sacks[27] has likened the use of randomized and historical controls to a diagnostic test (Table 7). He concludes that historically controlled trials (and by extension, to other weak methodologies) rarely conclude that a technology is ineffective when they are effective (high sensitivity), but that they have a high false positive rate (poor specificity). Therefore, a therapy that does not look favorable after a subexperimental study can generally be discarded. In contrast, RCTs rarely find a therapy effective when it is ineffective (high specificity) but have poor sensitivity in that they find therapies ineffective when in fact they are

Table 7
Clinical Trials and Clinical Errors

		Technology Effective	Technology Not Effective
Conclusion Inferred From Clinical Trial	Technology Effective	Correct a	False Positive Type I Error b
	Technology Not Effective	False Negative Type II Error c	Correct d

a) Randomized controlled trials tend to be specific (d/b + d) but lack sensitivity (a/a + c). Subexperimental methods tend to be more sensitive than specific. Therefore, randomized trials, if positive, tend to rule in a beneficial effect but are prone to producing false negative results. Subexperimental methods, if negative, tend to rule out an effective technology, but are prone to false positive errors.
b) The probability of drawing a false positive conclusion is expressed as the 'p' value. The risk of making a type II error is called 'beta'. The compliment of beta (1-beta) is designed as 'power'. Therefore, power represents the probability that a trial will detect a specified difference and find it to be statistically significant, if such a difference exists.

of benefit. The false negative rate of the RCT is not infrequently a function of sample size and inadequate statistical power.[28]

Sackett[29] has proposed a classification scheme to rank order evidence based on the study methodology. It has been used as a means of linking consensus statement recommendations to the strength of the available evidence.[29] The order of the following discussion corresponds to his scheme.

I. The True Experiment—The Randomized Controlled Trial. It is generally accepted that the randomized controlled trial provides the soundest evidence for demonstrating the value of a technology. The major advantages of the randomization process include: (1) the reduction of biases (both known and unknown) in the assignment of patients to treatment groups; (2) the opportunity for blinding; and (3) the provision of an experimental setting whereby assumptions underlying many statistical tests are approximated. Evidence from randomized trials is strongest when there is a low risk of either a false positive (type I) or false negative (type II) error (Table 7).[29]

Nonetheless, the randomized trial is not a panacea. There are many potential limitations that can threaten the internal and external validity of the study.[30–33] In general these trials are expensive and time consuming. Moreover, it would be impossible to perform an RCT on all interventions, tests, and procedures. In many instances, results cannot be produced fast enough. In some situations ethical, logistic, or economic considerations prohibit the conduct of a randomized trial (Table 8). Finally, generalizability (external validity or applicability) of the results is an issue as, strictly speaking, the results are limited to patients similar

Table 8
Limitations of Randomized Trials

Particular Clinical Circumstances
Multiple therapeutic candidates
Minor changes in therapy
Technology in 'flux' or development
Limited duration—lack of long-term follow-up
Studies of etiologic agents
Co-interventions among critically ill patients
Diagnostic technology

Adapted from Feinstein AR.[30]

to those included in the trial. A description of inclusion and exclusion criteria as well as those patients considered but not included are invaluable in allowing the audience to estimate generalizability. Some of these issues are of particular importance to the critical care setting.

Many technologies are "moving targets" because of technological advances and innovations. As a trial tends to be of a finite duration there runs the risk that the technology will be obsolete, or at least outdated, once the results are available. In some situations the trials are of insufficient duration to provide assurances that long-term adverse consequences will not occur. Some technologies are extremely sophisticated and require considerable expertise and experience. Trials are generally performed in specialized centers by dedicated physicians. Applied in a manner less rigorous than the controlled environs of the trial, the same technology may appear ineffective or even harmful. Finally, the critically ill patient is likely to have numerous therapies and interventions performed. Therefore, it will be important to minimize the confounding effect of co-interventions.

Diagnostic technologies have been less critically appraised than therapeutic technologies (Table 9). In part, this was because of the perception that these studies were too cumbersome or impractical to do. In addition, it was felt that the results would be impractical unless additional aspects of patient management were also evaluated. It is now clear that the same methodological rigour should be applied to diagnostic and therapeutic technologies, including the use of the randomized trial.

Prior to the performance of a randomized trial, the diagnostic tool will have to be assessed for its technologic capability and considered for its possible applications.[34] Currently, most studies on diagnostic

Table 9

Diagnostic Technology: Consideration of Difficulties and Impact

Difficulties	Possible Impact
Technological capability	On treatment plan
Range of possible uses	On the confidence of the health care provider
Diagnostic accuracy and precision	On the confidence of the patient
Observer variability and agreement	On health care costs
	On patient outcomes

Adapted from Guyatt GH et al.[45]

technologies concentrate on test performance characteristics and accuracy. Important considerations are the independent blind comparison against a criterion standard, the selection of a population suitable for study and adequately described to permit assessment of generalizability of the results, the inclusion of a wide spectrum of disease, and the assessment of intra- and interobserver variability.[27]

You consider the possible objectives for hemodynamic monitoring with the PA catheter[35]*:*

1. to assess left and/or right ventricular function pulmonary capillary pressure.
2. to monitor changes in hemodynamic status.
3. to guide treatment with pharmacological and non-pharmacological agents.
4. to provide prognostic information.
5. to assist in making a diagnosis such as right ventricular infarction, mitral regurgitation, or ventricular septal rupture.
6. and ultimately, to improve patient outcomes.

Important prognostic information is available in AMI patients from the results obtained from a PA catheter.[36] It has also been shown that, at times, the clinical evaluation of AMI patients is inaccurate and that the results of hemodynamic monitoring will lead to a change in therapy.[36] Nevertheless, there is also concern about the inaccuracies of the measurements and the lack of knowledge of the PA catheter.[37–44]

The cornerstone of patient management remains an accurate diagnosis but the purpose of a diagnostic test is no longer just to produce a test result. It is anticipated that the test will lead to a series of events resulting in an improved patient outcome.[45] Performance of the test itself is most unlikely to change outcomes. It is also appreciated, however, that the decision to change therapy may not hinge on one test result but on the consideration of many factors.

Between the extremes of patients outcomes and test performance characteristics, the diagnostic technology may have other intermediate impacts on management, provider and patient confidence (for example reduced anxiety and worry, enhanced satisfaction, and limiting disability), and the health care system.[45,46] In many instances these may be suitable enough goals to justify the use of the test in the absence of clear-cut benefit on altering patient outcomes.

Only one truly randomized controlled trial of the PA catheter has been completed to date and it suggested that the PA catheter did not improve prognosis.[47] *The mortality among controls was 9/17 (53%) as compared to 10/16 (63%) among those allocated the PA catheter, a 19%*

relative increase. Nevertheless, you are not sure how conclusive the study was. Only 33 patients were included and the trial was terminated early as funding was not renewed over concern about slow patient recruitment. The treatment that followed the insertion of the catheter was not adequately described. Because of the small study sample important mortality differences (in either direction) may have been missed; the 95% confidence intervals included an 81% relative excess and a 45% relative decrease in mortality with the PA catheter. There was considerable contamination in that 8/17 (47%) of the control patients crossed over to receive a PA catheter. The effect of this on the results is unclear. As Guyatt pointed out, seven of the eight died so they hardly could have done worse had they received the PA catheter.[47] *Nonetheless, perhaps they "crossed over" when the clinical situation was so desperate that no intervention could have made a difference. The major limitation of the study is the generalizability as many eligible patients were excluded due to the physician's impression that it was ethically imperative to insert the catheter. Moreover, only four patients with AMI (3 control, 1 PA catheter) were enrolled, limiting the generalizability of the results to your patient. At best, you feel that the results of this study are inconclusive and you seek other sources of information.*

A second trial was reported but only included post-operative patients. Nevertheless, it did suggest a mortality benefit with the PA catheter when accompanied by a therapeutic protocol.[48]

Subexperimental Methods

II/III. Cohort Study with Contemporaneous or Historical Controls. A cohort can be defined as persons grouped together or a group of persons with a common statistical characteristic. In a cohort study, a group of individuals who have been exposed to a technology are compared to another group who were not exposed and both groups are followed over time for the occurrence of an outcome of interest.[22] Controls can be either historical or contemporaneous. Generally, the studies are performed prospectively although the data can be obtained in a retrospective manner. The major limitation is that the exposure to the technology was not determined by random allocation but through a conscious decision of the physician and patient. Therefore, the groups may not be truly comparable either in important demographic and prognostic variables as well as the exposure to other technologies. Numerous other potential biases can occur including the reasons for selecting patients for the study and the rigour with which the outcome event is sought among unblinded clinicians. In the ICU setting the use of historical, as compared to contemporaneous, controls may lead to greater imbalances between groups because of the ever changing use of technologies and the strength of the evidence may be further reduced.

In a cohort study using historical controls, Rao and colleagues[49] were able to show that preoperative optimization of the hemodynamic status (including the use of a PA catheter) and prompt treatment of an aberration was associated with an improved outcome among patients with prior AMI. Tuman and colleagues[50] were unable to show improved outcomes with the use of the PA catheter among patients undergoing coronary artery bypass surgery in a cohort study using contemporaneous controls. Neither study is helpful in consideration of your patient.

Zion and colleagues[51] performed a cohort study using contemporaneous controls among patients in a registry for a randomized controlled trial of nifedipine versus placebo in patients 7 to 21 days following AMI. Although registry data was collected prospectively, data and outcomes for this ancillary substudy were collected in a retrospective manner. A higher in-hospital mortality was found in those receiving a PA catheter, likely because they were a sicker group of patients. Many important pieces of information were lacking because of the retrospective nature of the data collection; the missing data was not routinely collected as part of the protocol for the RCT. The description of important variables that could influence prognosis of AMI patients was incomplete and no mention was made of therapies that followed insertion of the catheter. Whereas one is not sure that the PA catheter necessarily increased mortality, there is no suggestion that it was beneficial.

IV. Case-Control Study

A somewhat weaker design than the above is the case-control study.[22] Subjects with the outcome of interest are identified and compared to "comparable" control subjects who have not had the exposure to some technology. As such they are relatively easy and cheap to perform especially with large administrative data sets. In addition, they may be the only real alternative method for identifying rare or long-term effects. Nevertheless, these studies are performed retrospectively and subject to numerous biases. Primarily, there is no guarantee that cases and controls will be "comparable" despite the use of techniques such as matching. Moreover, the source population from which the cases and controls are drawn is not always specified or clear. Because of the numerous problems, the results should not generally be trusted.

V. Case Series

This is essentially a collection of case reports or anecdotes although more planning in terms of data collection may have been undertaken.[22,52] Nevertheless, it has major limitations, the most important being the lack of comparison. It cannot control for the power of the placebo effect, the possibility of spontaneous regression of disease, and the inherent biases that may be introduced because of lack of blinding. Therefore, such studies may conclude that a technology can produce the desired effect, but there is no guarantee that it will.[24] Results of these studies may, at best, provide a hypothesis for further study.

Chatterjee and colleagues[53] *described the outcome of 43 AMI patients with severe pump failure who had a PA catheter inserted and were treated with vasodilator therapy. No control group was included. Hemodynamic status was improved on vasodilator therapy. Nevertheless 44% of the patients died in hospital and 24-month survival was only 28%. Whereas the vasodilators used in 1975 are not generally used for these purposes today, the concept of hemodynamically guided therapy is intuitively appealing. The lack of controls is a major limitation.*

Secondary Methods

Other methods for the assessment of technology exist. Apart from meta-analysis, it is unclear what level of evidence these alternate methods should hold. A well conducted meta-analysis with clear-cut results could strengthen the evidence from that of the individual randomized trials.[29]

Meta-Analysis

Meta-analysis is an attitude or way of looking at data analysis applied to quantitative summaries of individual experiments.[54–59] The major difference with overviews based on best evidence synthesis is that it places more evidence on statistics. It must be stated that a meta-analysis is not a substitute for a well designed randomized trial.[54] It can be used to increase the power absent from individual trials (particularly in subgroups), to possibly resolve uncertainty, to improve the estimate of effect size, and to pose new questions.

Like a randomized trial a meta-analysis requires a rigorous and well defined methodology. It is subject to problems of publication bias, poor quality studies, and heterogeneity of patients or treatments (comparing apples and oranges) among others.

As Wittes[56] states: "There is, however, no reason to assume that the pooling of RCTs can bail us out of the fundamental uncertainty that will accompany any situation where excellent clinical trials, the cornerstone of therapy evaluation, do not exist."

Nonetheless, despite their limitations, high-quality overviews or meta-analyses will continue to serve a useful role in medicine.

With only two trials of the PA catheter, there would be no value in a meta-analysis. Moreover, as the studies involved two completely distinct groups of patients, it is likely that they should not be pooled (mixing apples and oranges).

Decision Analysis

Decision analysis is a formal, inherently quantitative, method of decision making that uses stepwise analysis of the component decisions in solving a problem.[60–62] It involves breaking the problem into smaller, manageable parts and combining them in a logical way. It is of most value when there is incomplete information but a decision must be made. Whereas it has many uses, it is most applicable in the clinical arena to help create policy, guidelines, protocols, and algorithms applied to a group of patients with a specific condition. Less frequently, it is applied to individual patients.

It involves the construction of a decision tree that includes choices and the quantitative estimates of chance and outcomes (utilities). These are then combined to form an estimate of the expected value of each course of action, preference being given to the highest value. The initial assumptions can be varied through a range of expected values to see to what extent the optimum strategy is dependent on the initial assumptions in a technique called sensitivity analysis.

The major limitation is that disease processes are much more complex than can be developed in such models. This may be particularly true of the critically ill population. In addition, many analyses are restricted to a narrow scope of patients limiting the generalizability of the results. Nonetheless, decision analysis holds promise in the critical care setting both as a decision tool and as a means of focusing research to particular aspects of a problem.

The use of the PA catheter in the setting of complicated AMI could be assessed with decision analysis. The decision tree would be very complex but perhaps not as complex as the myriad problems facing these patients. Due to the paucity of evidence from randomized trials supporting various treatment options in these patients, the numerous assumptions would make the validity of the results somewhat tentative.

Consensus Development

The purpose of consensus development process is to develop guidelines that could be used to bring clinical practice in line with research evidence.[63] A number of formats exist and include the traditional committee, the National Institute of Health model (or variations thereof), the Delphi technique, and the Nominal Group Process.[64–69]

In general, the process involves the assembly of an expert panel to answer a specific question. In some variations public input is also sought. A large body of medical literature is collated and translated into a statement that is then released.

Shortcomings of the process are recognized and include the problem of excessive compromise (rather than consensus) to the detriment of the research evidence and the lack of impact on clinical practice.[63] As they tend to be endorsed by experts in the field, consensus statements have the potential to change practice. Readers can critically appraise the quality of the recommendations if there is an explicit link with the strength of the medical evidence.[70]

You have recently read statements concerning the use of hemodynamic monitoring from two authoritative bodies.[36,71,72] *The first concerned the issue of clinical competence as well as an outline of indications, contraindications, and complications.*[71] *They suggest that competence may be acquired after inserting 25 catheters and may be maintained by as few as 12 per year. The statements are opinion based and do not appear to be linked to any particular scientific evidence.*

The second involved more formal consensus building tactics such as the Nominal Group process and a modification of the Delphi technique.[72] It dealt only with the technical aspects of hemodynamic monitoring.

The third was entitled "Hemodynamic monitoring: A technology assessment".[36] A formal consensual process was used. They concluded that hemodynamic monitoring " . . . apparently provides diagnostic information in cases of acute myocardial infarction . . . However, much of the information can be gained by non-invasive means" and furthermore " . . . (hemodynamic monitoring) provides prognostic information in cases of acute myocardial infarction . . . and has been shown in some nonrandomized trials to lower death rates in certain patient groups." The latter were not clearly specified. They go on to say: "The therapeutic utility of hemodynamic monitoring is still unproven . . . " It was recommended that the use of the PA catheter be restricted to secondary and tertiary care centers and that further research be directed at the use of hemodynamic monitoring and patient prognosis.

Before-After Trials

There are perceived difficulties in performing RCTs on diagnostic technologies. An alternative methodology is the before-after trial where judgments concerning changes in patient management (further diagnostic or therapeutic plans) are assessed when before and after they are provided with the results of a diagnostic test.[73] The major advantages are that it is less expensive and logistically difficult as compared to the RCT. It may be particularly appealing to clinicians as all patients are tested with the new technology.

Before-after studies are restricted to added tests once the conventional work-up is complete, not substitutes. The latter would have to be compared with an RCT. Subconscious bias, either for or against the test, may still influence the results of the study although the direction and magnitude are difficult to predict. Moreover, what physicians say they will do and what they actually do may, in terms of treatment plan, not coincide particularly where the treatment is associated with considerable patient risk.[73] Similar to the RCT of a diagnostic test, the results will only be of value if it leads to a therapeutic change that improves patient outcomes.

As with other weaker study designs, results tend to be biased in favor of the new technology. Therefore, before-after trials are not an adequate substitute where an RCT can be undertaken and may have to be confirmed with an RCT. Nevertheless, this design may be particularly attractive to the ICU.

Outcomes Research—Observational and Administrative Databases

"Observational evidence is clearly better than opinion, but it is thoroughly unsatisfactory. All research on the effectiveness of therapy was in this unfortunate state until the early 1950s."[74]

Archibald Cochran

These types of studies are the foundation of outcomes research, which attempt to forge a link between outcomes and the structure, process, and costs of health care.[75–77] It has been likened to a "natural experiment" that occurs through the observed variation in practice patterns.

Observational databases entail the prospective collection of a structured data set that specifically describes baseline patient characteristics, treatment, and outcomes.[78–80] The major advantage to these studies is that it can assess a wider scope including a large number of patients as well as health care providers in various clinical settings. Not only can the number of patients be large but the spectrum or mix of patients is larger than that of a randomized clinical trial. This heterogeneity would enhance the generalizability of the results. The studies are continued longitudinally so that time dependent changes in the technology can be ascertained or so that temporal changes in case-mix may be assessed.

The major problem with databases is that physicians and patients have chosen a specific therapy for some reason, introducing a source of bias that is difficult, if not impossible, to control. Whereas statistical adjustments of differences in baseline prognostic variables can be undertaken, the treatment decision may not have been made based on these known factors. It is widely held that the retrospective adjustment for known prognostic factors cannot guarantee the elimination of bias. In addition, the database will only be as good as the data collected. Therefore, considerable effort is required to define the collection systems, to establish methods of standardization to ensure consistency, and to select the appropriate outcome measures as a means of ensuring accurate and complete data. Recently, a method of applying many of the principles of the RCT to enhance the quality of observational studies.[81] As it has only been applied in one setting, further research in this area is required.

This technique has been expanded to the use of databases that are already assembled such as administrative data sets.[75] Consequently, these studies tend to be relatively cheap to perform. It has all the limitations of other database methodologies. The data may be prone to greater inaccuracy as its collection is not structured for the purposes of answering many research questions. In general, there should be an a priori hypothesis to attempt to control for the problems of multiple hypothesis and multiple statistical testing.

"While databases can suggest problems and offer answers, they cannot prove them; database analyses must be followed by trials."[80]

The Worster Heart Attack Study is a community based study examining the trends in the mortality rates of acute myocardial infarction in a geographically defined area. Gore and colleagues[82] assessed the association of the PA catheter and mortality. The study was retrospective with all the inherent limitations. Complications were obtained by abstracting information from charts leaving some question as to their accuracy. The reason for the selection of patients for a PA catheter were not specified nor were the subsequent treatment plans.

Over the course of the study (1975–1984) there was a statistically significant increase in mortality with the use of the PA catheter. This was true for patients with congestive heart failure and hypotension. There was a small statistically insignificant benefit to the use of the PA catheter in patients with cardiogenic shock. It was clear that patients who received a PA catheter were more seriously ill than those who did not. Multivariate analysis to adjust for "several" potentially confounding variables failed to change their conclusions. Of course, such retrospective statistical adjustment will only correct for important variables that were measured, not for those that were not measured (a problem with retrospective studies) and cannot adjust for those variables that are not known (the advantage of randomization). Misclassification of complications (heart failure, hypotension, and cardiogenic shock) is also a concern when data is reviewed retrospectively and abstracted from charts. It is of interest that there was a slight mortality benefit (6%) in patients with cardiogenic shock; the definition of which may be less open to question as compared to heart failure, which required the presence of a third heart sound. Moreover, with only 231 patients in shock, this subgroup analysis lacked statistical power and a relative mortality benefit of as much as 20% may have been missed.

(Along the same line a small mortality excess cannot be excluded either.) If such a mortality benefit was proved, this would be a very effective strategy corresponding to the treatment of six or seven patients with cardiogenic shock to save one life.[83] While you are concerned about the results of the study you feel your patient is in cardiogenic shock, a group where it is less clear that the use of the PA catheter is associated with harm but it is clear that the mortality remains very high.

Surveys—Cross-Sectional and Surveillance Systems

Cross-sectional surveys capture a "snap shot" of a particular area of interest. It can take on the guise of a longitudinal study if respondents are contacted on more than one occasion. Its major advantages are the low cost and the prompt answers to questions. Inference and generalizability of the results are tentative depending upon the representativeness of the sample survey and how it was assembled.

Surveillance is a form of data collection best exemplified by the post marketing drug surveille, primarily relying on reports from a large number of physicians. Given the breadth of the database, it is possible to capture information on rare events but as with the case series, the magnitude of the risk cannot be estimated as the size of the numerator is not known.

As with other non-experimental methods, it is limited by the numerous biases inherent in observational studies. Both methods are applicable to critical care technology. Nevertheless, they are both best at identifying areas for further investigation.

N of 1 Trials

This is analogous to the RCT but applied to one subject.[84] Generally, the subject systematically undergoes a series of pairs of treatment periods; the order assigned by random allocation. The patient receives active treatment during one pair and no treatment, placebo, or alternate therapy in the other. The trial is continued until the effectiveness is proved or disproved. A suitable outcome measure is assessed at the end of each study period. The overall objective is to prove or disprove the effectiveness of treatment in that individual subject. Blinding can be used to enhance the validity of the study. Unfortunately, such trials are limited to conditions that are relatively stable in terms of disease activity and are not suitable for surgical trials or where the disease is self-limiting. Although it has been suggested that this type of trial may be applicable to some critically ill patients, it is probable that the severity of illness and the unstable nature of the patient's clinical course render the N of 1 trial unsuitable for the majority.[23]

The concern over the hemodynamic instability of a patient in cardiogenic shock makes the performance of an N of 1 trial impossible.

Anecdote

The anecdote is no more than a detailed observation of a clinical event. The major advantage is the low cost and that it can be applied to any subject matter. It can be valuable in identifying late or rare manifestations of a technology. Nonetheless, it is seriously limited because of incompleteness of data collection, nonstandard observations, and the fact that it is a numerator in search of a denominator. Most importantly, they are subject to recall bias, that is it stands out in our minds for a particular reason. It is best left as a method of generating hypotheses for further study.

You are aware of the large number of case reports recounting the numerous potential complications related to the insertion of the PA catheter.

Is it Something that Society Can or Should Pay For?

If the technology is found to be either efficacious or effective the economic impact should be addressed unless there is clear evidence that it is both more effective and less costly, an extremely rare combination. As Evans[85] logically points out, the demonstration of efficacy is a prerequisite: "Projects which do not work are not worth doing at any (positive) price . . . there is no point in the economic evaluation of a project for which efficacy has not been established . . . "

Economic evaluation is the comparative analysis of alternate courses of action in terms of both their costs and consequences.[86] They

Table 10

What Constitutes "Cost Effective" in Technology Assessment

No

Cost saving
Effective

Yes, but too restrictive

Cost saving, with an equal (or better health outcome

Yes

Having an additional benefit worth the additional cost, including:

a) less costly and at least as effective
b) more effective and more costly, its additional benefit worth its additional cost
c) less costly and less effective, the added benefit of the rival strategy not worth the extra cost

Adapted from Doubilet P et al.[90]

provide a means for assisting decision making when choices have to be made. Interested readers are referred to articles by the Department of Epidemiology and Biostatistics at McMaster University and Drummond and Davies for discussions on understanding economic evaluations and the methodological issues for conducting an economic analysis alongside a clinical trial.[86–88] Drummond[89] has extended these concepts to the economic evaluation of medical technologies.

Although the phrase "cost effective" is used in many different ways (Table 10), the definition that best describes its meaning is: "whether the additional benefit is worth the additional cost".[90] Other definitions slightly miss the mark. Effectiveness alone is an insufficient criterion as it does not include consideration of cost. Cost saving is too stringent and would exclude most technologies. Rather than cost saving, the issue remains whether the extra cost is acceptable.

As described by Stoddard and Drummond,[86] such analyses take the form of partial or full evaluations. The essential difference is that full evaluations are a comparison of two or more alternatives where both costs and consequences are examined. The spectrum of costs is dictated by the perspective of the analysis. In general, the main categories of costs include: health services costs; costs borne by patients and their families; and external costs borne by the rest of society.[91,92] It is important to make the distinction between average and marginal (or incremental) costs. The latter refers to the change in total costs for a change at the margin.

Partial Evaluations

These are purely descriptive.[86] They provide a description of the costs and/or consequences of alternate strategies but not a direct comparison. Alternatively, they provide a comparison of alternate strategies, but not the costs and/or consequences. Being descriptive they provide insufficient evidence on efficiency.

Full Economic Evaluations

There are four main forms of full evaluations (Table 11): cost minimization, cost benefit, cost effectiveness, and cost utility.[86] Relevant costs are identified and measured in similar ways in all analyses. It is the handling of the consequences or clinical outcomes that determines the type of analysis.

In a cost minimization analysis evaluations are performed only in terms of the competing costs as the effectiveness of competing programs has been shown, preferably with a randomized trial, to be equivalent.[92] Indeed, proof of equivalence is at times problematic and the major limitation of this form of analysis. In this scenario the least costly option is preferred.

In a cost benefit analysis, monetary value is placed on both the costs and the consequences.[93] Results are expressed as the net benefit or loss of one program over another. The major limitation is the valuation of clinical outcome events in monetary terms. Techniques are available to estimate this and are based on the value people attach to certain health outcomes.

A cost effectiveness analysis is appropriate when the consequences

Table 11
Types of Economic Evaluations

Approach	Assessment of Consequences
Cost-minimization	None, outcomes assumed, or shown to be equivalent
Cost-benefit	Money
Cost-effectiveness	Natural units, for example life years gained, mmol/L reduction in cholesterol
Cost-utility	Utility measures, for example healthy days, quality adjusted life years, healthy years equivalents

can be measured in natural or biological units.[86] They are then expressed as cost per unit of outcome. A common measure is cost per year of life. Nonetheless, as relatively few technologies impact on mortality the outcome of interest can be any intermediate outcome measure. Different technologies can be compared if the units of measure are the same. A specific form of cost effectiveness analysis incorporates the subjective level of well being in different health states, termed utility. Outcome is expressed as a single measure that captures both quantity and quality of life such as the quality adjusted life year (QALY) although other measures exist.[94]

Whereas a definition for cost effective can be agreed upon, what is considered to be cost effective (in units of money, or units of money per some health outcome) cannot. Frequently, interventions are ranked in a league table based on their estimated cost effectiveness ratios. Mason and colleagues[95] provide a discussion of the many pitfalls with this sort of ordering. Laupacis and colleagues[96] have advocated the grading of recommendations for the adoption and appropriate utilization of technologies based on strength of the evidence (methodological rigor of the study) and arbitrary cost utility ratios in dollars per QALY. Others have pointed out the numerous problems with this approach.[97,98] Consequently, to the present there is no definitive answer to: When is a technology cost effective? More simply, the results of a technology assessment can be viewed as a trade-off between costs and benefits (Table 12). It is along the diagonal where the tough decisions have to be made. Ultimately, the decision to adopt a technology will be based not only on issues of cost effectiveness but on political and ethical considerations as well.

In the absence of definitive data supporting the efficacy of a therapeutic strategy involving the insertion of the PA catheter there is no

Table 12
Potential Results of a Technology Assessment

		Costs		
		Increase	No Change	Decrease
Benefits	Increase	Trade-off	Good	Ideal
	No Change	Bad	Trade-off	Good
	Decrease	Terrible	Bad	Trade-off

need for a formal economic evaluation. Partial evaluations suggest that the PA catheter may cost as much as US$ 2 billion per year.[99]

Putting It All Together

The basic assumption underlying the assessment of any technology is that it will improve the health of a population.[100] For this to happen a critical chain of events must occur (Table 13).[100]

Foremost, a result or conclusion must be reached that has the potential to change the use of the technology. This requires high quality study methodology and is the role of the new technology assessment.[13]

A comprehensive approach to the clinical and economic evaluation of health care technologies is provided by Guyatt and colleagues.[101] A simpler approach outlining questions that may be asked in evaluating a technology is provided in Table 14. First, there is the consideration as to whether the play of chance can be eliminated as an explanation of the results. If the results are "statistically significant", the strength of the study methodology and the possibility of bias should be considered. Different tactics are required to assess various types of technology and questions regarding the validity of therapeutic and diagnostic studies are provided in the articles by Guyatt and colleagues and by Sibbald and Inman.[23,101] If the results are "not statistically significant" then further additional explanations should be considered. Was the technology applied correctly and to the right type of patients? Could other influences such as confounding, co-intervention, or contamination account for the results (Table 15)? Was the study too small (that is, lacking in statistical power) to exclude the possibility of a clinically important treatment effect?[28,102,103] If the study was too small, should it be consid-

Table 13
Technology Assessment: Altering Outcomes
Critical Chain of Events

1. A result or conclusion must be produced that will change the use of a technology
2. Some practitioners must change their use of the technology
3. A change must occur in the proportion of potential candidates who actually receive the technology
4. The change in the use of the technology must lead to changes in outcomes

Adapted from Eddy D.[100]

Table 14

Possible Steps in Evaluating A Technology Assessment

1. Has chance been eliminated as an explanation of the results?
   a) If yes ($P < 0.05$), consider:
      Was the study based on strong methodology?
      Could any biases in design or analysis account for the results?
   b) If no (P = not significant), consider:
      Was the study based on strong methodology?
      Could confounding, contamination or co-intervention account for the results?
      Was the intervention applied appropriately to the right type of patient?
      Could other biases account for the results?
      Was the study large (powerful) enough to exclude a clinically important difference?
2. Was the observed effect, if any, important?
   a) If yes, consider:
      Was both statistical and clinical importance considered?
      Were all clinically relevant outcomes assessed?
   b) If no, consider:
      Was both statistical and clinical importance considered?
      Were all clinically relevant outcomes assessed?
      Were the results considered in both relative and absolute terms?
3. Are the results potentially applicable to my patients and clinical setting?
   a) If yes, consider:
      Is it feasible?
      Is it practical?
   b) If no, consider:
      Why are my patients and practice so different that it would not be applicable?
4. Have both the costs and consequences been considered?
   a) If yes, consider:
      Was the methodology sound?
         If yes, is the additional benefit worth the additional cost?
         If no, was the methodology poor enough to render the results questionable?
   b) If no, consider:
      Is the technology both more effective and less expensive than the alternative?
         If yes, consider adoption of the new technology
         If no, should not an economic evaluation be performed?

Table 15
When Considering a Negative or Inconclusive Technology Assessment: The Three Cs

Confounding	An extraneous variable that wholly or partially accounts for the apparent effect or masks the true association. Prevent with random allocation of subjects. To be of importance, a confounder should be: 1) extraneous to the question posed 2) associated with exposure but not as a consequence of exposure 3) unequally distributed among exposed (treated) and unexposed (controls)
Contamination	Trials are most efficient when if all experimental and no controls receive the 'test' therapy. If controls receive it, this may systematically reduce any differences in outcomes.
Co-intervention	The performance of additional therapeutic procedures upon the experimental or control group. Prevent with 'blinding', if possible.

ered inconclusive and what was the chance of detecting a clinically important difference?[103]

Second, for the result to change clinical practice, the effect must be clinically meaningful and all clinically relevant outcomes must be considered. If the result does not appear important, they should be considered in other manners of presentation (relative or absolute risk reduction, number needed to treat)[82] and the relation of therapeutic efforts to clinical yield compared to similar technologies.[104–107]

Third, to be applicable in your setting the technology must be feasible and practical. Finally, both the costs and consequences of the technology assessment must be considered. Interested readers are referred to the excellent discussions of the methodological principles of economic evaluations that may be applied to technology assessments.[86–89,101]

Even in the face of the contradictory evidence about the use of the PA catheter a decision must be made. A non-invasive assessment of cardiac function is not available at the late hour. You feel that you do not want to miss a potentially treatable cause of cardiogenic shock such as one of the mechanical complications of AMI. The PA catheter is inserted without incident. The measured hemodynamics support your clinical impression of cardiogenic shock. More importantly, a significant oxygen step-up from the proximal to the distal port is found to be consistent with a large left-to-right shunt; you diagnose a rupture of the intraventricular septum. This sets in motion a series of steps that culminate in emergency cardiac surgery. Prior to surgery the information obtained from the PA catheter is found to be useful in optimizing various hemodynamic parameters using a combination of an intra-aortic balloon pump, vasodilators, and inotropic agents. The patient undergoes surgery and survives.

Can Technology Assessments Lead to Better Patient Outcomes?

Up to the present the evidence proving that technology assessments improve patient outcomes is lacking. Indeed, it is unlikely anyone will perform a trial comparing the new technology assessment with the traditional approach.[13] Nevertheless, the rationale behind these new assessments is strong and rooted in the new paradigm of evidence based medicine and justifies their use.[19] They will provide a basis for making more informed choices among alternative uses of resources than would otherwise be possible.[18] If results are based on strong scientific methodology: " . . . it is very unlikely that deterioration in care results from the evidence based approach . . . "[19]

In the absence of long-term data on the impact of technology assessments per se, intermediate measures such as the demonstration of effectiveness, cost effectiveness, and that the care delivered was appropriate, are regarded as suitable surrogates. The first two were addressed earlier in this chapter. Up to the present, there is no universally accepted scientific definition for appropriateness.[33] Jennet[12] has suggested a five point classification for the inappropriate use of technology (Table 16). The first two, unnecessary and unsuccessful, are the most absolute. All have relevance in the critical care setting. The use of unnecessary and unsafe technologies should be avoided. The unsuccessful inappropriateness is not uncommon in the ICU given the frequently far advanced clinical deterioration of a patient's condition, at times beyond the capacity to respond to many interventions. Similarly, the advances in medical technologies in the ICU occasionally lead to the prolongation of lives not worth living.[12] Finally, given the high costs of providing intensive care, it remains to be shown that it is technically and allocatively efficient.

There are many factors that affect the impact of technology assessments and that are perceived as reasons for non-acceptance (Table 17).[108] For an assessment to have an impact it is best if it is performed

Table 16
Technologies—Inappropriate Uses
The Five Uns

Unnecessary	where the patient's condition is not serious enough to justify the use of the technology
Unsuccessful	where the patient's condition is too advanced to respond to the intervention
Unkind	where life of poor quality is prolonged
Unsafe	where the expected complications outweigh the anticipated benefits
Unwise	where the use of the technology diverts resources from other health care activities (or other activities outside the health care sector) that would bring more benefits.

Adapted from Jennet B.[12]

early in the life cycle of the technology, based on high-quality evidence, endorsed by a reputable organization, and disseminated widely. With the rapid expansion of biomedical knowledge and the arrival of new technologies it is difficult for practitioners to assimilate the data and appropriately modify clinical practice.[109] Practice guidelines have been suggested as a means of optimizing medical practice based on the best existing data and focused on the improvement of the quality of care. Importantly, practice guidelines should not be regarded as equivalent to standards of quality or policies (Table 18).[109]

To be of value, guidelines must be current, comprehensive, specific, sensible, and must address important clinical questions.[109–111] Yet they must not be too restrictive as clinical judgment is essential in the management of an individual. Finally, the guidelines must be reevaluated in light of new information.

Table 17
Technology Assessments

Factors Affecting Impact	Reasons for Non-acceptance
Timing in life-cycle of the technology	Preconceived ideas
Quality of the evidence	Poor quality of error prone assessment
Constituency supporting the assessment	Inconsistent study results
Method of dissemination	Vested interest

Adapted from Gutzwiller F.[107]

Table 18
Guidelines, Standards, and Policies

Practice guidelines	Systematically developed statements to assist practitioner and patient decisions about appropriate health care for specific clinical circumstances
Standards of quality	Authoritative statements of: 1) minimal levels of acceptable performance or results 2) excellent levels of performance or results 3) the range of acceptable performance
Clinical policy	A definite course or method of action selected from among alternatives and in light of given conditions to guide and determine present and future decisions

Adapted from ref. 109

In general, the publication of guidelines is insufficient to influence the process of care unless introduced in the context of rigorous evaluations.[112–116] This is because there are numerous educational, administrative, patient centered, and economic barriers to their implementation. Other strategies to change patterns of clinical practice have resulted in inconsistent findings and are the focus of ongoing research.[115,116] Presently, no one method has been shown to be superior but a multifactorial intervention increases the likelihood of success.[116]

Later you reflect on the use of the PA catheter. You have the "impression" that hemodynamic monitoring was of value in this particular instance. You suspect that the local cynic will say that the diagnosis might have been made non-invasively with echocardiography. Unfortunately, it was not readily available at the moment when the patient was seriously ill. Moreover, you "know" that an echocardiogram would not have been of much help in attempting to stabilize the patient in preparation for definitive surgery. Yet, you find it curious that an expensive diagnostic technology that has been available for more than 20 years is somewhere between level 4 and level 6 in McKinlay's scheme.[14] *The widely disparate views on the PA catheter evoke a call for a moratorium on its use among some despite the fact that many physicians feel it is ethically impossible to withhold its use in many clinical situations.*[8,47]

Summary

Demonstrating that increasing the resources devoted to the critical care setting results in acceptable marginal returns or benefits will only be possible through the systematic assessment of the net costs and consequences of the technologies used. In the current resource constrained environment, this on-going process should improve our ability to provide efficient and quality health care.

References

1. Technology Subcommittee of the Working Group on Critical Care, Ontario Ministry of Health: The assessment of technology in Ontario's critical care system. Can Med Assoc J 1991;144:1613.
2. Grevnik A: The ICU in the modern hospital. In Miranda DR, Langrehr D (eds): The ICU—A Cost Benefit Analysis. Amsterdam, Excerpta Medica, 1986, p. 27.
3. Wagner DP, Wineland TD, Knaus WA: The hidden costs of treating severely ill patients: Charges and resource consumption in an intensive care unit. Health Care Financ Rev 1983;5:81.
4. Moloney TW, Rogers DE: Medical technology—A different view of the contentious debate over costs. N Engl J Med 1979;301:1413.
5. Miranda DR: Critically examining intensive care. Int J Technol Assess Health Care 1992;8:444.
6. Enthoven AS: Health Plan: The Only Practical Solution to the Soaring Cost of Medical Care. Reading, MA, Addison-Wesley, 1980.
7. Illich I: Medical Nemesis: The Expropriation of Health. Toronto, McClelland and Stewart, 1985.
8. Robin ED: Death by pulmonary artery flow-directed catheter? Chest 1987; 92:727.
9. Sibbald WJ, Sprung CL: The pulmonary artery catheter. The debate continues. Chest 1988;94:899.
10. Battista RN: Innovation and diffusion of health-related technologies: A conceptual framework. Int J Technol Assess Health Care 1989;5:227.
11. Donabedian A: The assessment of technology and quality. Int J Technol Assess Health Care 1988;4:487.
12. Jennet B: Assessment of clinical technology. Importance for provision and use. Int J Technol Assess Health Care 1988;4:435.
13. Fuchs VR, Garber AM: The new technology assessment. N Engl J Med 1990;323:673.
14. McKinlay JB: From "Promising Report" to "Standard Procedure": Seven stages of a medical innovation. Milbank Memorial Fund Quarterly 1981; 59:374.
15. Winkler JD, Lohr KN, Brook RH: Persuasive communication and medical technology assessment. Arch Intern Med 1985;145:314.
16. Anderson GM, Lomas J: Monitoring the diffusion of a technology: Coronary artery bypass surgery in Ontario. Am J Public Health 1988;78:251.
17. Banta HD, Thacker SB: The case for reassessment of health care technology. Once is not enough. JAMA 1990;264:235.
18. Fineberg HV, Hiatt HH: Evaluation of medical practices: The case for technology assessment. N Engl J Med 1979;301:1086.

19. Evidence based Medicine Working Group: Evidence based medicine. A new approach to teaching the practice of medicine. JAMA 1992;268:2420.
20. Grimes DA: Technology follies. The uncritical acceptance of medical innovation. JAMA 1993;269:3030.
21. Zelen M: A new design for randomized clinical trials. N Engl J Med 1979; 300:1242.
22. Sackett DL, Haynes RB, Tugwell P: Clinical Epidemiology. A Basic Science of Clinical Medicine. First Edition. Boston, Little Brown and Company, 1985.
23. Sibbald WJ, Inman KJ: Problems in assessing the technology of critical care medicine. Int J Technol Assess Health Care 1992;8:419.
24. Jaeschke J, Sackett DL: Research methods for obtaining primary evidence. Int J Technol Assess Health Care 1989;5:503.
25. Sackett DL. Bias in analytical research. J Chronic Dis 1979;32:51.
26. Sitthi-amorn C, Poshyachinda V: Bias. Lancet 1993;342:286.
27. Sacks HS, Chalmers TC, Smith H Jr: Sensitivity and specificity of clinical trials. Randomized v historical controls. Arch Intern Med 1983;143:753.
28. Freiman JA, Chalmers TC, Smith H, et al: The importance of beta, the type II error and sample size in the design and interpretation of the randomized controlled trial. N Engl J Med 1978;299:690.
29. Cook DJ, Guyatt GH, Laupacis A, et al: Rules of evidence and clinical recommendations on the use of antithrombotic agents. Chest 1992; 102(Suppl):305S.
30. Feinstein AR: An additional basic science for clinical medicine: II. The limitations of the randomized trial. Ann Intern Med 1983;99:544.
31. Horwitz RI: Complexity and contradiction in clinical trial research. Am J Med 1987;82:498.
32. Rabeneck L, Viscoli CM, Horwitz RI: Problems in the conduct and analysis of randomized clinical trials. Are we getting the right answers to the wrong questions. Arch Intern Med 1992;152:507.
33. Diamond GA, Denton TA: Alternative perspectives on the biased foundations of medical technology assessment. Ann Intern Med 1993;118:455.
34. Department of Clinical Epidemiology and Biostatistics, McMaster University Health Sciences Centre: How to read clinical journals: II. To learn about a diagnostic test. Can Med Assoc J 1981;124:703.
35. Voyce SJ, Goldberg RJ, Gore JM: Evaluation of right-heart catheterization: Where do we go from here? J Intens Care Med 1991;6:98.
36. Technology Subcommittee of the Working Group on Critical Care, Ontario Ministry of Health: Hemodynamic monitoring: A technology assessment. Can Med Assoc J 1991;145:114.
37. Steingrub JS, Celoria G, Vickers-Lahti M, et al: Therapeutic impact of pulmonary artery catheterization in a medical/surgical ICU. Chest 1991; 99:1451.
38. Komina KH, Schenk DA, LaVeau P, et al: Interobserver variability in the interpretation of pulmonary artery catheter pressure tracings. Chest 1991; 100:1647.
39. Tuchschmidt J, Sharma OP: Impact of hemodynamic monitoring in a medical intensive care unit. Crit Care Med 1987;15:840.
40. Fein AM, Goldberg SK, Walkenstein MD, et al: Is pulmonary artery catheterization necessary for the diagnosis of pulmonary edema? Am Rev Respir Dis 1984;129:1006.

41. Bayliss J, Norell M, Ryan A, et al: Bedside haemodynamic monitoring: Experience in a general hospital. Br Med J 1983;287:187.
42. Morris AH, Chapman RH, Gardner RM: Frequency of wedge pressure errors in the ICU. Crit Care Med 1985;13:705.
43. Iberti TJ, Fischer EP, Leibowitz AB, et al: A multicenter study of physicians' knowledge of the pulmonary artery catheter. JAMA 1990;264:2928.
44. Connors AF Jr, Dawson NV, McCaffree R, et al: Assessing hemodynamic status in critically ill patients: Do physicians use clinical information optimally? J Crit Care 1987;2:174.
45. Guyatt GH, Tugwell PX, Feeny DH, et al: A framework for clinical evaluation of diagnostic technologies. Can Med Assoc J 1986;134:587.
46. Sox HC Jr, Margulies I, Sox CH: Psychologically mediated effects of diagnostic tests. Ann Intern Med 1981;95:680.
47. Guyatt G, the Ontario Intensive Care Study Group: A randomized control trial of right-heart catheterization in critically ill patients. J Intens Care Med 1991;6:91.
48. Shoemaker WC, Appel PL, Waxman K, et al: Clinical trial of survivors' cardiorespiratory patterns as therapeutic goals in critically ill postoperative patients. Crit Care Med 1982;10:398.
49. Rao TLK, Jacobs KH, El-Etr AA: Reinfarction following anesthesia in patients with myocardial infarction. Anesthesiology 1983;59:499.
50. Tuman KJ, McCarthy RJ, Spiess BD, et al: Effect of pulmonary artery catheterization on outcome in patients undergoing coronary artery surgery. Anesthesiology 1989;70:199.
51. Zion MM, Balkin J, Rosenmann D,, et al: Use of pulmonary artery catheters in patients with acute myocardial infarction. Chest 1990;98:1331.
52. Bailar JC, Louis TA, Lavori PW, et al: Studies without internal controls. N Engl J Med 1984;311:156.
53. Chatterjee K, Swan HJC, Kaushik VS, et al: Effects of vasodilator therapy for severe pump failure in acute myocardial infarction on short-term and late prognosis. Circulation 1976;53:797.
54. Bulpitt CJ: Meta-analysis. Lancet 1988$_{\infty}$:93.
55. L'Abbé KA, Detsky AS, O'Rourke K: Meta-analysis in clinical research. Ann Intern Med 1987;107:224–233.
56. Wittes RE: Problems in the medical interpretation of overviews. Stat Med 1987;6:269.
57. Sacks HS, Berrier J, Reitman D, et al: Meta-analysis of randomized controlled trials. N Engl J Med 1987;316:450.
58. Bergarg ZB, Horwitz RI: Resolving conflicting clinical trials: Guidelines for meta-analysis. J Clin Epidemiol 1988;41:503.
59. Detsky AS, Naylor CD, O'Rourke K, et al: Incorporating variations in the quality of individual randomized trials into meta-analysis. J Clin Epidemiol 1992;45:255.
60. Goel V, the Health Services Research Group: Decision analysis: Applications and limitations. Can Med Assoc J 1992;147:413.
61. Thornton JG, Lilford RJ, Johnson N: Decision analysis in medicine. Br Med J 1992;304:1099.
62. Pauker SG, Kassirer JP: Decision analysis. N Engl J Med 1987;316:250.
63. Lomas J: The consensus process and evidence dissemination. Can Med Assoc J 1986;134:1340.

64. Dalkey NC: The Delphi Method: An Experimental Study of Group Opinion. Santa Monica, CA, The Rand Corp., 1969.
65. Dalkey NC, Rourke DL, Lewis R, et al: The Quality of Life: Delphi Decision Making. Lexington, MA, Lexington Books, 1972.
66. Delbecq A, van de Ven AH: A group process model for problem identification and program planning. J Appl Behav Sci 7:466,171.
67. Brook RH, Chassin MR, Fink A, et al: A method for the detailed assessment of the appropriateness of medical technologies. Int J Technol Assess Health Care 1986;2:53.
68. Merrick NJ, Fink A, Park RE, et al: Derivation of clinical indications for carotid endarterectomy by an expert panel. Am J Public Health 1987;77: 187.
69. Jacoby I: The Consensus Development Program of the National Institutes of Health. Int J Technol Assess Health Care 1985;1:420.
70. Hirsh J, Haynes B: Transforming evidence into practice: Evidence based consensus. ACP Journal Club (January/February), 1993;A-16.
71. A statement for physicians from the ACP/ACC/AHA Task Force on clinical priveleges in cardiology. J Am Coll Cardiol 1990;15:1460.
72. Technology Subcommittee of the Working Group on Critical Care, Ontario Ministry of Health: Guidelines for medical technology in critical care. Can Med Assoc J 1991;144:1617.
73. Guyatt G, Tugwell X, Feeny DG, et al: The role of before-after studies of therapeutic impact in the evaluation of diagnostic technologies. J Chron Dis 1986;39:295.
74. Byars DP: Why databases should not replace randomized clinical trials. Biometrics 1980;36:337.
75. Health Services Research Group. Outcomes and management of health care. Can Med Assoc J 1992;147:1775.
76. Roos LL, Sharp SM: Becoming more efficient at outcomes research. Int J Technol Assess Health Care 1988;4:555.
77. Greenfield S: The state of outcome research: Are we on target? N Engl J Med 1989;320:1142.
78. Byars DP: Problems with using observational databases to compare treatments. Stat Med 1991;10:663.
79. Rosati RA, Lee KL, Califf RM, et al: Problems and advantages of an observational database approach to evaluating the effect of therapy on outcome. Circulation 1982;(suppl II):II-27.
80. Temple R: Problems in the use of large data sets to assess effectiveness. Int J Technol Assess Health Care 1990;6:211.
81. Horwitz RI, Viscoli CM, Clemens JD, et al: Developing improved observational methods for evaluating therapeutic effectiveness. Am J Med 1990; 89:630.
82. Laupacis A, Sackett DL, Roberts R: An assessment of clinically useful measures of the consequences of treatment. N Engl J Med 1988;318:1728.
83. Gore JM, Goldberg RJ, Spodick DH, et al: A community-wide assessment of the use of pulmonary artery catheters in patients with acute myocardial infarction. Chest 1987;92:721.
84. Guyatt G, Sackett D, Taylor DW, et al: Determining optimum therapy—randomized trials in individual patients. N Engl J Med 1986;314: 889.

85. Evans RG: Strained mercy: The Economics of Canadian Health Care. Toronto, Buttersworth, 1984.
86. Department of Clinical Epidemiology and Biostatistics, McMaster University Health Sciences Center: How to read clinical journals: VII. To understand an economic evaluation (part A). Can Med Assoc J 1984;130:1428.
87. Department of Clinical Epidemiology and Biostatistics, McMaster University Health Sciences Center: How to read clinical journals: VII. To understand an economic evaluation (part B). Can Med Assoc J 1984;130:1542.
88. Drummond MF, Davies L: Economic analysis alongside clinical trials. Revisiting the methodological issues. Int J Technol Assess Health Care 1991;7:561.
89. Drummond M: Guidelines for health technology assessment: economic evaluation. Chap 7. In Feeny D, Guyatt G, Tugwell P (eds): Health Care Technology: Effectiveness, Efficiency and Public Policy. Montreal, The Institute for Research on Public Policy, 1986, p. 107.
90. Doubilet P, Weinstein MC, McNeil BJ: Use and misuse of the term "cost effective" in medicine. N Engl J Med 1986;314:253.
91. Robinson R: What does it mean? Br Med J 1993;307:670.
92. Robinson R: Costs and cost-minimisation analysis. Br Med J 1993;307:726.
93. Robinson R: Cost-benefit analysis. Br Med J 1993;307:924.
94. Mehrez A, Gafni A: Quality-adjusted life years, utility theory, and healthy year equivalents. Med Decis Making 1989;9:142.
95. Mason J, Drummond M, Torrance G: Some guidelines on the use of cost effectiveness league tables. Br Med J 1993;306:570.
96. Laupacis A, Feeny D, Detsky AS, et al: How attractive does a new technology have to be to warrant adoption and utilization? Tentative guidelines for using clinical and economic evaluations. Can Med Assoc J 1992;146:473.
97. Gafni A, Birch S: Guidelines for the adoption of new technologies: A prescription for uncontrolled growth in expenditures and how to avoid the problem. Can Med Assoc J 1993;148:913.
98. Naylor CD, Williams JI, Basinski A, et al: Technology assessment and cost effectiveness analysis: Misguided guidelines? Can Med Assoc J 1993;148:921.
99. Shoemaker WC: Use and abuse of the balloon tip pulmonary artery (Swan Ganz®) catheter: Are patients getting their money's worth? Crit Care Med 1990;18:1294.
100. Eddy DM: Selecting technologies for assessment. Int J Technol Assess Health Care 1989;5:485.
101. Guyatt GH, Drummond M, Feeny DH, et al: Guidelines for the clinical and economic evaluation of health care technologies. Soc Sci Med 1986;22:393.
102. Detsky AS, Sackett DL: When was a "negative" clinical trial big enough? Arch Intern Med 1985;145:709.
103. Miller DK, Homan SM: Graphical aid for determining power of clinical trials involving two groups. Br Med J 1988;297:672.
104. Naylor CD, Chen E, Strauss B: Measured enthusiasm: Does the method of reporting trial results alter perceptions of therapeutic effectiveness? Ann Intern Med 1992;117:916.

105. Forrow L, Taylor WC, Arnold RM: Absolutely relative: How research results are summarized can affect treatment decisions. Am J Med 1992;92: 121.
106. Braitman LE: Statistical, clinical, and experimental evidence in randomized controlled trials. Ann Intern Med 1983;98:407.
107. Braitman LE: Confidence intervals assess both clinical significance and statistical significance. Ann Intern Med 1991;114: 515.
108. Gutzwiller F, Chrzanowski R: Technology assessment: Impact on clinical practice. Int J Technol Assess Health Care 1986;2:99.
109. Health Services Research Group: Standards, guidelines and clinical policies. Can Med Assoc J 1992;146:833.
110. Brook RH: Practice guidelines and practicing medicine. Are they compatible? JAMA 1989;262:3027.
111. Battista RN: Clinical practice guidelines: Between science and art. Can Med Assoc J 1993;148:385.
112. Kanouse DE, Jacoby I: When does information change practitioners' behaviour. Int J Technol Assess Health Care 1988;4:27.
113. Eagle KA, Mulley AG, Skates SJ, et al: Length of stay in the intensive care unit. Effects of practice guidelines and feedback. JAMA 1990;264:992.
114. Grimshaw JM, Russell IT: Effect of clinical guidelines on medical practice: A systematic review of rigorous evaluations. Lancet 1993;342:1317.
115. Anderson G: Implementing practice guidelines. Can Med Assoc J 1993; 148:753.
116. Greco PJ, Eisenberg JM: Changing physicians' practices. N Engl J Med 1993;329:1271.

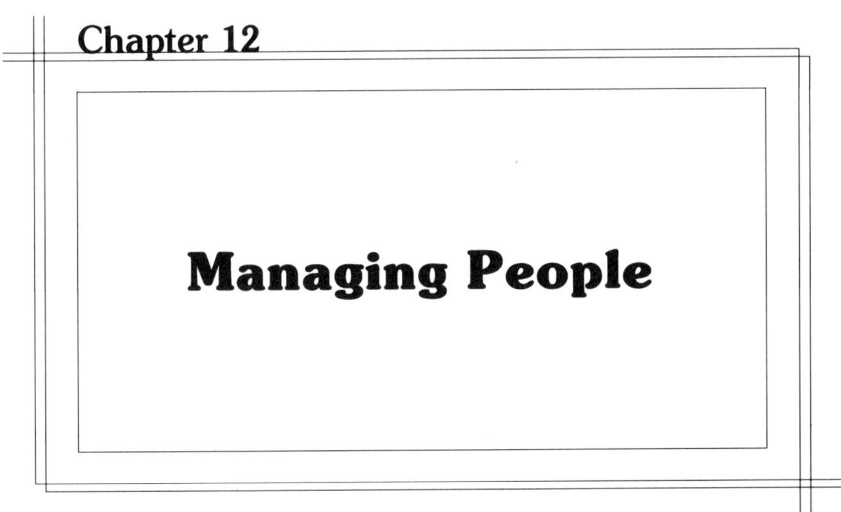

Chapter 12

Managing People

Sandy Whittall, R.N., B.A., B.ScN., M.B.A.

One phenomenon of critical care is that the complex patient needs require a cooperative environment with all disciplines participating in the ultimate outcome of the patient. Also, rapidly developing "leading edge" technology and medical knowledge set against decreasing resources forces justification of the utilization and demonstration of cost benefit for the expensive care. Faced with these realities, the staff must consciously strengthen the collaborative working relationships that already exist.

These essential relationships can be threatened, however, by a lack of understanding or respect among the disciplines. Mixed or unclear expectations can lead to conflict in this already tense and demanding environment. Without insightful management of the delicate balances, the quality of patient care will be the ultimate loser. These needs have a substantial impact on the human resource management styles of the leadership.

From: Sibbald WJ, Massaro T (eds.): The Business of Critical Care: A Textbook for Clinicians Who Manage Special Care Units. © Futura Publishing Co., Inc., Armonk, NY, 1996.

Literature in both the public and the private sector extol the benefits of a strong "team" for any successful operation. Most would agree that the distinct backgrounds and priorities of the critical care staff present unique challenges for the person or persons who choose to develop the winning team approach in this environment. But the rewards in terms of personal satisfaction and patient outcome make the effort worthwhile.

I want to acknowledge and encourage the trend toward shared roles in clinical management and especially within the critical care team. With this goal in mind, I will try to assist the readers' understanding of the values, priorities, and roles of the key players on the team and what it takes to successfully manage this unique group of professionals.

Factors that Determine the Management Approach

The approach that is necessary to manage a critical care unit (CCU) successfully is determined by multiple factors. These factors include individual personality traits and the environmental circumstances outside the CCU. Also included are the unique qualities of the CCU environment itself.

Vestal[1] discusses three contingencies or factors that contribute to the management style. These include psychological contingencies such as values, attitudes, and expectations. Second, are organizational contingencies, which involve the complexity of the business, technology, and the social climate. The third are environmental factors, which are the competitive pressures, the changing markets, and the changing regulations.

Values, attitudes, and expectations. As training and education programs are responding to the changes in the resource abilities and with increasing requirements to assume more responsibility, most health care professionals are experiencing dramatic shifts in their expectations of themselves, the system, and other practitioners in the system. This trend is forcing a responsiveness that no one learns in school. It is an adaptation that requires integration, cooperation, and communication.

The tie with the changing psychological contingencies has to do with how quickly our organizational contingencies are changing. Technological change in critical care in particular, has been dramatic with an ever increasing pace. The scope of knowledge and expertise that is needed to use the newest technology to care for today's critically ill patient requires a well coordinated and supportive environment.

In particular, the internal environment of the CCU presents operational implications for the management approach. Stahl[2] identified five unique realities of the CCU:

1. The technological advances require frequent educational upgrades.
2. Research development and application precipitate changing expectations for care delivery.
3. The rapidly changing environment requires flexibility with plan development.
4. There tends to be a characteristic pragmatic operating style that should be recognized and supported.
5. There should be methods in place to reduce the stress related to the environment.

The environmental contingencies are probably the biggest factor in the changes to our practice patterns. More and more accountability for our decisions is necessary. The introduction of continuous improvement techniques and expectations has provided very different ways to make decisions and take action. The practitioner can no longer have the singular objective of saving patients regardless of the cost. More and more, practitioners are finding the need to measure and evaluate efficacy to justify their clinical practice. As health care becomes more businesslike, clinicians will need to work more closely and effectively with the professional manager to develop the necessary evaluative measures.

All of these components must be acknowledged and understood to identify the necessary traits, qualifications, and styles needed to manage the CCU effectively. I propose that the current environment in health care and particularly in the critical care setting, supports a team or participative environment.

Support for the Team Approach

"If we are to compete effectively in today's world, we must begin to celebrate collective entrepreneurship, endeavours in which the whole of the effort is greater than the sum of individual contributions"—Reich.[3] While the business world has adopted this philosophy in earnest, the health care industry has been slower to adapt.

This delay can be attributed to multiple complex reasons. One reason is the traditional patriarchal relationship that has existed between medicine and the other health care professions. Another is the unique relationship between the physician practitioner and the health care system. Most notably is because health care participants have never perceived themselves to be in a competitive environment. However, the current economic climate with the corresponding funding changes presents a greater urgency to change old relationships and role expectations.

As our current environment forces us to look at the way we manage and the way that we relate to each other in the work place, one relationship of particular note is that between physicians and nurses. Even though the patient needs have forced a collaborative relationship to some extent, there is still a tendency for the professionals to see themselves as distinct entities with very separate contributions. Mutual expectations between physician and nurse need to be clearly articulated and understood. In some cases these will have to be negotiated. Both disciplines should be open to the changing nature of the roles and relationships. As the expertise required to care for the patients in the critical care setting increases, greater planning, cooperation, and coordination is necessary to provide optimal patient care. There must be a shift away from individual "stars" to a "team" of committed, equally appreciated members.

The critical care setting presents ideal circumstances to enhance and further develop some of the team relationships that already exist. Especially in the political environment in which the CCU finds itself, a well functioning team can identify strategies for advocating successfully for the unit better than any individual group.

Given the competitive field of recruitment and the limited resources to meet the demand, the successful unit must offer something better than the nearest competitor. Shared control might be considered a risk by the individual disciplines, but the reward is that this philosophy can attract the best and the brightest who are allowed to practice their profession in an enlightened environment.

The Manager

In order to understand how the team or participative approach can work in the CCU, it would be beneficial to discuss the role of the manager in this setting, and in particular how the role relates to "managing people". Management is defined " . . . as that process by which managers create, direct, maintain, and operate purposive organizations through systematic, coordinated, cooperative human effort."—McFarland.[4] The professional manager, by definition, is not directly involved with performing the activities of the organization but accomplishes the tasks of the job through the efforts of those who s/he manages. This requires the ability to influence and negotiate, with a major focus on fostering and maintaining effective interpersonal relationships.

As we consider the evolution of the management role in general, we are struck in particular, by the changes in the health care setting. Most practitioners relate to the traditional roles of the Head Nurse and the Medical Director. Management activities were usually associated with the professional discipline with the primary objective of providing patient care. With the changing environment, so have the expectations on these two groups of professionals changed. We have witnessed the emergence of the professional manager role in the health care setting. While the individual may or may not have a clinical background, different skills and knowledge are needed to successfully lead the staff in caring for the complex patient needs in the current environment. Strong clinical skills alone can no longer be the precursor to successful management ability. The critical care setting now requires thoughtful and expert coordination and support. It requires a different approach to accomplish the same patient care goals.

Worth understanding are the different orientations of the clinicians and the managers. Nugent[5] presents a discussion about the range of cognitive styles or thought preferences of individuals from the intuitive to the rational. "The more intuitive thinkers . . . provide the overall view and original ideas which the more rational thinkers help them to articulate, structure and test." While there is no absolute preference in any one individual, the analogous groups in the critical care setting are exemplified by the "intuitive" managers and the "rational" scientist physicians. Since these groups can provide complimentary perspectives, their roles can be developed to capitalize on the strengths. If the different orientations of these two groups are not acknowledged and directed, the team functioning and the unit operations can be compromised.

A better understanding of the multiple integrated "roles" that a manager must play and the essential human resource skills will provide insight into management as a "career" with a valuable contribution to the clinical setting. Johnson, Wagner, and Sweeney[6] have described desirable traits of a manager. They are well liked by their respective staffs and demonstrate good interpersonal skills. They possess strong communication skills in a variety of settings with the ability to freely express their opinions, feelings, and beliefs. They also possess the ability to see the other's point of view and be good listeners. They evidence self-motivation with the ability to initiate problem identification and solution and they demonstrate self-confidence while seeking appropriate guidance in uncertain circumstances.

Further, important managerial skills as identified by Mintzberg[7] include the ability to develop peer relationships, carry out negotiations, motivate subordinates, resolve conflicts, establish information networks and subsequently disseminate information, make decisions in conditions of extreme ambiguity, allocate resources, and above all, be introspective about his/her work so that s/he may continue to learn on the job.

It should be acknowledged that the nurse manager and the physician manager have chosen a perilous career path. In attempting to be the representative go-between for administration and the staff level, their loyalties and priorities are always under suspicion. The clinical staff rarely have the opportunity to observe the manager defend the critical care position among the multiple other stakeholders within the organization. Their understanding of the "politics" of the hospital environment is either limited or they reject the reality of the environment. Particularly in the critical care setting, both medical and nursing staff may hold the belief that a good manager must first be a good clinician. These groups are frustrated if the nurse manager does not have clinical expertise or does not help at the bedside. They resent the time commitments that the manager must make to administrative committees and responsibilities. The physician manager who actively participates with Medical Advisory or institutional committees is also seen to be a "traitor" by his or her colleagues. This betrayed attitude is especially felt when either manager must espouse a corporate position or philosophy. Education of both the administration and the clinical groups by the manager is critical to being successful in his/her role. It is important to emphasize that s/he can be an effective voice for the group and that s/he provides a unique understanding and synthesis of both perspectives.

The CCU manager must successfully develop confidence and a sense of purpose so that s/he can be influential in steering the direction of the unit. As leadership style can play an important role in the turnover rates, the effectiveness and the general morale of the unit, an effective manager is able to balance concern and interest in the staff as well as in the patients. S/he is able to acknowledge and recognize the frustrations of their situation and somehow assist them to see it in a larger perspective. "Effective leaders attract support and enthusiasm because they are positive, purposeful, and believe in what they are doing. People want to be part of that kind of organization"—Heckathorn and Smith.[8]

Definition of Participative Management

"Two truisms of management are: no one can do everything alone, and no one of us knows as much as all of us."—Heckathorn and Smith.[9]

With the introduction of the professional manager, have come relevant management theories. As discussed earlier, superior technical skill, knowledge, and expert leadership capabilities in the critical care environment are combined to support a participative or team management style.

If we look at how successful companies in the private sector use the employee participation model, we can draw comparisons to the critical care setting. Christopher[10] identifies the following characteristics:

1. They keep focused on fewer, well defined objectives.
2. They demonstrate trust in their employees ability to meet the objectives and give them ownership of the project or process.
3. This trust also allows them to allow employees to experiment or try different ways to accomplish the task.
4. They understand and promote the role of the manager as coach, facilitator, and mentor.
5. They value and show evidence of their value of the employees effort, commitment, and loyalty.

"One of the critical elements of the participative model involves goal setting. Goals should state clearly, who is responsible for their achievement, a measurable outcome, and a time period for accomplishing. Decision making is the next component. Then, once involved in the goal setting and decision making, participants can easily transfer this knowledge into the third component, problem solving"—Vestal.[12]

In the critical care environment, goal setting occurs during rounds when patient care management principles are discussed and established. Thus later, when the medical staff are not in attendance, there is clear understanding of the plan and subsequent responsibilities. In a critical care setting, one would acknowledge the need for consultative decision making about patient care management. As team members are allowed to participate in and understand the decisions, they are more able to work through the unpredictable problems and offer viable solutions. This then reinforces the ability to have control over their situation and work activities. The group at this level of participation is then best equipped to effect any change that is necessary. In the critical care setting, this might involve anything from a change in a patient's care plan to a change in policy or procedure. The empowered group would own the requirement to make a change that will ultimately impact their practice.

From the literature, Murtha and Regueiro,[13] and from my own experience, there are some key success factors for the critical care environment:

1. One common goal—Since the goals of the constituents can range from providing excellent or optimal patient care, acquiring leading edge technology, gaining international recognition, or some combination of these, the team must take the time to identify those that are most important to the collective group.
2. Clear role definition with each member understanding their own as well as the others'—Formalizing this aspect requires leadership and endorsement by all disciplines working in the critical care setting.
3. Trust and respect—Albeit, both trust and respect must be earned, the environment must be one without threat of intimidation or ridicule so that staff may participate in open and frank discussions about patient care management decisions. The advantage to the team is that understanding and consistency are enhanced.
4. Efficient communication—Without an extremely effective communication system, confusion and misunderstanding, which can impact the team function, can occur. There should be a clear communication strategy to ensure that all the information gets to all the right people in a timely manner.
5. Genuine care and concern for each other—No man is an island! For the times when all the effort in the world doesn't save a patient. For the times when there's not enough people to do the job. For the times when someone is still learning the ropes. For the times when a life is saved.

Developing and Managing the Team

Individuals who pursue a career in critical care share some similar personality traits. They share the ordinary needs of any individual for respect, loyalty, connection of goals, consistency, and clear expectations. But additionally, I have found that they seek a more demanding work environment and a higher degree of satisfaction from their accomplishments.

Regardless, there are unique challenges and stressors facing all of the critical care team members. Murtha and Regueiro[14] make the point that even though the physicians and nurses all have the best interests of the patient in mind, they still have their own distinct personalities and idiosyncrasies which "... requires a delicate blend of tact and diplomacy."[14] A better understanding of each member's specific needs could lead to developing the necessary supports for the most effective team.

"A conscious effort needs to be made to identify the personality traits as well as the developmental stages of each staff member as they work in the setting. It is important to encourage the development of and then to allow the staff to exercise their own clinical judgement in managing patient care but equally important is the educational support necessary to ensure that the team member's decisions are appropriate and thus that their judgement is respected. The effective manager uses positive reinforcement to help staff to develop the necessary skills and then encourages the staff to function at their optimum level"—Katzin.[19] In this way, each individual is recognized and appreciated for his/her own unique talent and expertise and the unique contribution that they can make to patient care. In encouraging and supporting this kind of behavior, the expectations and limitations must be very clearly communicated. Then the recognition provides a sense of accomplishment to the staff and gives them something to strive for and achieve.

"Another important aspect to identify and work within, is the work group's culture or norms and values"—Van Ess Coeling.[15] The culture has significant implications for hiring, orienting, implementing organizational change, and promoting learning. The manager needs to identify the group's attitudes toward rules for working together, the desire to follow established standards, their work organization and use of time, their psychosocial concerns, and the change rules.

It should be emphasized that there is no right or wrong. However, as previously discussed, if the manager and clinician have very different values, considerable change may need to occur before a successful team can be assembled. The manager should then understand the importance of how different interactions and communications can impact morale and should plan contingencies to address this aspect. The manager's "style must ... fit the nature of the work done there and the cultural habits of the people who perform its tasks and undertake its duties"—Uliss.[16]

Of particular note is that team membership has to be earned. The implications for the critical care manager is that new staff need guidance as they learn to understand the dynamics, the various roles and positions, and evaluate the abilities and knowledge base of the various members.

"In principle, all team members should take the time to learn about each other's educational background and experience and role. It is worthwhile to present a synopsis of the various roles in the critical care unit"—Murtha and Regueiro.[17]

The medical director or attending physician oversees patient care decisions made by the team members and intervenes as necessary to ensure optimal patient care. S/he liaises with the nurse manager to arbitrate conflicts among professionals and communicates with staff and families. S/he also acts in an administrative capacity to negotiate with hospital administration for resources, and with the Medical Advisory Committee for recognition and support for the unique environment.

The intensive care unit Fellow's responsibilities include the ongoing patient management by coordinating multiple clinical services for patient care. S/he also communicates with other staff and families and participates with the education of interns and residents. Administrative responsibilities such as making call schedules and identifying supply and equipment needs to the appropriate sources are included.

The nurse manager ensures nursing staff have the required knowledge and skill set to provide comprehensive patient care as well as ensuring the necessary resources—supplies, equipment, and staff—to provide patient care. S/he liaises with other departments and professionals to ensure proper support and arbitrates among professionals. S/he manages the budget, maximizing the utilization of available resources, and provides an important link with administration.

Nurses and allied health professionals provide direct patient care, coordinate and manage multiple demands, educate other professionals and families, communicate patient status to the appropriate person, and provide information and support to the family.

Although the roles may differ and in some cases overlap, the required skill set or personality traits that are desirable in all the team members are fairly constant: confidence, sensitivity, organizational skills, empathy, intelligence, patience, stamina, communication skills, negotiating skills, leadership, diplomacy, tolerance, delegation skills, and a sense of humor.

A critical element of managing the team is ensuring the viability of the team. Pattan[18] suggests that nurse managers or critical care teams should develop a formal nurse recruitment plan for each fiscal year.

He presents a model that suggests that the manager or team survey the current environment, start to predict future trends, and then attempt to match nurse work demand with nurse incumbent supply. This activity should not be restricted to the recruitment of nurses, as we are seeing greater competitiveness in attracting the brightest medical residents and fellows. What is necessary is the ability to see into the future, to identify trends, predict movement, and then position oneself to take advantage of the opportunities that exist in any changing environment.

After recruitment, retention is the next significant factor in maintaining a viable CCU. The use of such initiatives from the private sector industry as quality circles and other continuous quality improvement techniques allow the staff to have some control over the development of their work environment and provides incentives to remain in the setting. Other specific approaches and techniques for recruitment and retention of the critical care practitioner include such tactics as mentorship, flexible scheduling, and input into clinical decision making. Emphasis should also be placed on the caliber of the orientation program and the ongoing continuing education.

Of particular note is that the teams' input should " . . . address decision making from the perspective of potential impact at the bedside"—Sanford.[20] Thus, decisions that should include collaborative input include those related to patient care needs such as equipment, supplies, support staff, and procedures as well as those about capital equipment. "Further opportunities to provide collaborative input to joint practice committees fosters increased respect and credibility for the staff as they develop the necessary expertise"—Mottaz.[21] As discussed earlier, greater participation in decision making also fosters greater independence in accomplishing the tasks.

The type of manager that is required to manage the team described here is one that is able to act as coach and mentor rather than controller. In the participative model, first line supervisors or managers facilitate rather than direct; impart rather than practice their technical and administrative expertise; help workers develop the ability to manage themselves; and require stronger interpersonal skill and conceptual ability—Walton.[22]

Managing Conflict

Conflicting expectations from multiple constituencies presents unique challenges for CCU management. The CCU presents an environment where uncertainty about patient survival plus uncertainty about the random appearance of unpredictable clinical crisis causes anxiety and stress—Murtha and Regueiro.[23] In this setting, each individual's particular coping mechanism becomes apparent. Even as the nurse and the physician manager must respond to these different forces, they must somehow maintain mutual understanding and support for the benefit of the entire team.

Conflict in the critical care setting can occur for multiple reasons. There can be patient care issues where there is disagreement about patient management or about communications with families. The increased expectations for knowledge and responsibility at the bedside without the corresponding resources to accommodate the educational needs result in increased stress and sensitivity for the staff. Intra- and interdisciplinary conflict can be attributed to working with individuals with differing professional training and/or levels of expertise. There can be disagreements between patients/families and professionals and differing ethical values relative to patient care decisions may cause conflict. Often described is the stress related to heavy patient responsibilities and/or menial tasks and staff shortages requiring overtime work leading to fatigue and low tolerance. Also overriding is the threat and concern over legal liability for all members of the health care team.

To facilitate the resolution of conflict, the manager of the CCU must be an action oriented person. When a problem has been identified by any source, it should be investigated and resolved before misunderstandings, miscommunication, or significant patient sequelae occur. Ignoring problems can also destroy team building. The emphasis should be on "what" is right not "who" is right. Emphasis must be placed on removing the emotion from the conflict situation and reviewing the situation objectively. This means keeping focused on the issues and not making personal or professional attacks. It also means being persistent and assertive without resorting to aggressiveness. Sanford[24] recommends distinguishing between constructive and destructive conflict, with constructive being defined as "full airing of perspectives, opportunities to learn and appreciate the basis for differing views, and opportunities for development of solutions that simultaneously recognize and respect all players".

Heckathorn and Smith[25] provide an approach to conflict resolution or problem solving:

1. Do not become defensive—this only serves as a barrier to communication.
2. Try to separate fact from emotion—the individuals in conflict

need to verbalize their version of the events; allowing individuals to verbalize can bring out the underlying concern or frustration that may have triggered an outburst.
3. Some issues require documentation and intervention at a different level—this needs to be recognized appropriately.
4. Gather facts from both sides of a conflict situation—sometimes it is a matter of misunderstanding or misperception of intentions.
5. Deal with conflict in a timely manner—left alone a small misunderstanding can fester into a substantial unit demoralizer.

Most authors identify very similar steps for conflict resolution that are fairly practical to implement:

1. Carefully listen to understand how the conflict is perceived by the other person.
2. Share your interpretation or understanding of the conflict.
3. Allow the other person to specifically request a resolution.
4. Tell the person what you want.
5. Seek a compromise solution.
6. Agree on a solution.
7. Accept a role or responsibility with the solution and identify a follow-up time.

Conflict is part of the role of a manager and there will always be problems to solve. But conflict resolution does not have to have a negative impact on future relations and if dealt with effectively can serve to strengthen relationships. Effective techniques for managing conflict in the critical care setting are imperative to sustain the essential working relationships.

Summary

There is support for finding the most effective management practices for the critical care setting. As CCUs are being tasked to justify their resource utilization, more research is being done to identify the factors related to unit efficiency and improved outcomes of care. The National ICU Study discussed by Shortell et al.,[26] showed an association between the unit characteristics and processes with "greater efficiency of utilization, . . . lower nurse turnover, higher perceived technical quality of care and higher perceived ability to meet family member needs". These unit characteristics included variables such as culture, leadership, communication, coordination, and problem solving abilities of unit members. As models for evaluation and redesign are developed based on this kind of research, there will be even greater recognition of the important contribution that the professional manager can make to the critical care environment. Managing the "Critical Care Team" means managing in a changing environment. It means changes in roles and responsibilities as they respond to the corresponding changes in financial constraints and utilization accountability. The "team" will need leadership by people who understand and are effective change managers.

As these new roles continue to evolve for all team members, collaboration will no longer be a luxury—it will become a necessity.

References

1. Vestal KW: The participative pediatric nurse manager. J Pediatr Nurs 1987; 2:201–204.
2. Stahl LD: Demystifying critical care management Part 2. J Nurs Adm 1985; 15:14–21.
3. Reich RB: Entrepreneurship reconsidered: The team as hero. Harvard Business Review, 1987, May-June.
4. McFarland DE: Management: Principles and Practices. New York, NY, Macmillan Publishing Co., 1974, p. 6.
5. Nugent PS: Management and modes of thought. J Nurs Adm 1982;12:19–25.
6. Johnson EP, Wagner DH, Sweeney JP: Identifying the right nurse manager. An objective selection process. J Nurs Adm 1984;14:24–30.
7. Mintzberg H: The manager's Job: Folklore and fact. Harvard Business Review, 1975, July-August.
8. Heckathorn K, Smith SA: Management. AACN Organization and Management of Critical Care Facilities. Saint Louis, MO, The C.V. Mosby Co., 1979, p. 155.
9. Heckathorn K, Smith SA: Management. AACN Organization and Management of Critical Care Facilities. Saint Louis, MO, The C.V. Mosby Co., 1979, p. 155.
10. Christopher K: Striving for excellence—unlocking staff potential. Dimensions, 1985, February.
11. Reich RB: Striving for excellence—unlocking staff potential. Dimensions, 1985, February.
12. Vestal KW: Striving for excellence—unlocking staff potential. Dimensions, 1985, February.
13. Murtha MF, Regueiro L: Joining the Team. Part II: People p. 175.
14. Murtha MF, Regueiro L: Ibid.
15. Van Ess Coeling H, Wilcox J: Understanding Organizational Culture: A Key to Management Decision-Making. J Nurs Adm 1988;18:16–23.
16. Uliss D: What leadership style best suits critical care nurses? Nurs Management, 1991;22.

17. Murtha MF, Regueiro L: What leadership style best suits critical care nurses? Nurs Management, 1991;22.
18. Pattan JE: Developing a Nurse Recruitment Plan. J Nurs Adm 1992;22: 33–39.
19. Katzin L: Great head nurses. Am J Nurs 1989;89:42–47.
20. Sanford S: Critical Care at Risk. p. 389.
21. Mottaz CJ: Work satisfaction among hospital nurses. Hosp Health Serv Adm 1988;33:1.
22. Walton RE: From control to commitment in the workplace. Harvard Business Review, 1985, March-April.
23. Murtha MF, Regueiro L: From control to commitment in the workplace. Harvard Business Review, 1985, March-April.
24. Sanford S: From control to commitment in the workplace. Harvard Business Review, 1985, March-April.
25. Heckathorn K, Smith SA: From control to commitment in the workplace. Harvard Business Review, 1985, March-April.
26. Shortell SM, Zimmerman JE, Gillies RR, et al: Continuously improving patient care: Practical lessons and an assessment tool from the National ICU Study. QRB 1992;18:150–155.

Chapter 13

Creating and Managing High Performance in the Intensive Care Environment

Alexander B. Horniman, M.B.A., D.B.A., Thomas A. Massaro, M.D., Ph.D.

A critical care unit is an organization defined by people, skills, and equipment established in a specific location to deliver high-technology care to acutely ill patients. Critical care physicians coordinate and direct this process. As a result, intensivists are atypical among subspecialists in that a significant fraction of their professional energies is routinely devoted to administering their units and directing the people in them. This chapter focuses on the management strategies required to deliver highest quality care and the organizational structure in which they can be found. We assume that although the delivery of health care has many unique features, principles of effective organizational management learned from the study of other industries are relevant to hospitals and particularly to intensive care units (ICUs). Indeed, as health care reform continually expands, the influence of "corporate

From: Sibbald WJ, Massaro T (eds.): The Business of Critical Care: A Textbook for Clinicians Who Manage Special Care Units. © Futura Publishing Co., Inc., Armonk, NY, 1996.

medicine'', and the importance and relevance of these lessons are becoming even more important.

Organizational management is similar to clinical management in that the tension between research (empirical and theoretical) and practice drives the evolutionary changes in the field. The design and management of organizations in the public and private sectors has changed over time to reflect changes in current theory and practice. Presumably as our understanding of organizations and their environment improves, so does our potential for managing them more effectively.

This chapter begins with a summary of organizational theory and its relation to the health care setting. Next, we describe the nature of high-performing organizations and extend that framework to the ICU environment. We conclude by outlining the implication of these concepts for intensive care physicians and their practices.

Organizational Theory and Practice: A Brief Historical Summary

Conceptual models tend to influence the way organizations are designed and managed. Thus, an appreciation for the different basic theories and their consequences is important for the practicing manager.

Around the turn of the century, students of management began to ask: How can we design an organization to function effectively? Weber,[1] Taylor[3] (famous for the time and motion studies that preceded the mass production revolution of the early part of the century) and others[2,4] responded by development of a mechanistic model that characterized organizations in logical but impersonal terms. The model assumed that if the roles and role relationships were well defined and integrated, then people would function in an orderly and highly efficient fashion. Emphasis was on line and staff, spans of control, locus of authority, chain of command, and centralization versus decentralization. Structure, roles, and relationships between roles dominated the writings. It was assumed that if the design was appropriate, *rational* people would *logically* function in efficient ways. People were viewed as means to organizational ends. If the design was effective the variability in people did not matter. This perspective continues to be a major factor in the design and management of many contemporary hospital systems.

At about the same time, others[5] known as the Principles of Management Group began asking a related question: "What do people who manage organizations do?" Not surprisingly, their answer was slightly different: "They plan, organize, direct, control and staff". These tasks became accepted as basic management functions. The premise was that if these functions were executed capably, the organization would be well managed and able to achieve its goals and objectives, i.e., management tasks competently performed ensure the effective functioning of organizations.

Whether one describes management in terms of functions, roles, or tasks, these early approaches stressed the needs of the organization rather than the people who met these needs. The human psychological dimensions were subordinated, if not ignored. Structure and function were emphasized rather than the individuals who lived and worked in these environments. Over time, this focus on form and function created organizations that valued policies and procedures above all else. We call these rule based organizations bureaucracies.

As the size and complexity of organizations grew and new technologies were introduced to improve efficiency, the question became: "How do people and technologies interact?" Responses[6–9] began to incorporate the human dimension describing organizations with concepts that contrasted organic and mechanistic environments and introduced social technical systems relationships. However, even this group tended to minimize the intra- and interpersonal complexities of people and instead focused on systems.

Bennis,[10] Schien,[11] Athos,[12] Argyris,[13–15] and Tannenbaum[16] expanded the consideration of individual human behaviors. The uniqueness of people and their potential became the primary focus and the organizational context in which they behaved secondary. Structure, organization, and technology were seen as relevant because they influenced human activity and not as ends in themselves.

Today we have, in a sense, come full circle from the mechanists and are asking "How do we build organizations that improve and develop the human element?" People are central to the success of the organization and the organization should be structured to maximally encourage the contribution of the individuals involved. This approach has brought us to an emphasis on quality, process, and learning systems. Concepts such as empowerment, stakeholder ownership, systems thinking, and team deployment have become central to achieving both human potential and organizational effectiveness. Juran,[17] Demming,[18] Senge,[19] Athos,[12] and Pascale[12,20] did not abandon the previous approaches but made people and process equal, if not more important than structure or system. They raised the questions of high performance and how people in organizations could achieve extraordinary outcomes.

The Present Hospital Situation

Hospital design and management strongly reflect the rational perspective of the early theories. The emphasis on functional specialization, departments, extensive and specialized role training, protocols, and systems, clearly reflect the best in rational logical design. Hospitals operate with clearly delineated rules and rituals. The structure and management systems of the hospital are often viewed by physicians as a necessary evil that must be tolerated. We often speak of the "hospital bureaucracy" in negative terms as though it was something imposed on them by a mysterious force. Although the policies, procedures, rules, and rituals were intended in the best mechanistic tradition to ensure the most effective delivery of health care, they are oftentimes perceived as cumbersome if not inhibiting. This rational and functional structure is being severely challenged by the present rapid, and most likely continuing, change. These changes are occurring as a result of a different level of expectations that now exists in the society and the marketplace.

A History of Good Enough

Table 1 shows a range of possible performance expectations (poor to fair to good enough to very good to excellent). The assumptions and actions of the past several decades were sufficient to make most hospital systems "good enough." In fact, good enough may be a logical consequence of any system that places greater emphasis on structure, systems, and technologies than it does on the people who are central to its operation.

"Good enough" means the delivered protocols, procedures, skills, and abilities meet the requirements of the system. Good enough is not

Table 1
Performance Range

Poor	Marginal	Good Enough	Very Good	Excellent (Outstanding)

marginal or inadequate performance. Quite the contrary, it defines a state that is clearly satisfactory in many dimensions.

The Nature of High Performance

"High-performance" organizations strive for excellence at all times. They regularly meet or exceed the expectations and requirements of their multiple stakeholders. High performance is a significant departure from the past. High performance is a dynamic notion based upon an assumption of continuous learning and improvement. Good enough means the delivered protocols, procedures, skills, and abilities meet the requirements of the system and satisfy the expectations of the primary stakeholders (e.g., doctors, nurses, patients, technical, administrative staff, and others). The conditions represented by the very good and excellent zones are clearly distinguishable by those stakeholders most valued with the organization. To reach the very good and excellent high-performance zones requires the effective integration of the concepts of team management.

High-performing organizations are people centered, team focused, technology driven, information, and process supported. High-performance thinking represents a significant departure from the traditional bureaucratic model in that it is squarely centered on the worth and dignity of the individual.

Particular emphasis is placed on selecting highly qualified and competent people who are also capable of being effective team members. High-performing organizations utilize teams as the dominant organizational element. High-performing team members possess a unique set of skills, not the least of which is the capacity to subordinate one's ego to the process and objectives of the team. Continuous learning at the individual and team level is a necessary dimension of sustainable high performance.

Leadership in high-performing organizations represents an interesting variation on the rational, logical principles model that focused on direction and control. First of all, high-performing organizations require powerful people, not always the formal leaders, to focus, energize, and support the high-performance process. A powerful person is one who is capable of being engaged in the situation in such a way that not only are they personally inspired, they inspire others through their engagement. High-performance organizations are built around teams of powerful people both in the formal (managerial) and informal, personal and interpersonal sense. High-performing team leaders need to begin to lead and follow and then lead again. This is not an easily acquired skill.

High-performance organizations benefit from a clearly articulated vision and a set of strategies, goals, and objectives to both guide and inform the visioning process. The creation of a powerful vision provides an organizing and inspiring perspective, which can be internalized by the people who must make things happen in extraordinary ways. It takes a great deal of energy to sustain high performance and having a powerful vision contributes to the generation of energy.

Technology is a major element in the high-performance mosaic. Just as individual competence and continuous learning are essential so, too, is technology. There is a technology-competency dynamic that finds technology driving the need for personal competence and personal competence pushing the technology to its limits, and this is a continually repeated cycle.

The use of information and information technology in high-performing organizations tends to be quite different than found in the more traditional rational control-type organizations. Information becomes the organizing and integrating vehicle. Not only is the information technology (hardware and software) an essential element in the high-performance environment, its extension to and use by all members of the organization is a necessary attribute that both inspires and informs. As a consequence, high performance is often grounded in innovative information technology applications. In the private sector, these tend to be applications that provide a competitive advantage. In the public sector they are applications that move the organization to a level of performance and service that is easily recognized by the various stakeholders as distinctive and worthy of emulation.

All members of a high-performance organization are provided with all relevant information that they need. Information is open and available to all participants and consequently becomes a vehicle for informing and empowering people throughout the organization. This is in direct contrast to typical (good enough) organizations where information is collected and dispensed as a basis of power and control.

High performance requires continuous learning as a mind and action set for all involved. Most organizations reflect some degree of learning, for without that, they would fall out of the zone of "good enough." High-performance organizations require both "single loop" and "double loop learning" as articulated by Argyris.[14–16] Single loop learning is the development of personal skills and knowledge of individuals. Double loop learning describes how an organization takes advantage of personal development and absorbs the added skill base into "system". It goes beyond individual competence and becomes the basis for developing a true organizational learning capability. Not only do individuals learn, but these same individuals invest time and energy learning about how they learn and transferring that learning to others. Presumably, if an organization's members can't achieve the second loop stage of "learning about" they probably cannot sustain, or for that matter, reach a state of high performance. There is a great deal being written about learning organizations, and at the heart of these discussions is the notion that organizational learning is more than a collection of individual competencies. It is a process that becomes assimilated as a capability. As a capability, it transcends any single individual and becomes part of the mindset of the organization, no matter how extraordinary the individual mindset may be.

High performance also requires an ethical/moral platform to be sustained. A culture of trust must be developed. A culture of trust is one where all people are valued and their distinctive competencies are supported by technology, inspired by a vision and reinforced by continuous learning. Trust is the currency of high performance and is a consequence of very specific behaviors that include telling the truth and keeping promises. Individuals are respected and treated fairly. They are clearly regarded as ends of worth and dignity, not as mere means to accomplish the organization's ends.

There are three basic questions that people in high-performing organizations ask of each other:

1. Do we care about each other?
2. Can we trust each other?
3. Are we each committed to excellence?

If the answers to any of these questions is no, high performance cannot be achieved and sustained.

It is important to return to an issue introduced above, i.e., the difference between the *high-performance achievement* of individuals and a *high-performing organization*. Competent people acting alone can produce excellence. Collections of competent people, even when their efforts are not interdependent, can generate outstanding outcomes. We argue, however, that even though the accomplishments are laudable, unless a culture of trust exists, supported by the moral/ethical behavior described, it is unlikely that high performance can be sustained, can migrate, or can grow in organizations as complex and interdependent as ICUs or hospitals.

The Health Care Scene

The multiple and often conflicting demands of the 1990s have created profound challenges for health care organizations, especially those that are anchored in the old traditional ways of operating and managing. It is no longer sufficient to define hierarchies, roles, relationships, and routines. People working within these parameters cannot be expected to cope with the changes that are presently occurring and respond with performance beyond the level of "good enough". High performance represents a significant departure from the past and a necessary step forward if the health care systems are to be responsive to the changing times. The intensive care environment, with its multiple stakeholders, is a natural setting for this type of high-performance thinking, action, and outcome.

The Intensive Care Unit As A High-Performing Organization

ICUs are unique both from the critical nature of their efforts and the whole patient perspective that organizes the units' attention. These units are ideally constructed to embrace the high-performing elements previously discussed. Their missions of providing intensive care creates a focus and an urgency that is not present in most organizations, whether private or public. Critically ill patients require far more than a specialist intervention or series of procedures. Many of our patients push our technologies to their limits, the best skills and competencies of individuals and a kind of care that can only be provided by a highly trained, well integrated, disciplined team.

It is certainly possible and probably likely that, if all the members of an intensive unit did their tasks as assigned, the care provided certainly would be adequate and "good enough." In fact, given the level of training and the background of most people who work in intensive units, a good enough outcome is almost assured. The issue is not "good enough". The issue is "high performance" and it is with this challenge in mind that the following ideas are presented.

Intensive units provide a wonderful setting and structure for inviting all the members of the unit to contribute in ways that go beyond their respective disciplines, specific areas of competence, and the necessary protocols. Intensive care is an opportunity for all involved to share not only sets of particular skills and abilities but to exceed these and contribute insights and observations that might well not be elicited in more traditional, functional hospital settings. High performance requires a more engaged participation by all concerned in ways that transcend the necessary routine and protocols.

This full engagement of all personnel becomes a central theme for the intensive care environment. Simply doing one's job in a competent fashion is not enough. It is contributing with others so as to bring out the best (the extraordinary) from everyone that is the issue. This degree of engagement is essential. The people involved must be invited and feel personally obligated to contribute in ways that go well beyond what is usually expected and required. *The linking of invitation and obligation is not coincidental.* The leaders of ICUs must be prepared to invite people to become engaged more deeply than their traditionally defined professional and institutional roles. By the same token, individual members must feel a sense of obligation and invitation to be engaged through their insights, observations, and skills in ways that go beyond what is normally expected. This process does not mean that the leaders of intensive units abdicate making the necessary and often difficult decisions. It does mean that, where and when appropriate, leaders must invite more people to share their ideas and insights and incorporate them into the decision making process.

Powerful leaders engage people in ways that make them more powerful, ultimately resulting in better outcomes. The term "powerful leaders" implies a willingness and an ability to go beyond the traditional parameters used to define the role of the director of an intensive unit. Powerful implies a behaved philosophy that is centered on caring for and about people and being committed to bringing out their full potential. This is a process that requires both an individual and team focus, and yet it is done in a very demanding environment. The underlying assumption is that if the leader values his/her team members, they will value each other more and consequently add more value to the patients for whom care is provided. This goes far beyond the traditional structured and stereotypical relationships that were the results of the mechanistic approaches.

The high-performing director must find ways to engage people as a team, which in turn has members learning and motivating themselves. It is at this point that the high-performing intensivist takes on a significant new role. Medical competence is necessary but not sufficient to deliver this leadership role in a highly effective fashion. It requires redefining the role into a more personal engaging and challenging perspective.

The intensive unit and the people who comprise it must be capable of double loop learning if they are to truly become a high-performing unit. The generation of new technical information and the development of corresponding skills and abilities to apply this knowledge is a never ending process. A learning organization uses continuous technical knowledge acquisition as a platform for building interpersonal processes and routines allow them to assess what they have learned from their experiences and from each other. The first loop (technical learning) is easier for many than the second loop (psychological-social adaptation). The second loop is learning about the learning and its application to the intensive setting and the challenging of assumptions that are often at the heart of this process. These processes are essential to high performance.

Information and the maximum sharing of that information in all its forms provides the essential core to high-performing patient care. It is the open effective dissemination of this information that is so important. The more that people are informed, the more they are invited to contribute. The more people are engaged in defining reality, the richer the definition will become.

ICUs demand a team perspective and team work capability on the part of all members. ICUs must be staffed by people who are capable of personal specialization and, at the same time, contribute to a unique interpersonal integration around the patient's needs and requirements. The major orientation is for highly trained people working together to create a high-performance team. These are not teams of equals reaching decisions by consensus but rather teams of specially trained people who are willing and able to subordinate their personal egos when necessary in the spirit and interest of high-performance patient care. This implies that the more traditional roles and boundaries of physician, nurse, and technician are less appropriate than the need to be a highly effective team member. This team dimension requires an intensive culture that fosters respect for all individual team members.

This team dimension is also based on trust. Trust, in turn, is an earned outcome of a number of behaviors over time. There is a confidence that each team member will do his/her part in the overall care of the patient. When trust is established, the full use of technology, the effective delivery of skills and ability, and the full use of necessary information is possible, and patients are cared for in a superior fashion. When trust is missing or weak, high-performance outcomes are not possible.

The ICU can at times be physically, intellectually, and emotionally draining. Because of the stress, the need for support, reinforcement, and celebration is perhaps higher than in the more traditional, functional areas of the hospital. Those intensive units that have created ways to support and reward each other and celebrate outstanding efforts have gone a long way toward recognizing and sustaining high performance.

A high-performing ICU may exist in a hospital environment that is often quite different in form and function. The ICU leadership serves as a buffer between the intensive unit and the other divisions within the hospital. This buffering role is not well articulated in the management literature, but in the daily operating routines of the hospital it is an essential element in ensuring the effective functioning of the unit. The director shields the other members of the team from pressures and, at times, the distractions that flow from the other parts of the organization. This relates to the effective integration of the team based high-performance culture into the more traditional, functional divisions that can make up most of the rest of the hospital system.

Conclusion

High performance and intensive care seem to fit well together. Although imbedded in the more traditionally defined and control focused management system, the intensive unit provides numerous opportunities to model and extend the high-performance attributes described in this chapter. The people systems and processes that define the intensive environment should provide examples for the rest of the hospital system.

The questions that motivated theorists to move from the traditional models to those of high performance now include: "How can we build continuous learning, people centered structures that sustain extraordinary achievements for the benefit of our patients and the hospital systems in which they care or reside?"

References

1. Weber M, Parsons T (eds): The Theory of Social and Economic Organization. New York, NY, Free Press, 1947.
2. Fayol H: General and Industrial Management. New York, NY, Pittman Publishing Company, 1949.
3. Taylor FW. The Principles of Scientific Management. New York, NY, Harper and Brothers, 1939.
4. Gulick L, Urwick L (eds): Papers on the Science of Administration. New York, NY, Institute of Public Administration, 1937.

5. Mooney JD: The Principles of Organization. New York, NY, Harper and Brothers, 1939.
6. Follett MP, Metcalf HC, Urwick L (eds): Dynamic Administration: The Collected Papers of Mary Parker Follett. New York, NY, Harper and Brothers, 1941.
7. Koontz H, O'Donnell C: Principles of Management. New York, NY, McGraw Hill, 1959.
8. Rice AK: The Enterprise and its Environment. London, Tavistock Publications, 1963.
9. Katz, Kahn, Emery FE, Trist EL, et al. (eds): Sociotechnical Systems in Management Sciences, London, 1960.
10. Burns T, Stalker GM: The Management of Innovation, London, Tavistock Publications, 1962.
11. Woodward J: Management and Technology: Problems of Progress in Industry, No. 3. Report of Department of Scientific and Industrial Research, 1958.
12. Bennis WG: Changing Organizations. New York, NY, McGraw Hill, 1966.
13. Schein EH: Organizational Culture and Leadership, San Francisco, CA, Jossey-Bass, Inc., 1985.
14. Pascale RT, Athos AG: The Art of Japanese Management. New York, NY, Simon & Schuster, 1981.
15. Argyris C: Integrating the Individual and the Organization. New York, NY, Wiley, 1964.
16. Argyris C, Schoen DA: Theory in Practice: Increasing Professional Effectiveness. San Francisco, CA, Josey-Bass, 1974.
17. Argyris C, Schoen DA: Organizational Learning. Reading, MA, Addison-Wesley, 1978.
18. Tannenbaum R, Schmidt HW. How to choose a leadership pattern. Harvard Bus Rev 1958;36(2):95–101.
19. Juran JJ: Managerial Breakthrough. New York, NY, McGraw Hill, 1964.
20. Demming WE: Out of Crisis. MIT Center for Advanced Engineering Study, Cambridge, MA.
21. Senge PM. The Fifth Discipline. New York, Doubleday Currency, 1990.
22. Pascale RT: Managing on the Edge. New York, NY, Simon & Schuster, 1990.

Chapter 14

Managing the Strategic Planning Process

Jeannette A. Eberhard, B.Sc., M.B.A.

Planning is not a new concept in medicine. Clinical practice is centered around patient care plans that follow a continuous cycle of information gathering, evaluation, diagnosis, and treatment. These same basic concepts, transferred from the bedside to the board room, and cloaked in business jargon, are those used in the strategic planning process. While the physician obtains the patient history and test results, the manager gathers information on the business environment, current activities, and performance. The physician determines a diagnosis and treatment aimed toward measurable change in health status for the patient. The manager sets goals for company performance and a business plan by which to achieve those goals. Both return to their information gathering and analysis periodically to evaluate progress toward their goal and to make changes in their strategy as appropriate.

Despite these apparent similarities in their training and practice, health care providers rarely embrace the process of strategic planning

From: Sibbald WJ, Massaro T (eds.): The Business of Critical Care: A Textbook for Clinicians Who Manage Special Care Units. © Futura Publishing Co., Inc., Armonk, NY, 1996.

as much as their counterparts in the board room. Three reasons may explain this. First, there may be a feeling of discomfort with the jargon or a lack of previous experience. Second, it may be difficult to transfer tactical or short-term decision skills to the level of strategic planning and thinking. This chapter will address these two impediments by describing the content and process of strategic planning in the sections "What is a strategic plan?" and "The strategic planning process."

The third reason is less one of mechanics than one of commitment. Physicians may perceive little merit in a strategic planning exercise that consumes their time while offering few rewards. Simply put, it is not worth the investment. Changing this perception is the more difficult task. It is addressed in the section "Why plan?"

What is a Strategic Plan?

A strategic plan provides a road map of where you are today, where you want to be in the future, and the steps you must take to get there.

A strategic plan provides a long-term vision for the future of your institution, department, or program.

A strategic plan provides a consistent, predetermined framework in which to make operational decisions.

Strategic planning is the process by which a group of key decision-makers develop, implement, and continuously evaluate their strategic plan.

A strategic plan should not be a voluminous document adorning the shelf between undergraduate text books and clinical procedure manuals. It should not be your office "coffee table" book dusted off yearly to impress accreditation boards. It should be a document well worn by periodic review and consultation, a guidebook to the operational decisions faced by your department, program, or institution.

Why Plan?

Creating an effective strategic plan requires the commitment, time, and effort of busy professionals. In a health care environment, these same people are barraged by operational tasks from bedside patient care, to scheduling staff or balancing budgets. Using any portion of that time to invest in strategic planning must clearly be justified by the benefits. That being the case, what are the benefits of strategic planning and what investment should participants expect to make?

Business embraced strategic planning as a means by which to gain competitive advantage, as did its military predecessors. Henderson[1] stated in the Harvard Business Review, "Strategic competition is not new of course. Its elements have been recognized and used ever since humans combined intelligence, imagination, accumulated resources, and coordinated behaviour to wage war."

The need for strategic planning to gain competitive advantage may seem more appropriate in countries with a private medical system than those with socialized health care. But competition exists in both systems. In the private system, hospitals compete for business from private insurers. In the public system, programs compete for scarce public funding. Both systems compete for academic recognition and qualified human resources. All departments compete internally for their share of budget resources. The rising cost of health care and limits to spending in both systems will only serve to accentuate the need for competitive strategies in health care.

Physicians in critical care practice cannot escape these realities. Their practice is among the most resource intensive in a time when technological advances have begun to outstrip the resources available. Agencies that fund the system, consumers of their services, fellow health care workers, and administrators will no longer settle for the physician who defends expenditures or new treatments by saying "trust me."

Physicians in this resource intensive specialty must be better prepared to make difficult decisions or someone else will make them. They must be prepared to defend the merit of their practice to a new audience who may speak in different terminology than their physician colleagues. They must collaborate with other disciplines to evaluate their changing environment, the demands on their service, and their ability to provide appropriate care. They must create a vision for their programs that includes sound analysis, measurable objectives, and a structured implementation plan.

At the operational level, the benefits of developing a strategic plan are to be found in the earlier definitions. Consider this first . . . .*"a road map of where you are today."* Experience would suggest that most health care programs find it difficult to describe their services in quantitative terms. Measurable descriptions of current activities, whether it be nursing turnover ratios, morbidity and mortality statistics, basic admission and length of stay, or an inventory of physical plant and equipment, enables your program to monitor progress in the future. How can your group evaluate the costs of nursing turnover and the effect of retention programs if no measures exist by which to gauge the current status and future progress? How can you justify the upgrade of capital equipment if there is no record of the number, cost, and risk associated with current failure rates? How can you measure the results of quality improvement programs if baseline morbidity and mortality statistics are not available? How can you plan for improved utilization management if information does not exist to describe current admissions, practice, and resource utilization? Answering the question "where you are today" forms the first part of a strategic planning document called the *situational analysis*.

All of this is obviously background to taking action as captured in the second part of the definition *"where you want to be in the future and the steps you must take to get there."* In Lewis G. Carroll's classic tale, Alice encountered the cheshire cat at a fork in the road and asked which road to take. Upon confession that she did not know where she wanted to go, the cat replied "Then it doesn't really matter which road you take!" Should you spend limited nursing dollars on more educational programs or nursing retention strategies? If your strategic plan identifies quality improvement goals that require higher qualification levels for your nursing staff, then the decision to invest in educational programs makes sense. If future goals include a reduction in morbidity related to cross-patient infections, then the capital investment in physical plant to incorporate more private rooms may take priority over improved office space for consultants. If your goals include a commitment to excellence in medical research, then resources must be in place to provide protected time for your attending physicians.

These examples may seem simplistic or obvious, but many an hour is spent in meetings arguing about such operational decisions. On the other hand, consider a program in which decision-makers agree in advance to strategic goals and the steps required to achieve them. Choices about where to invest resources would be decided in advance and meeting time channelled toward dealing with external obstacles rather than creating internal ones. Commitment to a strategic plan means that operational decisions can be evaluated objectively by asking "Will this bring us closer to achieving our agreed upon goals and objectives?" A strategic plan answers the question "where do you want to be" by presenting *strategic directions*. The plan outlines "how you will get there" with a step-by-step *action plan*.

The cost of strategic planning is a tangible commitment of scarce time and the effort to learn new skills. Benefits, on the other hand, accrue subtly, bit by bit, in the daily ability to make efficient decisions, implement effective progress toward agreed-upon goals, and to measure the success of your efforts. Managed properly, these benefits far outweigh the investment. If that is enough justification of the theory, the rest of the chapter will deal with the practical aspects of creating a strategic plan.

The Planning Process

Strategic planning is usually attempted in two steps—assemble the task force and write the plan. A more comprehensive list of tasks in the planning process includes the following:

1. Establish expectations.
2. Assign a working group.
3. Develop a written plan.
4. Implement the plan.
5. Measure progress and re-evaluate.

Each of these will be discussed in more detail.

Establish Expectations (What Do We Expect to Achieve?)

Be wary of participants in a strategic planning process who believe that a written strategic plan will solve all of their problems or none. The answer lies somewhere between the two extremes. Before a representative task force is struck to develop a written document, an inclusive group of stakeholders should agree on their expectations for the process. At the institutional level, each division should be consulted. In a department, each discipline (medicine, nursing, allied health, administration) should begin the process. In an academic program, this circle should include each institution and the sponsoring university. Expectations set by the inclusive group will provide a framework for the smaller task force. At the end of their work, members of the task force must satisfy themselves, and the larger group, that they have successfully met expectations.

Setting expectations for the process should not be confused with setting goals for the program. Rather, discussion should revolve around the question "What prompted this planning process?" (Having read this chapter is not a sufficient answer!) Planning strategically makes good sense for the reasons presented earlier. However, your program may be aware of specific problems or opportunities that must be addressed. There may be external pressures on your group from competing programs, internal or external, to your institution. You may find it increasingly difficult to meet operating budgets. Morale within your program may be low if opinion is constantly divided among your staff on capital investment decisions. You may need to prepare for the impact of decisions made by other programs to expand or contract.

With those concerns on the table, your group should be able to state "What do we expect to achieve?" You should quickly be able to arrive at answers that sound like these: A program that is threatened with closure may want "a better understanding of our strengths and weaknesses relative to competing programs and the steps we must take to maintain sufficient funding levels"; A department facing budget cuts should look for "a predetermined consensus of our patient care priorities as a basis by which to allocate scarce resources"; A surgical intensive care unit may want to "develop a better understanding of the relationship between surgical case type and resource consumption" if the department of surgery plans to add operating room capacity. Specific priorities will change over time with the ebb and flow of your external environment.

Each division or discipline may have different expectations. An open discussion of these expectations will enable participants to appreciate the others' perspective and eliminate the potential for hidden agendas. As you write, implement and evaluate your strategic plan, don't forget to ask if these expectations have been met.

Assign a Working Group (Who Will be Involved?)

There are three decisions to be made. One, who will form the working group. Two, who will be consulted. Three, who will lead the process and write the report. The working group should be representative of the leaders in your larger group. These tasks should not be delegated to junior people. Junior staff in the program will be part of the process as they assist in the preparation of background material, statistics, and trends requested by the working group.

In the case of a stand-alone unit or department, the working group should include medical, nursing, and administrative staff with responsibility for patient care, and operational and capital decisions. If critical care spans multiple units, each should be represented in some capacity. In the case of an academic program, the group might expand to include members of the academic faculty and may include multiple institutions. Temper the inclusive nature of these recommendations with a limit on the total working group of no less than four and no more than twelve people who can commit to meeting on a predetermined schedule.

The core working group will want and need to consult with others. In addition to operational information and concerns filtered up by their staff, the working group should consult people with relevant information outside the program and those who will be affected by the strategic decisions the group may consider. These stakeholders may include other hospital departments, the community groups that depend on your services and services upon which you depend. Planning documents from your institution, academic health complex, or regional health care governing bodies should also be reviewed.

The program chair or departmental director may seem the obvious candidate to lead the planning process as that person will bear responsibility for the success of the plan. Temper that obvious choice by the need for participants to feel comfortable introducing new directions and to participate without intimidation. Another member of the team may help to accomplish these goals more readily than the existing leader. Outside facilitators or consultants may also become involved. Consultants can contribute skills, time, or an impartial perspective that may not be available within the working group. This may be especially true if the program is working through the process for the first time, if issues are controversial, or if time is constrained for information collection and assimilation by staff.

Develop a Written Plan

The specific contents of any strategic plan will vary depending on the size and scope of activities in your hospital, program, or department, and the issues that surface during the planning process. That is to say, there is no "rubber stamp." In spite of these comments, all documents should cover three broad areas: the situational analysis; strategic directions; and an action plan. Consider your audience when preparing your plan. Describe your activities and plans in language that is readable by someone outside your department or the medical field. Justify your conclusions to a reader who may have reason to question priorities. If external parties play a role in allocating the resources you need, they will be more amenable to investing in something they can understand. Table 1, the Strategic Planning Check List, will serve as a guide for your discussions and the preparation of a written document.

Table 1
Strategic Planning Checklist

1. Establish Expectations (What do we expect to achieve?)
   Why are we taking the time and effort to (re)develop a strategic plan?
2. Assign a Working Group (Who will be involved?)
   Who will be on the working group?
   Who else will be consulted or involved?
   Who will lead the process?
3. Develop a Written Plan
   a) Situational Analysis (What are we doing? How well are we doing?)

      Internal

      What clinical, educational and research services do we offer?
      How do we organize ourselves to deliver those services?

      External

      What is the present and expected future demand for our services?
      With whom do we compete and what are their relative strengths and weaknesses? How might that change in the future?
      How will factors or trends in the environment affect our programs? Consider political, technical, social, economic and international factors.

      Implications

      What are our relative strengths and weaknesses?
      What problems, opportunities and uncertainties do we face?
      What are the implications of this and what issues must be addressed by our future strategies?
   b) Strategic Directors (What do we want to do?)
      What is our overall mission?
      What are our broad goals?
      What are the specific, measurable objectives required to achieve each goal?
      How will stakeholders be involved in or affected by this strategy?
      What factors will be key to the successful achievement of these goals and objectives?
      How does the plan minimize our weaknesses, reinforce our strengths and address the problems and opportunities identified in the situational analysis?
   c) Action Plan (How will we do it?)
      What specific steps must be undertaken by the end of one, three and five years to achieve our objectives?
4. Implement the Plan (Let's go!)
5. Measure Success and Re-evaluate (Have we achieved our goals and objectives?)
   How well are we doing compared to stated objectives? Should we adjust our action plan?
   Has anything changed in our environment to warrant a re-evaluation of our goals and objectives?

Situational Analysis (What Are We Doing Now? and *How Well Are We Doing?)*

A Situational Analysis describes the structure and activity of existing programs, the environment in which your program operates now, and a best estimate of how that environment will change in the future. The background necessary for the development of a realistic and successful strategic plan is an understanding of the current situation, pressures, and demands, how well current strategies address this situation, and implications for future direction.

Many strategic plans omit this section or give it brief mention, assuming the information to be common knowledge. The breadth of your current activities, your successes, and the pressures under which your program operates may not be well understood by the external audience who will sanction your future plans and allocate resources. Many arguments among your team about future priorities arise because there is no consensus on the problems and opportunities you face! A descriptive and, where possible, quantitative assessment of the current situation enables the measurement and evaluation of future strategies to invoke change or improvement.

The situational analysis answers two questions "What are we doing now?" and "How well are we doing?" for an audience who may, or may not, be familiar with critical care in general or your program in particular. Answering the first question provides a description of what is happening now—both internally and externally to your program. Analysis is required to turn data into information, to paint a clear picture of the problems, opportunities, and implications for your program. Both steps are necessary to provide the "set up" required to justify your conclusions.

Internal Analysis: The internal analysis provides an overview of the structure and activity of your program; the way in which you supply your services. Describe your internal structure using diagrams or descriptions of your internal organization, governance, planning, budgeting, evaluation processes, and payment/reward schemes. Provide a qualitative and quantitative description of the clinical, educational, and research activities of your program. Strive to find objective rather than subjective measures. Clinical service descriptions might include number of admissions, length of stay, morbidity, and mortality. Where possible, stratify or segment this analysis by diagnosis and source of referral over time. Educational programs can be quantified by describing number of graduates and the positions they now hold. Research programs can be quantified by the dollar value of grants, industrial contracts, and papers published. Use these measures as examples, but do not be limited by them. Ask yourself, "How do we measure how well we do?"

External Analysis: The external analysis outlines the environment in which your program operates. Describe the current and future demand for your services. Consider the programs with which you compete. What is their focus and their relative strengths and weaknesses using the same criteria by which you measure your own success? Evaluate the factors or trends that will affect your program in the future. Be sure to mention political, technological, social, economic, and international factors of importance.

Implications: This is your opportunity to set the stage for future strategies. Summarize your relative strengths and weaknesses. Discuss the problems, opportunities, and uncertainties facing your program. Describe the implications of this analysis and present the issues to be addressed by future strategies.

Strategic Directions (What Do We Want to Do?)

The Strategic Directions describe the path your program will take in the future. The strategy begins with a statement of overall mission or vision translated into a few long-term goals appropriate to the mandate of the program within your institution, community, and/or teaching center. Each goal is assigned specific, measurable objectives required to achieve that goal and to address the problems, opportunities, and issues identified in the situational analysis. The reader should see a focused vision with consistent goals that move from the general to the specific. Lest this task seem too mechanical, the reader might prefer Mintzberg's[2] image of a potter *crafting* strategy instead of senior managers *planning* strategy. In his metaphor, managers are craftspeople who bring an intimate knowledge of their work to the materials at hand as they address corporate capabilities and future opportunities.

Some people find it easy to conceptualize an overall mission as a first step. Others find it similar to writing the abstract before the contents of a research paper. If your group is having difficulty getting past obvious mission statements that sound like "Our mission is to provide critical care services" you may want to try a different approach. You may find that a more effective route is to start in the middle with some tangible goals. Draft three to six broad goals that encompass the range of services important to the future of your program. How far in the future should you project? A useful exercise is to ask your group "What might we look like in 10 or 20 years? In order to be ready, what should we aim for in 5 years, 3 years, next year?" Draft goals that are both tangible and intangible. In their book "Strategic Analysis and Action", Fry and Killing[3] describe "hard" goals as measures of economic performance and position and "soft" goals as those used to describe the values that drive a business. In the case of health care, hard goals are measurable achievements in clinical outcome, resources utilization, or status of education and research programs. Soft goals should be expressed as the values inherent in the patient care relationships or of the academic programs provided. It is more difficult to define soft or intangible goals in measurable terms. Ratings by trainees or from patient satisfaction questionnaires may be a reasonable way to develop such measures.

Now return to the task of drafting a mission statement in three to four sentences. Your goals should suggest a "bigger picture." Collins and Porras[4] suggest that a "vision consists of two major components—a *Guiding Philosophy* that, in the context of expected future environments, leads to a *Tangible Image*." The "Guiding Philosophy" represents the values and principles of a company, or in this case, a program. The "Tangible Image" creates a vivid description of the mission that is alive and engaging. What underlying values does your program espouse? What vivid image will distinguish your program from other programs? What priorities or limitations exist in terms of the population you will serve or the services you will provide? The mission of a regional referral center will naturally differ from a community hospital, an academic program will emphasize different aspects than even its member institutions. Try to capture this uniqueness in your mission statement. The development of a mission statement and goals will be an iterative process. Read the mission statement followed by your goals. They should "fit" each other. They should capture the vision you have for your program. You should feel confident that achieving the stated goals will create the program described in your mission statement.

Associate with each goal a list of specific, measurable objectives or short-term goals. Where possible, set a time line by which to achieve each objective. Measurable objectives provide targets of achievement and a means by which to evaluate your success. Written, measurable objectives create an immediate commitment to their achievement. Adding target dates increases the tendency for action! Instead of "improve management of nursing personnel", state your intentions to "reduce nursing turnover from 20% to 10% in 1 year". At year end your team could argue about whether or not nursing was improved, but there will be no doubt as to whether turnover reached 10%. Research objectives can include targets for agencies to be approached, number of grants to be written, and dollar amounts to be received. Educational programs may want to implement a new course, increase number of trainees, or raise the score on their internal reviews. When you encounter problems achieving short-term goals it will help to focus on your long-term goals. When the long-term goals seem unattainable, the achievement of short-term goals will provide reassurance.

Of greatest importance, and often most difficult to measure, is the commitment to improve patient care or reduce resource utilization. Programs that keep their own statistics on morbidity, mortality, and resource consumption may find it difficult to compare changes over time without a reliable adjustment for patient acuity. Even more difficult is finding a gold standard to compare performance against your peers. Where no standards exist, create ones with meaning for your program. An interim goal of your program may be the development of such quantifiable measurement tools for use in the future.

The document should also include a description of the factors that will prove key to the successful achievement of the objectives. These "key success factors" represent obstacles to be overcome or avoided, the commitment of resources, or simply the cooperation of others. At this point, the working group is wise to share a draft of their strategic directions with the other stakeholders. This provides an opportunity for helpful feedback and a way to obtain early commitment from a wider audience.

As a final check, return to the expectations prepared in advance of the planning process and the issues described in the situational analysis. Have expectations been met to the best of your abilities? Have issues been addressed in a practical way? If not, why? Did the planning process raise new issues that were more important or should your group rethink their proposed strategies?

Your mission statement and goals describe a path by which to address the needs of your community and uses your strengths and minimizes your weaknesses. The objectives provide a clear and measurable interpretation of the goals to facilitate implementation and a means by which to measure success. Strategies should answer the question "What do we want to do?"

Action Plan (How Will We Do It?)

Don't stop now. Pinpointing a destination is only the first step in completing the journey. In order to map out your route, you must determine the specific steps to be undertaken by the end of 1, 3, and 5 years to achieve the objectives. The working group can invite those responsible for implementation to assist in the development of the implementation plan. A thorough action plan must address:

1. time frame and priorities,
2. person(s) responsible for tasks,
3. resource requirements including staff, skills, and operational and capital budgets, and
4. re-evaluation and measurement of progress against stated objectives.

An action plan establishes a list of priorities for the implementation and periodic evaluation of the progress made in achieving the objectives. The action plan answers the question "How, when, and by whom, will our goals and objectives be achieved?"

Implement the Action Plan (Let's Go!)

The action plan will outline a list of specific steps to be accomplished over the course of the upcoming year, over the next 3 and 5 years. Depending on the breadth of your specific goals and objectives, the assignment of tasks may vary. In some manner, however, the leader of your program should be able to identify an individual or team responsible for each objective, the process by which it will be achieved, the time frame for its completion, and a means by which to measure progress throughout the year.

The leader of your working group or program should meet with individuals or the team periodically to review completion of the action plan and to deal with any problems or changes that may be necessary.

It would be unrealistic to suggest that simply writing a plan will make it so. Obstacles will arise; many of which are predictable. Understanding these obstacles and developing predetermined steps to manage them will facilitate the achievement of your goals and limit the frustration of those in charge of achieving them. Further reinforcement is required for the dogged determination to follow through with your plan. Any means by which your team can visualize the rewards of achieving your goals will assist in creating and constantly reinforcing the desire to move step by step through your action plan.

Measure Success and Re-evaluate (Have We Achieved Our Goals and Objectives?)

A strategic plan should be reviewed on a yearly basis before capital or operational budgeting time. As mentioned before, understanding what you have achieved last year and what you want to achieve in the upcoming years will facilitate budgeting and operational decisions. A complete redraft of your original document is not required every year unless your environment changes dramatically. A yearly review should produce a brief addendum for the situational analysis as necessary. The bulk of the yearly review will be a report on achievements in the preceding year and a restatement of the strategic directions with a revised 1-, 3-, and 5-year action plan.

Summary

A commitment to move continuously through the cycle of strategic planning is not a task for the faint of heart. For the physician it means new language, new skills, and new partnerships. For all participants it is "front-end loaded" with a commitment of time and energy. The rewards come from a team satisfied when worthwhile goals are achieved and united in the pursuit of a common vision to meet the needs of its community, institution, and staff in an effective and efficient manner.

References

1. Henderson BD: The Origin of strategy. Harvard Bus Rev 1989;67(6):139.
2. Mintzberg H: Crafting strategy. Harvard Bus Rev 1987;65(4):66.
3. Fry JN, Killing PJ: Strategic Analysis and Action. Second Edition. Scarborough, Ontario, Prentice-Hall Canada Inc., 1989, p. 4.
4. Collins JC, Porras JI: Organizational vision and visionary organizations. California Management Rev 1991, Fall.

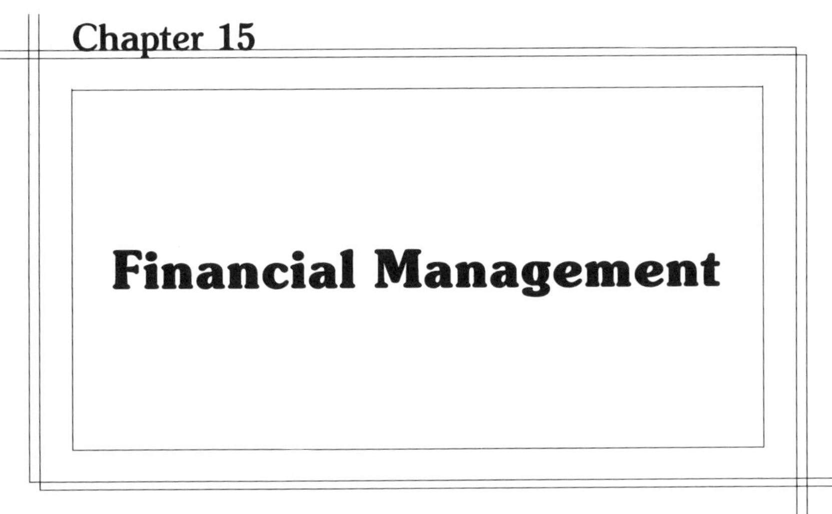

Chapter 15

Financial Management

E. Richard Brownlee II, C.P.A., B.B.A., M.B.A., Ph.D.

To be effective in the current health care environment, critical care unit CCU managers must have an appreciation of the financial consequences of their decisions. Most intensivists understand the need for relevant financial information at both the system and the unit level, but, in general, they do not have the background to deal with the types, quantity, and level of detail of financial data that can be required. The purpose of this chapter is to provide a fundamental framework of financial concepts and applications germane to the management of CCUs in the present climate.

It is important at the outset to acknowledge the limitations of financial information as it pertains to the decision-making process. This is particularly true in areas such as acute care medicine where decisions can have direct and immediate personal implications. This chapter does not attempt to posit quality of life or other personal issues in financial

---

From: Sibbald WJ, Massaro T (eds.): The Business of Critical Care: A Textbook for Clinicians Who Manage Special Care Units. © Futura Publishing Co., Inc., Armonk, NY, 1996.

terms, but rather it takes the position that health care management requires numerous complex and difficult decisions, many of which can be enhanced by informed financial analysis.

The Need For Scorecards

Suppose that late one sunny summer afternoon you and a group of colleagues decide to go to the stadium to watch the Blue Jays play the Yankees. You have a few things to finish at the office, so you tell the others to go on ahead and you will meet them at the ballpark. You don't get away as early as you planned, and the Toronto traffic is worse than usual. You arrive at the stadium about 15 minutes past game time. Once inside, the first thing you do is check the scoreboard. Why? Because you want to know what happened before you arrived. Of course, the only things you can learn pertain to the number of innings played and the number of runs, hits, and errors attributable to both teams. But, at least it's a start.

Fortunately, you are seated right next to someone who enjoys keeping the detailed scorebook contained in the printed program. Thus, she is able to give you a detailed description of everything that has occurred prior to your arrival. You thank her and ask her why she keeps the scorebook. She replies that it helps her see aspects of the game that she otherwise wouldn't notice and it contains information that she finds useful as the game proceeds. You ask her if it's difficult to learn how to keep the scorebook. Her reply surprises you a little, for she says that it isn't hard at all once you understand the game.

There are, in fact, a number of different scorecards being kept at the stadium that evening, all of which are designed to serve the information needs of a variety of different users. The most detailed scorebooks are, of course, those kept for the most sophisticated and interested users—the team managers. Those scorebooks will contain whatever historical data the managers believe might be useful to them. Sportswriters will be keeping somewhat different scorecards intended to provide the basis for a subsequent article that describes the entire game in a manner that is both factual and interesting. Obviously, some data, such as the final score, are of such importance that they will appear on all of the various scorecards. The extent to which additional data are recorded depends on the information needs of various parties, some of whom will use the data to assist them in making future decisions.

Like baseball managers, medical directors of ICUs need scorecards that not only provide an accurate account of the past, but are also useful in making decisions that will help shape the future. The number and types of scorecards maintained are constrained only by the availability of data and the costs associated with data collection. At some point, the benefits derived from additional data are simply not worth the additional costs that would be incurred. Also, at some point, information overload occurs. The next section discusses three different but related types of business scorecards written in a health care context.

Understanding the Scorecards

Hospitals are comprised of many different types of resources: buildings, equipment, physicians, nurses, and technicians are but a few examples. From a management perspective, all hospital resources can be thought of as falling into one of three categories: physical resources, human resources, and financial resources. It is the financial resources that provide the means for obtaining the physical and human resources. Hospitals obtain financial resources through donations, selling equity interests (i.e., some type of ownership), borrowing, or profit retention. Because all resources have an identifiable source, the following fundamental relationship exists:

$$\text{Resources} = \text{Source of Resources}$$

Organizational resources are commonly referred to as assets, and the two principal resource sources are debt (i.e., liabilities) and equity. The three most important types of hospital equity are donations, ownership capital, and earnings that have been retained and reinvested. Thus, the previous equation can be restated as follows:

$$\text{Assets} = \text{Liabilities} + \text{Equity}$$

This fundamental relationship provides the basis for understanding a hospital's financial position and how it is affected by a variety of daily activities.

Traditionally, most organizations have periodically prepared three basic financial statements as a means of assessing the financial consequences of their activities. These are the *balance sheet* (also called the statement of financial position), the *income statement* (also called the profit and loss statement, or the statement of earnings), and the *cash flow statement*. Although these financial statements were originally intended primarily for interested external parties such as creditors, investors, or governmental entities, they also contain information of consid-

Table 1
Hypothetical Hospital: Balance Sheet, December 31 ($000)

Assets	1994	1995	Liabilities	1994	1995
Cash	$ 1,200	$ 1,400	Accounts Payable	$ 1,900	$ 2,200
Accts. Rec.	$ 2,400	$ 2,100	Accrued Liabilities	$ 2,500	$ 3,300
Inventory	$ 1,000	$ 950	Long-term Debt	$10,000	$10,000
Land	$ 1,500	$ 1500	Equity		
Bldg and Equip. (Net)	$19,200	$20,000	Capital Stock	$ 8,000	$ 8,000
			Retained Earnings	$ 2,900	$ 2,450
Total Assets	$25,300	$25,950	Total Liab. & Equity	$25,300	$25,950

erable relevance to management. As a means of providing a framework for explanation, simplified financial statements are presented in Tables 1–3.

The balance sheet shown in Table 1 is intended to present the financial position of Hypothetical Hospital as of December 31, 1994 and December 31, 1995. In essence, a balance sheet presents a snapshot of an organization as of a particular point in time. In doing so, it shows both the nature and the dollar amounts of an organization's assets, liabilities, and equity. *Assets* are items that have value to the organization,

Table 2
Hypothetical Hospital: Income Statement, Year Ended December 31, 1995 ($000)

Gross Revenue		$22,000
Less: Contractual Allowances and Uncollectible Accounts		$ 3,300
Net Revenue		$18,700
Operating Expenses:		
Salaries and Wages	$10,800	
Other Personnel Costs	$ 500	
Medicines and Supplies	$ 1,100	
Equipment Rental	$ 600	
Depreciation-Bldg. & Equipment	$ 800	
Utilities	$ 400	
General and Administrative	$ 3,250	
Total Operating Expenses		$17,450
Operating Income		$ 1,250
Less: Interest Expense		$ 800
Income		$ 450

Table 3
Hypothetical Hospital: Statement of Cash Flows, Year Ended December 31, 1995 ($000)

Income	$ 450
Add: Non-cash Expenses	
Depreciation	$ 800
Net Income Adjusted	$1,250
Change in Balance Sheet Account Balances:	
Inc. in Accounts Receivable	$ 300)
Inc. in Inventory	$ (50)
Dec. in Accounts Payable	$ (300)
Dec. in Accrued Liabilities	$ (800)
Decrease in Cash	$ (200)
Add: Beginning Balance	$1,400
Ending Balance	$1,200

Decreases in cash are shown as ( ).

primarily because they have purchasing power, will be sold, or will be used in the process of providing goods and services. Cash and accounts receivable are shown at amounts representing their net realizable values (i.e., estimated uncollectible accounts have been excluded from the accounts receivable balance, which is the reason for the use of the term "net"). Inventory and land are shown at historical cost. Buildings and equipment are shown at original cost less the total amount of depreciation expense recognized since they were acquired. So, the term "buildings and equipment-net" means original cost minus total accumulated depreciation. More will be said about the concept of depreciation later in this chapter.

Notice that the balance sheet does not show any asset that represents physicians, nurses, technicians, or any other human resources, even though these resources are believed to be the ones that are the most important. The reason for this omission is that they are not owned by the hospital. They are used by the hospital, however, and represent operating expenses to be shown in the hospital's income statement. Because employees have the right to seek employment elsewhere, they cannot be considered as assets of the hospital where they presently work. If somehow an attempt were made to show human resources in the balance sheet, the difficult issue of determining the appropriate dollar amount would have to be resolved. The exclusion of human resources from traditional balance sheets is a good example of the type of limitations that are inherent in traditional financial statements.

Liabilities are debts or obligations of an organization that are usually settled through the payment of cash, the delivery of products, or the performance of services. Most organizations also have a number of potential liabilities that may arise in the future as a result of past occurrences. These are referred to as contingent liabilities and are not shown in the balance sheet until such time as they appear to be both probable and estimable. Guidance for the presentation of contingent liabilities and for all other types of financial statement and financial reporting issues can be found through reference to "generally accepted accounting principles" applicable to a particular country. The concept of establishing "generally accepted international accounting standards" has widespread support but its implementation is a long way off.

Equity refers to the investment that the owners have made in an organization either through the purchase of ownership shares (i.e., capital stock) or through the retention of profits (i.e., retained earnings). Non-profit hospitals often refer to their equity as *surplus*. The relationship between an organization's debt and its equity is referred to as financial leverage. The larger the debt/equity relationship, the more highly leveraged an organization becomes. The tax deductibility of interest makes debt a desirable source of assets. A key management issue, then, is determining the appropriate level of debt, because too much leverage can lead to financial disaster.

The income statement shown in Table 2 is intended to present a representative measure of profitability for Hypothetical Hospital for the year ending December 31, 1994. Another way of stating it is that an income statement portrays the financial affects of operational activities that increase and decrease an organization's equity. The income statement contains two major categories: revenues and expenses. Revenues are increases in an organization's net assets (i.e., assets less liabilities) resulting from the sale of products or the delivery of services. For hospitals, this would include billings for such things as medicines, food, rooms, physicians, nurses, technicians, and testing. Revenues are considered to be earned (and, therefore, should be reflected in the income statement) as soon as products are sold or services are rendered. Notice that revenue will frequently be recognized prior to the actual receipt of cash. This approach is referred to as the *accrual basis* of revenue recognition and provides a fairer representation of revenue than would be the case if revenue were recognized on a cash basis.

Expenses are decreases in an organization's net assets that occur in connection with the revenue generation process. For hospitals, these would include the costs associated with providing medicines, food, and rooms, with performing tests, and with the costs associated with physicians, nurses, and technicians. Expenses are also recognized on an accrual basis, meaning that they are recorded at the time they are incurred, which is frequently at a different time than when actual cash is paid. Thus, an organization's income or loss as presented in its income statement is calculated on the "accrual basis of accounting." Over the entire life of an organization, accrual-basis income and cash basis income will be identical. Nevertheless, the timing of the periodic income recognized, can be substantially different under the two methods. For purposes of measuring ongoing financial performance, the accrual basis provides the fairest representation.

The lack of usefulness of cash-basis accounting for periodic income determination should not be interpreted as suggesting that periodic cash flow data are not useful. The notion of "don't run out of cash" is one of considerable importance to managers of all organizations. It is for this reason that the statement of cash flows is prepared. As illustrated in Table 3, traditional cash flow statements begin with income as shown in the income statement (using accrual accounting) and end with the ending cash balance shown in the balance sheet. Depreciation expense is added back because it was deducted in calculating the $450 income figure, but depreciation does not cause a corresponding cash outflow. Therefore, as a non-cash expense, depreciation is added for the purpose of calculating a type of cash basis income, called net income adjusted in Table 3. The additional adjustments reflect the effects that other balance sheet account changes have on the ending cash balance. Note that increases in assets cause the cash balance to decrease and that decreases in liabilities also cause the cash balance to decrease. Therefore, the overall change in the cash balance for Hypothetical Hospital during 1995 was a decrease in the amount of $200. Notice that the balance sheet, income statement, and cash flow statement are interdependent and represent three ways of looking at and understanding an organization. The balance sheet shows financial position at a point in time, the income statement reflects profitability over a period of time, and the cash flow statement portrays cash sources and uses over the same time period. All three statements contain useful information.

Before concluding this section, some explanation is needed regarding the process by which organizational activities are reflected in the financial statements. Generally speaking, activities can be classified into two categories: events and transactions. *Events* are activities that, for a variety of reasons, are viewed as not affecting an entity's assets, liabilities, or equity and, consequently, do not receive financial statement recognition. Examples include employment contracts, short-term leases, and purchase and sales commitments. *Transactions* are activities that affect an entity's net assets and, therefore, do receive financial statement recognition. Examples include purchasing supplies, obtaining a bank loan, and providing medical care. When transactions occur, the resulting effects on an entity's net assets are reflected through changes in its balance sheet. The income statement and the cash flow statement may or may not also be affected. Stated differently, some transactions affect only the balance sheet, some the balance sheet and income statement, some the balance sheet and cash flow statement, and some affect all three financial statements.

The fundamental process through which transactions are recorded in the accounting records of organizations is actually rather logical, and it is based on the equation: Assets = Liabilities + Equity. The mechanism used to record transactions is called an account, and in its simplest form it resembles the letter "T". Thus, each account has a left side and a right side. Just as there are useful rules and techniques for keeping a baseball scorebook, the same is true for "keeping the books" of organizations. The overall system is called the double-entry system of accounting, and it requires that every transaction be recorded such that equal amounts are placed on the left side of some accounts and on the right side of other accounts using the following convention:

Asset Accounts		=	Liability Accounts		+	Equity Accounts	
Left	Right		Left	Right		Left	Right
Increases	Decreases		Decreases	Increases		Decreases	Increases

For example, a $50,000 10% interest bank loan would be recorded as follows:

Cash (A)		Bank Loan Payable (L)	
Left	Right	Left	Right
$50,000			$50,000

This transaction affects both the balance sheet and the cash flow statement, but it does not affect the income statement. If the loan plus interest were paid off a year later, it would be recorded as follows, with the $5,000 decrease in equity representing interest expense:

Cash (A)		Bank Loan Payable (L)		Equity	
Left	Right	Left	Right	Left	Right
	$55,000	$50,000		$5,000	

This transaction is one that affects the balance sheet, the income statement, and the cash flow statement.

useful to managers. Perhaps the most widely applicable concept, particularly where a decision requires cost benefit tradeoffs, is that of relevancy. This involves the identification of both relevant benefits, including revenues, and relevant costs. Relevant benefits and costs are those that result from a specific decision or course of action. In essence, they result from managerial choices. An important component of relevant cost analysis is understanding the cost behavior patterns of the costs under consideration. The two major cost behavior patterns are fixed and variable. Fixed costs remain constant over relatively large increases in volume or output. Thus, the greater the volume, the less the cost per unit of output. For example, suppose the monthly rent for a building serving as a hospital annex is fixed at $1,000. If 100 patients are cared for during the month, then rent expense per patient is $10. If, however, 200 patients are cared for, then the net expense per patient becomes $5. So, costs that are fixed over a specific time period become variable when expressed in per unit terms.

Variable costs increase in total with increases in volume or output. Expressed on a per unit basis, however, true variable costs remain constant. For example, suppose the cost of a certain medication is $20 per vial. If 10 vials are used, then the total cost is $200. If 50 vials are used then the total cost of medication is $1,000. The cost per vial, however, remains constant at $20.

In reality, fixed costs are more appropriately thought of as consisting of a series of cost levels that remain constant for a while and then increase to a new level for a while. Thus, the terms semifixed, or step, costs are used.

Understanding how costs are expected to behave at different levels of output or service is critically important in analyzing the financial consequences of alternative courses of action. Although both fixed and variable costs can be relevant to management decisions, frequently fixed costs are not relevant to shorter-term decisions because they won't be affected. It should be mentioned that, for ease of explanation, the terms cost and expense are being used interchangeably. Technically, however, cost usually refers to the amount paid to acquire an asset. As the asset is used or consumed, part of the cost must be recognized in the income statement as an expense. For example, if a hospital purchases new equipment and pays $2 million, then the cost assigned to the equipment is $2 million. If management estimates that the equipment will have a useful life of 10 years, then the annual depreciation expense (calculated on a straight-line basis) is $200,000. From a financial reporting perspective, the concept of depreciation is one of allocating the cost of an asset to an expense to be deducted in calculating operating income. In essence, the concept of depreciation allows the costs associated with long-lived assets to be allocated as expenses to all of the time periods during which they are used. The other options would be to expense the entire cost when a long-lived asset is purchased, expense the entire cost of the end of the asset's useful life, or not expense it at all. Accrual accounting takes the position that all costs associated with providing goods and services should be deducted from the revenues earned in a manner that results in a true and fair reflection of periodic income. For long-lived assets, this means gradual expense recognition through recording depreciation. The resulting *book value* amount shown in the balance sheet (book value is the original cost less the total amount of depreciation recognized) is *not* intended to be an approximation of the asset's fair market value. Thus, depreciation can be thought of as a process of cost allocation and not as a process of asset valuation.

Costs are also categorized based on their linkage to products or services. Those that are readily associated with and traceable to specific products and services are called *direct* costs; those that aren't are called *indirect* costs. Some costs are easily classified into these two categories, and some costs are not. The importance of thinking in terms of direct and indirect costs comes from the realization that, in order to determine the "full cost" of producing a specific product or providing a specific service, some means of allocating the indirect costs to individual products and services must be established. Thus, another important cost related concept is that of allocated costs. *Allocated* costs are those indirect costs that management has assigned to specific time periods (e.g., depreciation) or to specific products or services based on some predetermined, rational allocation method. More will be said about the importance of and approaches to cost allocation in the next section on activity-based costing.

Of all of the different costing concepts, none are more important than the final two discussed in this section. These are sunk costs and opportunity costs. *Sunk* costs are those that have already been incurred and, therefore, can't be changed. Therefore, they have no relevance to any subsequent management decision. To repeat, sunk costs should never influence a decision. The problem is that they often do, and the reason they do is that the decision makers have a psychological attachment to them.

Opportunity costs are those that represent the current fair market values associated with certain decision alternatives. Thus, opportunity costs are relevant to management decisions. To illustrate, suppose that you own 100 shares of stock in a publicly-traded company and that you paid $75 per share. You find that you have a need for additional cash, and one option is to sell your stock. You check the current market price and discover that the stock is selling at $60 per share. Your immediate reaction is that you shouldn't sell your stock because if you do, you will suffer a loss of $15 per share, which adds up to a total loss of $1,500. You have now become a victim of the "sunk cost trap." You can't change the fact that you paid $75 per share (even though you wish you could—but remember, you thought $75 per share was a real bargain when you bought the stock), so it represents a sunk cost and, except for calculating any tax consequences on the sale, has no relevance whatsoever to your decision. The current market price of $60 per share represents an opportunity cost and is extremely relevant to your decision. By deciding not to sell the stock, you are foregoing an opportunity to receive $6,000. Another way to look at it is that by deciding not to sell, you are deciding to invest $6,000 in that particular stock.

Now it may be that buying 100 shares of that stock for $60 per share would be a fantastic investment, but you won't know that unless you assess the true appreciation potential of the stock and then compare that investment with other investment options, including your current need for cash. Thus, the only logic for not selling the stock is that you honestly believe that the best $6,000 investment you could make is to buy 100 shares of that stock. The chances are good that you wouldn't reach that conclusion. So, the truth is that you have become psychologically attached to the $75 per share that you paid (i.e., the sunk cost) and it has become the major factor in your decision. As managers, this is an easy trap to fall into. In a hospital setting, an example would be an unwillingness to consider the purchase of new equipment because, unaware that substantial improvements in the equipment were forthcoming, similar equipment with fewer capabilities was recently purchased. Another example pertains to research and development expenditures, and it has to do with the temptation to continue to go forward with the project because "we have already spent millions of dollars" which will be lost if the project is cancelled. The appropriate analysis involves realistic estimates of future expenditures that will be necessary to complete the project and realistic estimates of the expected benefits.

Activity-Based Costing

One of the important lessons learned from the competitive environment of the 1980s was that many organizations did not have internal costing systems that provided them with accurate information regarding what it really costs to produce individual products or provide individual services. The costing systems used did provide accurate data regarding the total cost of all products or services, or regarding groups of products or services, but simply weren't adequate at the individual product or service level. When competitive pressures brought about the need for accurate product-specific or service-specific cost data, many cost systems were found to be deficient.

A new approach to cost information systems known as activity-based costing (ABC) has emerged in response to the need for more accurate cost data. Initially developed for manufacturing settings, ABC has proven to be equally useful for service environments.* The focus of ABC is on indirect costs (i.e., those not easily traceable to individual products or services). Notwithstanding, that many indirect costs are relatively fixed in the short-term, ABC takes a long-term perspective and accepts the position that, over time, indirect costs can be changed and, therefore, be a focus of management attention.

Although not limited to these, ABC has two primary benefits in a hospital setting: it provides accurate information about the costs that are incurred in providing each of the numerous patient services; and it motivates administrative and management personnel to think differently and in ways that should lead to more efficient and effective health care. A key concept of ABC is that of an "activity". ABC uses activities as the basis for allocating indirect (i.e., support) costs to individual patient services. By identifying the links between performance of particular activities and the demands those activities make on a hospital's resources, managers can focus their attention on eliminating non value-added activities and on improving the value-added activities that consume substantial resources. Value-added activity improvements come from improved patient care, the ability to serve more patients, and more effective utilization of capital resources.

There are three essential steps in establishing an ABC system: (1) Identify the individual outputs (i.e., services) and the activities that support them; (2) define the links between activities and outputs; and (3) develop the costs associated with each activity. A hospital's outputs can be thought of as a patient's stay and associated services. Patients are billed for some services separately, and some services are included in the daily room charge. Generally, different daily room rates are

---

* This section is based on a more comprehensive discussion of activity based costing contained in "Activity-Based Costing in Service Industries," William Rotch, *Journal of Cost Management*, Summer 1990.

charged based on the type of room (e.g., single or double) and the type of care (e.g., critical care). Within each different unit (e.g., critical care or obstetrics), all patients are typically charged the same daily rate for the same type of room. Frequently, however, the amount of nursing care needed by patients within the same hospital unit can vary significantly. By treating the service output as "a patient day's stay in the hospital," the hotel, feeding, and nursing costs were all aggregated and billed as a single amount, one that represented some type of overall average. ABC would define at least two types of service output; nursing service for a specific acuity level, and hotel and food. This would require each unit's head nurse to rate based on some type of relative scale (say from 1 to 5) the amount of nursing care expected to be needed by each patient in the unit. Nursing charges would then be billed according to the acuity level designated and would appear as a separate daily hospital charge. Thus, nursing care is treated as a distinct activity and is not aggregated with hotel and food. A key component of implementing such an ABC system is an in-depth analysis of the types of nursing skills required in each unit, the frequency with which these skills are needed, and the costs associated with the nurses processing them. These types of cost data allow management to identify ways of making the units more cost effective, enhance managements' ability to prepare flexible budgets (discussed in the next section), and result in more representative patient charges.

Budgeting

Although there are many different types of budgets, all of them can be thought of as "written plans for the operation of an organization, stated in quantitative terms, that cover a specific period of time." Budgets are normally expressed in terms of dollars, but other measures of volume or activity are sometimes used. They represent agreed upon plans and are based on decisions made and conclusions reached as part of a comprehensive planning process. Thus, the budgeting process is not a stand-alone activity but one that must be linked to an organization's goals and strategies.

This section presents a brief overview of three types of budgets that are commonly prepared by hospitals: Operating budgets, cash budgets, and capital budgets. Of these, operating budgets and capital budgets have particular relevance to ICUs. An *operating budget* is a projection of expected revenues and expenses for all or part of an organization for a specified time period. Frequently the time period is a year, and it is usually subdivided into months. Sometimes operating budgets prepared by segments or units of an organization will contain only estimated expenses based on a predetermined level or previously predetermined levels of activity. Budgets that show expected expenses for a single activity level are called fixed or static, whereas those that contain expected expenses for multiple activity levels are called flexible budgets.

The preparation of an operating budget requires input from numerous people within the organization or part thereof. In fact, one of the most important benefits of the budgeting process is the internal communication and coordination it requires. Operating activities must be examined and planned in considerable detail before an operating budget can be completed. In many ways, then, the budgeting process brings a discipline to the entire planning process. Operating budgets also serve as guides for subsequent actions and as means of communicating the financial consequences expected to result from the implementation of agreed-upon operating plans. Once adopted, operating budgets sometimes represent the authority to spend the amounts specified, and they also provide a basis for analyzing how actual operations compare to plans. Thus, budgets are an important part of a management control system. Still, the most useful aspect of any budgeting process is its impact on future decisions and not its "after the fact" comparisons.

Cash budgets are projections of future cash inflows and outflows for a specified period, typically a year subdivided into months. They are based on and reflect the cash flow consequences of planned activities represented in the operating budgets. The most common type of cash budget is one that contains a listing of expected cash receipts and cash disbursements. Another type of cash budget takes the form of the cash flow statement discussed earlier in this chapter. The only difference is that it presents projected rather than historical data.

Capital budgeting is the process of identifying desirable investments in long-lived assets such as buildings and equipment. Capital budgets are also an outgrowth of operating budgets, and capital budgeting decisions are some of the most important decisions an organization makes because the amounts involved are usually large and the long-term consequences are usually significant. Not surprisingly, most organizations have a well-defined and tightly-controlled capital budgeting process that requires extensive documentation, analysis, and top management approval.

Probably the two most common criteria for evaluating capital expenditures proposals are payback and return on investment (ROI). *Pay-*

back is the length of time (usually expressed in number of years) it is estimated it will take to recover the cost of the investment. The primary focus of payback analysis (and other types of capital expenditure analysis) is on projected cash flows. For taxpaying organizations, the focus is on after-tax cash flow. Thus, capital budgeting requires that numerous estimates and judgments be made regarding both the amounts and the timing of the cash benefits expected to result from alternative investments.

The *return on investment calculation* incorporates the concept of the "time value of money" and is commonly referred to as discounted cash flow (DCF) analysis. This concept is based on the notion that, because cash can always be invested at some positive rate of return, it is better to receive cash sooner rather than later. Another way of stating it is that the present value (i.e., the value today) of cash received sooner (say in 1 year) is greater than the present of the same amount of cash received later (say in 2 years). This means that a project that is expected to result in large cash inflows beginning far out in the future may be less desirable than another project that is expected to result in smaller cash inflows that begin in the very near future. To elaborate on the concept present value, suppose you invested $1,000 in a bank of an interest rate of 10%. At the end of 1 year, you would have $1,100 in your bank account. Another way to look at the same situation is to say that the present value of receiving $1,100 1 year from now, if you desire a 10% return on your money, is $1,000. It can also be said that the rate of return that equates receiving $1,100 1 year from now with $1,000 today is 10%. The 10% can be thought of as the ROI of investing $1,000 for 1 year, at which time $1,100 is received in return.

Calculating the ROI of capital investment proposals requires the following five steps:

1. Determine the cash cost of the project.
2. Determine the expected life of the project. This means estimating the appropriate time period over which to perform the financial analysis.
3. Determine the amount and the timing of estimated cash benefits resulting from the project.
4. Determine any terminal value estimated for the project at the end of the time period used in the analysis.
5. Using DCF analysis, calculate the ROI for the project.

This discussion is not intended to be so comprehensive as to provide the basis for performing capital budgeting calculations, for this can be done by the financial personnel within an organization. It is, however, intended to provide an overview of the capital budgeting process. With that in mind, there are a few other managerially-relevant points that need to be made. The first is that consideration needs to be given to some point to the risk of a project. As used here, risk means the likelihood that the projected cash benefits will be realized. Projects that carry greater risk should usually be expected to provide a greater return. The second point is to be clear just why a project is being proposed. It is expected to result in better services and will the better services mean additional cash benefits? It is intended to result in cost reductions? Is it a defensive investment needed to "keep up" with the competition? The point here is that the reason for the proposed project needs to be well-defined.

The third and last point has to do with the time period over which to perform the financial analysis. This can be particularly difficult for hospitals trying to make a decision regarding the purchase of new equipment when the type of equipment under consideration is subject to rapid technological change. Perhaps the initial question to be answered pertains to the extent to which the capabilities of the new equipment over and above those of the existing equipment are really needed. It is easy to get caught up in the technological revolution and lose sight of just what capabilities are really essential. Next, the temptation to "wait for the next generation" must be resisted. Certainly consideration must be given to future price reductions or enhanced capabilities, yet, unless they can be identified with reasonable certainty, they probably should not influence the time horizon over which a proposed piece of equipment is evaluated. Avoid trying to incorporate "risk of obsolescence" into the analysis simply by shortening the expected useful life of a proposed project. As the time horizon shortens, so does the project's ROI. Generally speaking, next generation equipment is longer in coming, costs more than expected, and doesn't do all that was expected.

As a final thought, the capital budgeting process described here deals only with the quantitative aspects. There are usually important qualitative dimensions that also must be considered before any decisions are reached. Sometimes the qualitative aspects dominate the decision, particularly in settings such as hospitals where personal welfare concerns are paramount.

Chapter 16

Managing the Educational Process

Brenda L. Morgan, R.N., CNCC(c), B.ScN(cand), William J. Sibbald, M.D., FRCP, C.H.E.

The delivery of competent care depends upon adequate knowledge and training of caregivers, with education being an essential element of any critical care unit (CCU). One of the greatest challenges is to develop a program that not only provides for the information needs of staff, but actually contributes to improved patient outcomes. An ideal educational program facilitates the transfer of knowledge into clinical practice, promoting life-long learning. If a spirit of inquiry is encouraged as an essential ingredient to any unit's culture, education will be fostered. The end result will be a high standard of care and low patient morbidity.

Many educational programs are discipline specific, developed and presented by members of a given discipline to colleagues in the same area of practice. However, the multidisciplinary nature of CCUs requires members of the team to not only acquire a solid grasp of their own

From: Sibbald WJ, Massaro T (eds.): The Business of Critical Care: A Textbook for Clinicians Who Manage Special Care Units. © Futura Publishing Co., Inc., Armonk, NY, 1996.

unique roles, but to develop a thorough understanding of the specialty services provided by other members of the team. Critical care medical education must integrate the expertise from all subspecialties to ensure effective care for individuals with complex multi-organ insults.[1,2]

This need to integrate expertise from other subspecialties also applies to the various health disciplines represented in the CCU. While discipline specific education is important to develop mastery within that particular scope of practice, education should also promote the sharing of knowledge and skills in order to encourage collaboration and teamwork. The ability to draw from other specialties is vital to the provision of optimal holistic care.[3]

A relationship has clearly been demonstrated between positive patient outcomes and units where true collaboration exists.[4] The abilities to collaborate and communicate effectively, are almost as important as the mastery of clinical skills. Knowledge and expertise will not improve patient outcome if that knowledge is misinterpreted as a result of ineffective communication, or an inability to work efficiently as a team exists. Strategies to promote and foster collaboration and partnership development, are essential parts of any educational program.

Collaborative environments have also been shown to increase staff satisfaction and reduce turnover rates.[5] Given the high cost of training, programs which encourage long-term commitment and retention of experienced staff are essential in today's economy. When considering affordable programming, be wary of quick fix training; it may not be cost effective if staff are inadequately prepared or unsatisfied with their level of training.

There is a need to focus beyond the diagnostic and physiological treatment approach when dealing with the patient and family. For example, a lack of attention to the development of interviewing or psychosocial skills may leave new graduates from medical programs ill prepared to deal with ethical dilemmas or family crisis.[6] The complexity of the patient population in critical care requires caregivers to acquire skills in family support, and develop confidence when dealing with ethical challenges.

While education is essential to the development of expertise, the principles taught in any training session must be reflected in the clinical practice. A teaching session that describes a procedure or technique that is neither supported nor expected at the bedside is unlikely to impact favorably on actual practice. For education to alter outcome, content must be reinforced within the clinical setting.

The ever changing environment with a constant influx of new technologies and associated knowledge, necessitate continuous staff development. While introductory and basic critical care training may provide the infrastructure, the desire for continuing education must be a fundamental value of the unit environment to truly impact practice. One strategy to foster this culture is to approach education as a continuum of several components, which are linked together interdependently. These components include critical care theory development, skill acquisition, unit orientation, ongoing education, development of teamwork skills, and the promotion of a spirit of inquiry. The adequacy of each component must be continually evaluated and modified to ensure quality management is in place. Keeping in mind that the customers of any educational program include the learners, as well as the patients, attention to program design is as important as program content. The relationship between these components promotes a comprehensive educational program depicted schematically by Figure 1.

This chapter will introduce an approach to education within critical care that emphasizes learning as a continuous process. At the end of this chapter, the reader will be exposed to a number of strategies to

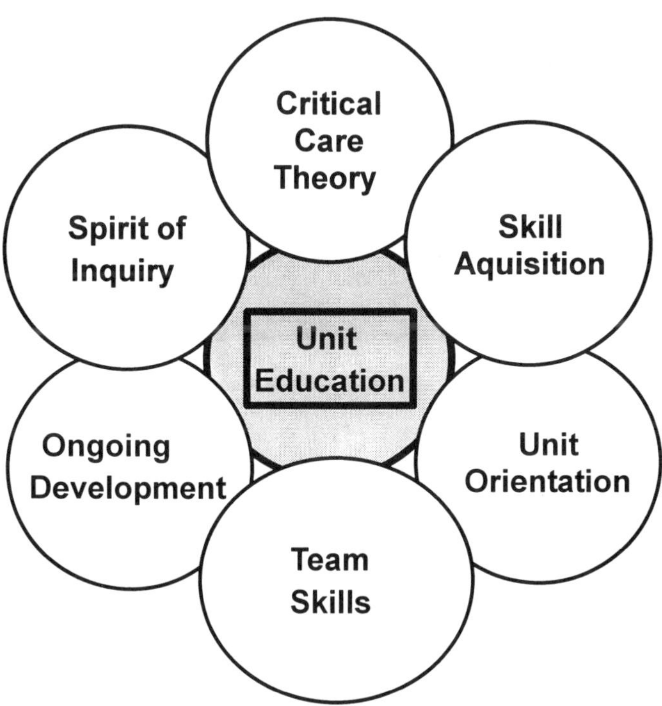

Figure 1.

Table 1
Unit Education

Component	Key Focus
1. Critical Care Theory	Basic critical care curriculum Formalized teaching content Combines classroom instruction with clinical application Program design will be influenced by past experience of learner and unit specific needs Provides foundation for critical thinking and successful skill application
2. Skill Acquisition	Period of developing mastery with critical care skills follows theoretical understanding of expected standard Facilitated by supervised clinical practice
3. Unit Orientation	Defines unit specific policies and procedures Introduces unit culture and norms Identifies supporting structures and lines of communication
4. Team Skills	Must be reflected in all training sessions Need to be demonstrated in the clinical environment Educational sessions to assist staff in role clarity and team building Promoted through multidisciplinary activities
5. Ongoing Development	Variety of mechanisms needed to ensure identification of staff development needs Needs to be directed by the learner Should provide opportunities to develop staff as educators
6. Spirit of Inquiry	Needs to be fostered through all aspects of unit activity Resources and support systems to encourage staff to challenge practice are important An environment where staff are free to question practice without risk is critical

promote enthusiasm for learning and foster a culture where ongoing development is a way of life (Table 1).

Critical Care Theory

Developing a critical care curriculum for new staff is often the starting point for education in any unit. The considerations outlined can be modified as needed to suit a unit's structure, the focus or discipline of the learner, and past training and experience. For example, new staff may obtain basic critical care theory by taking a mandatory certificate program as a prerequisite to hiring. Curriculum requirements will identify the minimum expectations for new members of the team; experienced individuals who demonstrate desired outcomes should be supported through curriculum modifications. The following aspects of curriculum development are not restricted to the initial critical care theory alone, but should be incorporated into all unit education.

Program Organization

Curriculum can be defined as a systematic group of "courses, sequence of subjects, and planned experiences".[7] The organization of program content should provide a logical flow of information that promotes integration of content into clinical practice. The curriculum can be organized to fit unit philosophy or specific models of practice. It is important that all relevant educational needs are included and the curriculum is organized to ensure prerequisite learning occurs in an orderly fashion. For example, it would be inappropriate to review interventions or treatment modalities for ARDS before ensuring that baseline knowledge of respiratory and cardiovascular physiology is sound.

Needs Analysis

The first step in developing any educational program is to perform a careful needs analysis. This will allow the program developer to establish content for the curriculum. Whether developing a new program or revising an existing one, it is important that the following needs are addressed.

An inventory of unit specific requirements is one of the first points to consider. For example, if your unit does not provide neurosurgical services, your unit training will be different from a unit that does. The admission criteria and technology interface need to be evaluated from a list of knowledge and training specifications. Once unit needs are established, a compilation of practice expectations should be formulated.

The next process of developing a training program is the identification of any standards for clinical practice or education related to the

Table 2
Examples of Standards for Care Givers in Critical Care

Standard	Author
Standards for Critical Care Nursing Practice	Canadian Association of Critical Care Nurses (1992)
Objectives of Specialty Training Requirements in Critical Care Medicine	Royal College of Physicians and Surgeons of Canada (1993)
Standards for Nursing Care of the Critically Ill	American Association of Critical Care Nurses (2nd 1989)
Outcome Standards for Nursing Care of the Critically Ill	American Association of Critical-Care Nurses (1990)
Guidelines for Program Content for Fellowship Training in Critical Care Medicine	Society of Critical Care Medicine (1992)

specific disciplines involved. Practice standards for nursing[8–10] and medicine[11,12] in critical care are defined and any unit curriculum should be consistent with these standards (Table 2). While modifications may be made to curriculum based on the experiences available within a specific unit, it would not be appropriate to develop an educational program where expectations for practice fall below the standard outlined by a given discipline. One test of a highly developed critical care program would be the ability of candidates to qualify for any national critical care specialty or certification program.[13–15] Advanced Cardiac Life Support is an example of a specific training expectation that might be required.

Development of Goals and Objectives

Each aspect of the course curriculum needs to be developed further with specific goals for training established. For example, if one of the unit needs involved care for patients with an intra-aortic balloon pump (IABP), the goal may be defined as "to provide safe care for a patient using an IABP". This goal would then be developed further into specific program objectives, clearly outlining what the expectation of the training will be. For the same IABP example, objectives might state that by the end of the training, candidates will be able to: identify indications for the use of the IABP; describe balloon pumping physiology; discuss complications; and demonstrate the use of the console. This intricate detailing of course content will promote consistency from program to program, and ensure that everyone involved in the process has a clear understanding of the training expectations.

Competency-Based Program

Pike states that "learning has not taken place until behavior has changed".[16] The observation of the behavior associated with training is the basis of competency-based programming. While many references for competency based orientations come from nursing curriculums,[17] competency based design can easily be adapted to the training for any discipline.

Competency-based programming focuses on the outcome of education rather than the process of learning. Transfer of training is described as "the effective and continuing application, by trainees to their job, of the knowledge and skills gained in training".[18] Simply instructing methodology or presenting information in no way guarantees that transfer will occur. Since the ultimate goal for any educational program is the optimization of performance, it makes sense that curriculum design should emphasize outcome or performance rather than process.

Competency statements are similar to behavioral objectives. They differ, however, because they specifically focus on the action the individual will carry out rather than the knowledge associated with it (Table 3). For example, a behavioral objective might state that a learner will "describe" the pathophysiology of angina, whereas, a competency statement would indicate that a learner will intervene to reduce symptoms of angina. One of the concepts behind measuring competencies is that knowledge can exist without being able to apply it to practice, whereas, knowledge is demonstrated by successful clinical application.

Competency based programs are particularly advantageous in critical care training. Each competency statement clearly defines what the expectation for clinical practice should be, so new staff can quickly perform a self analysis. This also simplifies evaluation and provides an easy mechanism to develop a program for experienced staff. Competency based programs identify clear criterion for what successful performance looks like, and may include concise checklists for clinical skills. This helps new learners to articulate each successful step in a process.

In addition to the ability to develop programs to match the level of previous experience, competency based programs permit individual-

Table 3
Examples of the Contrast between Goals and Objectives and Competency Statements

Goals	Objectives	Competency
To provide competent care in the management of the patient with angina.	Discuss signs and symptoms of myocardial ischemia. Describe interventions to reduce myocardial ischemia	Assesses the patient with angina. Intervenes appropriately to improve oxygen balance to the myocardium.
To provide endotracheal intubation.	Discuss the signs and symptoms of respiratory failure. State three indications for endotracheal intubation. Describe method of maintaining oxygenation and ventilation prior to intubation.	Recognizes the signs of respiratory failure. Assesses indications for endotracheal intubation. Intubates a patient while maintaining oxygenation and ventilation.

ized speed of movement through the program. The pace for movement through the curriculum will obviously have some limitations, for example, a new resident may only be in the CCU for 3 months, or a new staff member may be required to reach independent practice within a specific length of time.

Accrediting agencies view competency-based programs very positively when reviewing curriculum design. Quality management requires an emphasis on outcome and this provides an added bonus to competency-based design.[19]

Method of Instruction

Individual learners do not all integrate information in the same manner. Learning styles refer to the "typical ways a person behaves, feels, and processes information in learning situations".[20] Effective curriculum design needs to provide for the variation in learning styles. For example, one individual may learn best from a lecture format, while others may prefer self-study. A number of tools to assess learner styles are available. However, from a practical point of view, unless you are able to provide individualized one-on-one programming, it is a difficult issue to satisfy.

One of the most practical solutions to address learner style variance is to provide diversity in instruction by adding variety to the format. Provision of variety can be achieved by: using a holistic approach (involving learner's emotions, intellect, physical, and spiritual selves); by varying the program length; by using different mediums for teaching (e.g., overhead, slides, models, or flip charts); by changing the intensity of the experiences (a mixture of very intense or emotional content with content that is lighter and less energy draining); and through variation in techniques (e.g., lecture, group discussion, individual problem solving drills).[21] Short presentations followed by some hands-on application or group activity can help to reinforce information as well as provide variation in style. Varying instructional methods also provides a break to help reduce monotony.

Self-instructional programs can be developed to allow individualized pace setting and provide educational opportunities at times convenient to the learner. Examples include written information packages or computer-based programs, and can provide cost effective educational alternatives. In an effort to reduce the costs of training, recommendations for the development of self-instructional programs are often made. While this method of training can be very effective in the right situation, it is not the best solution for all training situations or learners.[22,23] While the increased access to educational support may be advantageous, the inability to critically analyze or discuss options can prove to be a limitation.

The Role of Facilitators

Traditionally, the bulk of teaching is facilitated by instructors from the same discipline as the learner. With a tremendous focus on multidisciplinary care models, partnerships in practice can be promoted if training is provided by instructors who demonstrate collaboration in their educational programs. While many programs allow for isolated lectures to members of one discipline from members of another, collaboration can be promoted even further. When patient care interventions are being discussed, strategies that encourage the integration expertise of other team members, helps to demonstrate partnership development. For example, care of a patient with pneumonia that promotes medical therapies, pharmacological agents, nursing interventions, physiotherapy maneuvers, nutritional support, and respiratory therapy, demonstrates activation of a true multidisciplinary plan of care.

One of the challenges faced when promoting multidisciplinary practice is the need to demonstrate mutual respect for the unique and joint contributions of the various members of the team. Collaborative programming is much more than physicians lecturing to other disciplines; collaborative programming should apply universally. If the expertise for developing knowledge and skill related to mechanical ventilators is highest in the respiratory therapy group, have them provide this training to all other disciplines. Or if experienced nursing staff have developed particular expertise with hemodynamic monitoring, their involvement in the training of new residents could be very beneficial. If the various members of the multi-disciplinary team are to work effectively together and demonstrate mutual respect, these relationships need to be nurtured from the beginning.

Training Partnerships

In order to influence outcomes through educational programming, methods that promote the transfer of training into the clinical setting are critical. Although education provides a foundation to support clinical decision making, alone, education does not guarantee changes to practice. Bard and Newstrom[24] describe the manager as the most significant player in the transfer of training. While information can be provided regarding the desired standard of care, unless that standard is expected in the clinical setting, training may not alter practice. A commitment to and support for education by the manager in any area is essential.

The role that the manager plays in ensuring that standards of care are maintained cannot be emphasized enough. The manager is also central to the identification of educational needs related to practice issues. As a cautionary note, it is important to differentiate between problems of compliance and knowledge deficits; education alone will not solve all practice issues.

In addition to the importance of managerial support to training, a commitment by the learner is also critical. One recognizes the saying about leading a horse to water; this truly applies to education. Being in a classroom does not ensure learning takes place. Prior to acceptance to a program, an agreement or learning contract from the trainee can help to enhance training as a partnership. This contract can be easily obtained by having learners identify their personal goals and objectives for the training session in consultation with the trainer.[25] If a competency-based curriculum is in place, learners can quickly review the program and readily identify their training needs.

Learners

Appreciation for the unique considerations of adult learners is important when developing programs. Knowles principles of andragogy (the art and science of helping adults learn) includes a set of assumptions that provide a framework for the training of adult learners (Table 4). These principles are outlined in Table 1.[26]

The "readiness to learn" principle values that critical opportunities exist when learning can be impacted. For example, individuals may have had little interest in learning how to use intraventricular drains, however, the need to learn may become critical the moment insertion of a drain is imminent. This demonstrates a valuable role for mentors or preceptors in a clinical setting. The presence of these experts at the time when critical learning needs arise, can significantly augment the educational process.[27]

Programs that incorporate realistic scenarios and case presentations assist learners to value the information presented as relevant to their area of clinical practice. Allowing learners to work through cases in a classroom setting encourages practical application of knowledge.

A final consideration when providing educational sessions for adults is a need for the physical environment to be conducive to learning. Adults need comfortable chairs, suitable room temperatures, and a relaxed learning environment. Simple things such as coffee and light snacks can heighten learning.

Table 4

Knowles' Principles of Adult Learning

Knowles' Principles of Adult Learning
Adults have a need to know why they should learn something.
Adults have a deep need to be self directed.
Adults become ready to learn when they experience in their life situations a need to know or be able to do something to perform more effectively and satisfyingly.
Adults enter a learning experience with a task-centered, problem-centered, or life-centered orientation to learning.
Adults are motivated to learn by both extrinsic and intrinsic motivations.

Mentoring

The transfer of knowledge to clinical practice is supported when combined with role models or mentors who are committed to nurturing new staff and assisting them in mastering skill application. Preceptorship programs also provide formalized instruction to mentors to help them to deal with learner style variations. Selection of preceptor candidates should be done carefully as these individuals set the standard for junior staff. Many individuals are excellent care providers, but have little patience with new learners. Others may provide efficient care, but have poorly developed communication skills. Identification of preceptors who possess a balance of these skills can be essential to successful mentoring.

In addition to the role played by preceptors, other members of the team should be expected to promote a supportive environment for new staff. According to Maslow's hierarchy of needs, individuals cannot self-actualize unless basic needs are met. These include a need for individuals to feel safe, sense that they belong, and have the ability to develop self-esteem.[28] An environment that supports and nourishes these needs will be more likely to reap the rewards of competent, committed caregivers.

Skills Acquisition

Skill acquisition is not separate from critical care theory; rather the two aspects of training are complementary. Skill acquisition is the application and mastery of techniques presented in initial training programs. Successful skill development depends on a solid knowledge base to guide problem solving and practice decisions.

Demonstration

The first step in skill acquisition is observation of a competent demonstration. Once the theory and principles have been defined, observation of a skilled role model will help to solidify the concept for the learner. This also provides a method of reinforcement and variation on teaching technique.

Practice

In order for proficiency with any new skill to develop, learners need opportunities to practice the skill with the aid of experienced mentors. For some skills, particularly where significant risk to a patient exists, mock situations in a lab setting may help to develop proficiency under less stressful circumstances.

Once competency in a lab situation has been demonstrated, opportunities to practice the skill in the clinical setting are required. Past clinical experiences and learner confidence will influence the amount of support and mentoring needed before independent practice is safe. New staff can be set up to fail or develop substandard practice if left to acquire skills with inadequate support. The level of support needed may be as simple as having an experienced mentor present to confirm that the skill is done well.

Criterion

The simplest method for assisting new staff to successfully achieve skill acquisition, is to provide clearly defined criteria that measures competency.[29] If each desired action or step in a new skill is outlined by measurable behavior, new staff can clearly identify how their practice should look, and take appropriate steps to ensure that they meet the standard. Expectations should be objective and criteria should be supported by current literature findings. This enables the development of objective evaluation tools.

Nursing has for many years used criterion evaluation when developing advanced practice skills, utilizing simple checklists to confirm successful completion of each step of an identified skill. Checklists can easily be adapted to training situations for any discipline in a CCU. The procedure for central line insertion or endotracheal intubation are examples where checklists could be easily applied (Table 5).

Unit Orientation

Unit orientation is essential for all new employees regardless of past experience, discipline, or level of competence. Staff need to know the practice standards, lines of communication, resource location and back-up support, in order to practice safely. Unit orientation answers

Table 5
Examples of Competency or Skill Checklist

Procedural Step	Successful Completion
Insertion of an Intravenous	
Washes hands	√
Collects equipment	√
Identifies potential site	√
Applies tourniquet	√
Distends vein	√
Preps skin	√
Secures vein	√
Inserts needle bevel up	√
Identifies blood return	√
Advances cannula	√
Removes needle	√
Connects IV	√
Evaluates flow	√
Secures and dresses site	√

the basic question, "how and why we do it here". Failure to provide appropriate direction may leave new staff feeling abandoned or confused. Institutions can be at risk for liability if adverse occurrences can be linked to failure to adequately educate staff regarding policies or procedures. Accrediting bodies have very clear expectations that new staff are provided with a unit orientation.

Team Skills

As already described, the importance of collaboration and teamwork in a multidisciplinary environment cannot be overstated. The value of partnership development and shared goals for patient outcome must be reflected in the philosophy, strategic planning, and everyday practice. In addition to ensuring a collaborative theme in basic critical care training, ongoing education and procedure development should include a multidisciplinary approach. While collaboration has become the "buzz" word of the 1990s, it is often easier to talk about than put into action. Every member of the team must constantly work towards its development; each individual must constantly strive to remedy situations that threaten teamwork.

Invariably, human beings bring to every situation an assortment of past experiences, values and beliefs which may interfere with team effectiveness. When obstacles develop, strategies need to be in place to assist team members to work through challenges and achieve positive outcomes. Mutual respect and honesty needs to exist in order for this to happen.

Through quality management monitoring strategies, variances in unit processes will occur from time to time.[30] These variances should be dealt with promptly to ensure optimal level of care. Often, analysis of the process will show breakdown within team efficiencies. Variances may stem from communication failures, unsuccessful conflict resolution, or ambiguity in role delineation. Educational programs can be directed towards these specific areas.

Ongoing Development

To keep up with the rapid change in information, learning must be continuous. Providing front end training that stops once staff meet entry level standards fails to recognize ongoing educational needs. The most important component of ongoing education is the need to have in place mechanisms to identify staff development needs.

Applying the principles already discussed for adult learners, staff development needs should involve the learners, provide clear rationale for the training, build on existing knowledge, and demonstrate respect for existing expertise. One of the greatest challenges in a clinical environment is to incorporate training opportunities during patient care delivery. Access to teaching rooms and reference material close to the work place can provide a setting for short or informal educational sessions. A major downside of training during working hours is that learners are rarely able to completely divorce themselves from the clinical setting. With this in mind, intense or long training needs are best addressed away from the patient care setting.

Identification of learning needs can be validated by utilizing a number of different strategies. Informal mechanisms such as suggestion boxes or staff meetings can often provide important feedback loops. Occasional formal surveys can provide additional information. Obvious training needs may develop when new procedures or technologies are introduced. However, periodic reviews may be warranted for infrequently applied skills, or those which are particularly complex. Audit results, family/patient satisfaction questionnaires, and incident reports provide additional sources for collection of data.

In addition to providing information and supporting clinical development, ongoing unit education can offer opportunities for staff who wish to develop their teaching skills. Encouraging interested staff to research and present information to colleagues, helps direct their own learning, gain confidence with presentation skills, and become more comfortable reviewing pertinent literature. Staff who have participated in unit education often gain an increased respect for fellow presenters. In addition, development of presentation skills can help to prepare staff to submit abstracts for oral or poster presentations, which provide recognition for the unit and institution.

As with all unit programs, ongoing education should maintain a multidisciplinary focus. Inservice programs should strive to demonstrate how the team approach to care delivery is enacted.

Spirit of Inquiry

The promotion of a spirit of inquiry is pivotal to ensuring that unit practice continually evolves and improves. To assure that practice remains state-of-the-art, every member of the team must be free to question existing policies, procedures, and practice and be encouraged to explore new options. To truly advance practice, a climate must be created where team members who actively pursue new avenues are recognized, valued, and supported.

Forums for dialogue and exchange of ideas are important mechanisms to stimulate the spirit of inquiry. Journal review clubs, article of the month files, and channels for reporting new findings from conferences can be invaluable to shift or change existing paradigms.

In addition to opportunities that promote and encourage staff to review practice, programs to develop literature search and article review skills can prove helpful. The ability to decipher valuable research from questionable data is important if changes to clinical practice are at stake.[31]

A unit where staff are free to table any innovative idea or strategy without risk of adverse consequence can provide the catalyst for creativity. Team members whose hypotheses are sanctioned by support and encouragement from colleagues and managers are more likely to feel committed to the pursuit of excellence.

Evaluation

Evaluation of any educational program is important to ensure that training goals are met. Abruzzese's model for educational evaluation looks at five specific levels. The minimal level of evaluation reviews process. This involves assessment of the overall satisfaction rating for the program design and presentation, and the degree to which the learner's objectives for the session were met. Content evaluation provides a more concise measurement by testing actual knowledge or skill at the end of a training experience. Outcome evaluation moves the process of interpretation to a higher level by assessing the degree of change in practice, or outcome of training in the clinical setting. Impact evaluation considers institutional results by looking at cost benefit factors, turnover, or quality of care. The highest level of evaluation measures congruence of goals and accomplishments of total educational programs.[32]

Complete evaluation of the educational process in critical care involves not only a critique of the curriculum design, but necessitates careful evaluation of the trainee. Review of the trainee's practice at the end of training is mandatory due to the ramifications of unsatisfactory clinical performance. If inadequacies are identified, appropriate remedial education and supervision is essential. As long as there are human beings in the health care system, human errors will continue to be made.[33] Patient care rounds, morbidity and mortality reviews, and isolated observations will from time to time identify situations where practice has varied from expected standards. While paying careful attention to the learner's self-esteem, errors must be dealt with. A training situation must never disregard the obligation to ensure safe patient care. Careful monitoring, appropriate supervision based on the level of demonstrated competency, and education as required, are important factors for ongoing development and quality management.

Summary

A comprehensive educational program for any CCU is much more than just entry level training. Training must demonstrate strategies to promote collaboration and support for the multidisciplinary philosophy, as well as targeting and promoting optimal standards for care. Education must continue beyond formal training sessions and be reflected in day to day practice, through the expectation that the team will continually strive for the highest standards of care. A unit culture that promotes respect among its team members, fosters the desire for continuing education and development, and encourages self-evaluation and inquiry, is critical to ensuring quality care.

References

1. King G, Sibbald W: Training and certification of critical care medice in the United States (editoral). Chest 1988;93:1122.
2. Weil MH, Shoemaker MD, Rackow EC: Training and certification of critical care medicine in the United States. Chest 1988;93:1122–1123.
3. Merrow S, Selegman M: Nurse-pharmacist collaboration in clinical nursing education. Nursing Connections 1989;2:55–62.
4. Baggs JG, Ryan SA, Phelps CE, et al: The association between interdisciplinary collaberation and patient outcomes in a medical intensive care unit. Heart Lung 1992;21:18–24.
5. Mitchell P, Armstrong S, Simpson TF, et al: American Association of Critical-Care Nurses demonstration project: Profile of excellence in critical care nursing. Heart Lung 1989;18:219–237.
6. Reuben D: The transition from residency to practice . . . A focus for change. Brown University Program in Medicine, 1989.
7. Good CV (ed): Dictionary of Education, Third Edition. New York, NY, McGraw-Hill, 1973.
8. Canadian Association of Critical Care Nurses: Standards for critical care nursing practice. Can Assoc Crit Care Nurs, 1992.
9. American Association of Critical Care Nurses: Standards for nursing care of the critically ill, Second Edition. Am Assoc Crit Nurs, 1989.
10. American Association of Critical-Care Nurses: Outcome standards for nursing care of the critically ill. Am Assoc Crit Nurs, 1990.
11. Royal College of Physicians and Surgeons of Canada: Objectives of specialty training requirements in critical care medicine, 1993.
12. Society of Critical Care Medicine: Guidelines for program content for fellowship training in critical care. Crit Care Med 1992;20:875–882.
13. Canadian Nurses Association: Blueprint for the critical care nursing certification examination. Can Nurs Assoc, 1994.
14. Alspach JG: Core Curriculum for Critical Care Nursing, Fourth Edition. Philadelphia, PA, WB Saunders Company, 1991.
15. Royal College of Physicians and Surgeons of Canada: Objectives of specialty training requirements in critical care medicine, 1993.
16. Pike R: The Creative Training Handbook. Minneapolis, MN, Lakewood Publications, 1989.
17. Alspach JG: Competency based orientation program for medical/surgical ICUs. Crit Care Nurs, 1990.
18. Broad ML, Newstrom JW: Transfer of Training: Action-packed Strategies to Ensure High Payoff from Training Investments. Reading, MA, Addison-Wesley Publishing Co. Inc., 1992.
19. Abruzzese RS, Quinn-O'Neal B: Nursing Staff Development. . . Strategies for Success. St. Louis, MO, Mosby, 1992; p. 259.
20. Stephen L: Assessing your learning style. In Bard R, Bell CR, Stephen L, et al. (eds): The Trainer's Professional Development Handbook. Jossey-Bass, 1987.
21. Cooper S, Heenan C: Preparing, Designing, & Leading Workshops . . . a Humanistic Approach. Van Nostrand Reinhold, 1980, pp. 21–24.
22. Resko D: Self-learning in critical care: A debate. DCCN 1991;10:230–234.

23. Billings D: Advantages and disadvantages of computer-assisted instruction. DCCN 1986;5:356–362.
24. Broad ML, Newstrom JW: Transfer of Training: Action-Packed Strategies to Ensure High Payoff from Training Investments. Reading, MA, Addison-Wesley Publishing Co. Inc., 1992.
25. Tobin H, Yoder Wise P: The Process of Staff Development. Components for Change, Second Edition. St. Louis, MO, Mosby, 1979, pp. 150–151.
26. Avillion A, Abruzzese R: Conceptual foundations of nursing staff development. In Abruzzese R (ed): Nursing Staff Development . . . Strategies for Success. St. Louis, MO, Mosby, 1992, pp. 30–34.
27. Avillion A, Abruzzese R: Conceptual foundations of nursing staff development. In Abruzzese R (ed): Nursing Staff Development . . . Strategies for Success. St. Louis, MO, Mosby, 1992, pp. 30–34.
28. Poole D: Changing behaviour. In Tobin H, Yoder Wise P (eds): The Process of Staff Development . . . Components for Change. St. Louis, MO, Mosby, 1979, pp. 87–88.
29. Avillion A, Abruzzese R: Conceptual foundations of nursing staff development. In Abruzzese R (ed): Nursing Staff Development . . . Strategies for Success. St. Louis, MO, Mosby, 1992, p. 257.
30. Dagher M, Lloyd R: Managing negative outcome by reducing variances in the emergency department. QRB 1991;(January):15–21.
31. Chambers L, Stoddart R, Sullivan B: Continuing education for health professionals and administrators: Workshop on becoming a critical user of health care research. Can J Public Health 1985;74:29–34.
32. Avillion A, Abruzzese R: Conceptual foundations of nursing staff development. In Abruzzese R (ed): Nursing Staff Development . . . Strategies for Success. St. Louis, MO, Mosby, 1992, pp. 238–248.
33. Butler M: Education in the critical care setting. CCQ 1984;75–78.

Chapter 17

Research in Critical Care: Its Scope, Methods, and Organization

James E. Calvin Jr, M.D., Joseph E. Parrillo, M.D.

Introduction

For no other reason than the tremendous expense of intensive care and relatively high morbidity and mortality of critically ill patients, all sectors in the society have a vested interest in finding better strategies of patient evaluation and treatment for the critically ill. Such efforts must span the breadth of all health care research encompassing biological sciences, epidemiology of the critically ill, utilization of new technologies, and other health care resources.

Research is essential to the future of critical care. Without it, government intrusion and regulation will influence care without a counterbalanced reason and rationale advocacy based on sound science. What future can we expect without strong research advocacy and commitment? Unfortunately, we are left with only blind acceptance of today's

---

From: Sibbald WJ, Massaro T (eds.): The Business of Critical Care: A Textbook for Clinicians Who Manage Special Care Units. © Futura Publishing Co., Inc., Armonk, NY, 1996.

therapeutic and diagnostic limitations, our own frailties, and the loss of hope for many of our patients.

The purpose of this chapter is to review the organization of clinical research within critical care units (CCUs) to support the advancement of knowledge essential for the care of the critically ill. In 1991, the Research Division of the Society of Critical Care Medicine published a statement summarizing the present status of critical care research. Its purpose was to define the scope of critical care research, and its goal was to identify important areas of research not receiving sufficient attention by researchers and funding agencies.

The statement published by the Research Division of the Society of Critical Care Medicine highlighted four important areas of research. These areas included:

1. Natural history, risk, and outcomes research.
2. Intensive care unit (ICU) technology and therapeutic intensive research.
3. Optimal personnel and resources research.
4. Disease entity research.

A brief review of each of the above provides an overview of the potential span of research questions requiring attention.

Natural History, Risk, and Outcomes Research

This area of research involves the development of accurate disease criteria, acuity scoring,[2–4] and the analysis of outcomes based on diagnosis and severity of illness. The development of these methodologies support not only quality assurance but also allow for better prognostication and aid in clinical research design. Although these tools predict patient population outcomes well, they have not yet been proven to be helpful in managing the individual patient.

Intensive Care Unit Technology and Therapeutic Intervention Research

The goal of this area is to assess the cost benefits and cost effectiveness of sophisticated technologies and treatments available to critically ill patients. Many of these are expensive, and their value is largely unproven. Much of this technological and treatment assessment has been retrospective, uncontrolled, unblinded, and unrandomized. Over time, many technologies have lost popularity after growing awareness of ineffectiveness. Unfortunately, much cost and little benefit has been the result. The goals of technology assessment have been summarized[5] previously and include: (1) the technology's feasibility; (2) its efficacy; (3) its effectiveness; and (4) its economic impact.

Understanding all of the necessary components of technology assessment highlights the importance of avoiding ineffective "in house" studies that do not answer the important question of cost effectiveness of a given technology but rather serve to enhance diffusion of an unproven one.

Guyatt et al.[6] have described a multi-step process for the assessment of diagnostic technologies to be undertaken before an economic evaluation including:

1. the demonstration of technological capability.
2. the potential range of uses.
3. the accuracy of the technology in comparison to a gold standard.
4. the effect upon the health care provider in terms of the importance, uniqueness, and timeliness of the information provided.
5. the impact of the technology upon changing therapy.
6. the impact of the technology upon changing outcome.

In general, most technologies utilized in critical care have completed the first three stages.[5] Rarely, some technologies have completed steps 4–6.[7,8] In part, the failure to complete higher levels of evaluation is related to expense. Furthermore, outcome assessments for certain technologies such as hemodynamic monitoring are difficult to evaluate because they only provide information, and their efficacy depends upon how the information is used and the effectiveness of the treatment strategy.[9]

Subsequent economic evaluations include cost benefit analysis, cost effectiveness analysis, and cost utility analysis. Cost benefit analysis is used to measure in dollar amounts the difference between costs and benefits resulting from an activity. Cost effective analysis compares strategies with similar outcomes. It helps to demonstrate the most efficient method of achieving a particular health care objective. Cost utility analysis replaces money with cost utility as a measure of economic desirability. It compares the cost of a program with health improvement attributable to the program where health improvement is measured in quality adjusted life years gained.

Optimal Personnel and Resources Research

Any lack of access to new proven treatments undermine their potential effectiveness as a health care advance. Necessary infrastructure and resources must be ensured for adequate access and availability of effective treatments. Human resource studies are needed to ensure adequate staffing, not only in hospitals, but cities, states, and regions. Data on optimal training and evaluation of practice guidelines are also necessary.

Diseases Entity Research

The goal of this area is a better understanding of the pathophysiology of disease entities commonly treated in the ICU. In the last 25 years, a greater understanding of the physiological derangement of organ failure has been integrated into the treatment of a variety of disorders. The use of vasodilators to reduce left ventricular afterload has resulted in improved mortality in patients with chronic congestive heart failure.[10] The use of thrombolytic agents in acute myocardial infarction was based on the knowledge that acute coronary occlusion with thrombus was the basis of this clinical entity.[11] This strategy has reduced mortality along with other treatment such as aspirin and beta blocker.[12]

In the future, a better understanding of the pathophysiology of disorders at a cellular and molecular level holds bright promise to further reduce morbidity and mortality. The interaction of the basic scientist and clinicians skilled in methods of clinical research will be necessary for this promise to become a reality.

Clinical Trials

To ensure research of the critically ill is valid, a sound knowledge of experimental design, statistical techniques, and demonstration of organizational skills is mandatory.

To understand the organizational design of research activities within CCUs, a brief review of study design is necessary. The clinical trial[13] is the most robust model of study design and is defined as a prospective study in human subjects comparing the effect and value of an intervention against a control. A clinical trial is the most definitive method of determining whether an intervention has the postulated effect. In addition to using a control group,[14] the other important characteristics of a clinical trial are: (1) that it is prospective; (2) that there is a clearly defined intervention and clear endpoint to be tested; (3) that the treatment is randomized; and (4) that both patient and doctor are blinded where possible.[15]

It is important to review some other important elements of a clinical trial:

1. Prospective studies require "a priori" definition of the inclusion and exclusion criteria and follow patients longitudinally forward from the initiation of the intervention.
2. The intervention, which may be a drug, device, test, or strategy must be applied in a standard fashion.
3. The control group is an integral part of the trial and should be comparable in all important aspects to the test groups.
4. Randomization is processed so that all subjects have an equal chance of being assigned to the treatment or control group. This procedure protects against bias in the allocation of subject to one group or another, ensures comparable groups and the validity of the statistical methods.
5. The process of blinding is to guard as much as possible against bias by patient or investigator.
6. There is a clearly defined endpoint that determines the success of the trial.

These elements make it apparent that a clearly written protocol is a necessary prerequisite of the clinical trial acting as an agreement between investigator, subject, scientific community, and funding source. The protocol must contain the background, the objectives, and hypothesis to be tested, and the design and organization of the trial. It must be developed prior to the beginning of the trial and is a major portion of both grant applications and requests for approval by the Institutional Review Board.[16]

The protocol must also contain the inclusion and exclusion criteria of the study population, sample size estimates, process of enrolling subjects including informed consent, baseline examinations, and group allocation, description and schedule of intervention, follow-up schedule, ascertainment of response variables, and study organization.

This overall organization has particular relevance when determining whether a center should initiate a single center trial or participate in a multicenter trial. Description of inclusion and exclusion criteria and calculation of sample size helps determine the feasibility of being able to recruit sufficient patients in a specific unit of time. A center with a special expertise may be able to participate by providing specialized diagnostic or analytical services for all centers. A center providing such a core laboratory usually does not participate in patient recruitment.

The issue of patient recruitment is probably the most important question to be addressed when considering participation. One has to ask whether it is realistic to recruit enough patients, based on the best estimate from medical records and available databases. At this point, expanding the trial to other centers may be necessary to accomplish this task. It is quite obvious that considerable organizational assistance is necessary to not only gather necessary data for recruitment estimates but also to screen potential test centers.

Patients who are possible subjects can be identified by standard screening techniques. Considerable care must be extended to keeping accurate and complete records. To accomplish this, staff must often be available on off-hours or during vacation periods. Quality checks must be performed periodically. Missing data is often used as an indicator of the quality of the research and must be minimized.

Other Forms of Studies

In addition to randomized clinical trials, other forms of investigation are available.[17]

Nonrandomized concurrent control studies can be utilized, but their major criticism in that the groups may be dissimilar and bias towards treatment allocation may exist. Historical series have been used as a control and permit all new subjects to receive a new therapy. Again, groups may be dissimilar, there is vulnerability to bias and outcomes may be secondary to confounded variables. Cross-over designs are popular because smaller sample sizes can be used, but one cannot use this design to test treatments where the effects of the first treatment period may carry over to the second treatment.

Databases[18] are often used to assess an experience with a treatment technology. However, these reviews are usually retrospective and often are lacking in necessary information because of the lack of "a priori" planning.

Organization of the Study

Very little has been written about the organizational structure of research enterprises within the hospital, let alone the CCU. However,

Table 1
Composition of Management Staff for a Large Multicenter Trial

Investigator(s)
Coinvestigators and assistant investigators
Members of Institutional Review Board
Professional consultants
Regulatory agency reviewers
Trial coordinators
Trial monitors
Monitoring committees
Project champions
Project managers
Supervisors of data processors
Statistical reviewers
Executives of sponsoring institutions
Data analysis committee members
Independent auditors of diagnoses, laboratory data, trial conduct
Independent review committee of trial results and interpretation

Adapted from Management Styles, Staff and Systems in Guide to Clinical Trials, ed Spilker B, Raven Press, New York, NY, 1991, pp. 953–960.

a great deal has been written about the organizational structure of multicenter clinical trials,[19–23] and this offers a starting point for our discussion about the organization of critical care research within our institution.

Table 1 lists the composition of the management staff for a large multicenter clinical trial.[23] The number of people involved in this endeavor can be enormous, although a few specific roles are common to all trials. In particular, the principal investigator provides the leadership necessary to organize a sufficiently large and skilled enterprise to answer the major hypothesis tested. In concert with the study statistician and coinvestigators, he coordinates prestudy organizational meetings that select the hypothesis to be tested, determines the inclusion and exclusion criteria, and estimates the sample size and power calculations. An administrative or executive committee can be formed at this point whose first job is to determine which test centers will be involved. Other staff listed in Table 1 may be specific to the sponsoring agency, the study center, or may be part of organizational committees or core laboratories.

Quality assurance of data collected by multicenter trials involves ensuring standardization of patient eligibility criteria, diagnostic classification, and assessment of the effects of treatment. To perform this function, an independent group or committee is formed that is not directly involved with actual patient recruitment or study execution. Such a committee can also act as a safety monitoring committee with preset rules for stopping the trial if there is evidence of harm occurring to either treatment or control groups.

The interpretation of specialized tests should also be performed by individuals not directly involved with patient recruitment, and these individuals should remain blind to patient treatment. By organizing such individuals as a central committee, variability can be assessed and reduced.

Other administrative committees are often necessary including executive, data and safety monitoring, data analysis, writing, and external advisory committees. A representative outline of such an organizational structure is depicted in Figure 1.

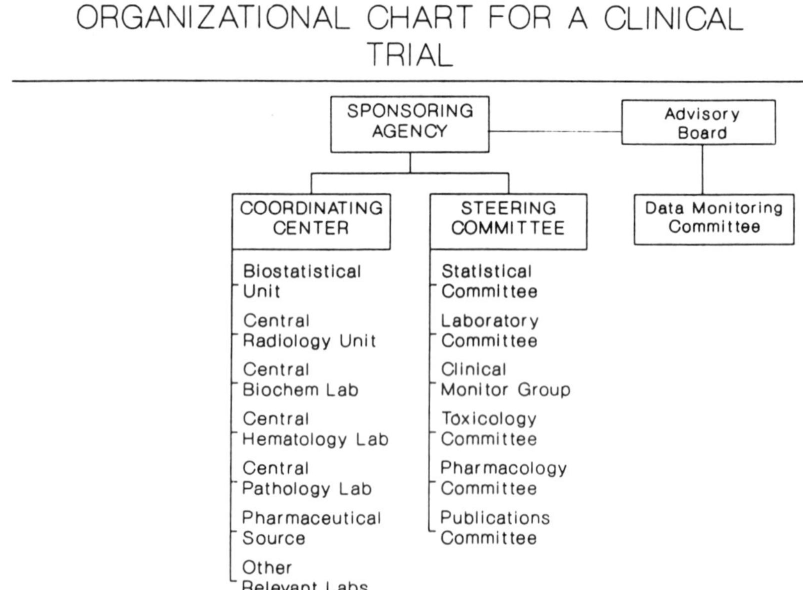

Figure 1. Organizational chart for a clinical trial. This is a representative model with coordinating and steering committees answering to the sponsoring agency. This model includes an Advisory Board and a Data Monitoring Committee. Other committees and core laboratories are established to handle various facets of the trial. In general, core laboratories answer to the coordinating center and organizational committees answer to the steering committee.

Organizational Structure Within the Institution

The organizational structure of research with an individual center recognizes the accountability that must exist to the funding agency and multicenter administration committee. However, accountability within the institution needs clarification.

In the simplest case scenario (Figure 2), the principal investigator of a single study is accountable to either the funding agency or executive committee of a multicenter trial. Staff fully dedicated to the project are responsible to the principal investigator. The principal investigator is also responsible to his section director or department head as representatives of the institution. This implied matrix is necessary to protect interests of the study, the patient, and the institution.

Often, several small projects are ongoing at the same time. The workload of each either is not enough for full time personnel and there

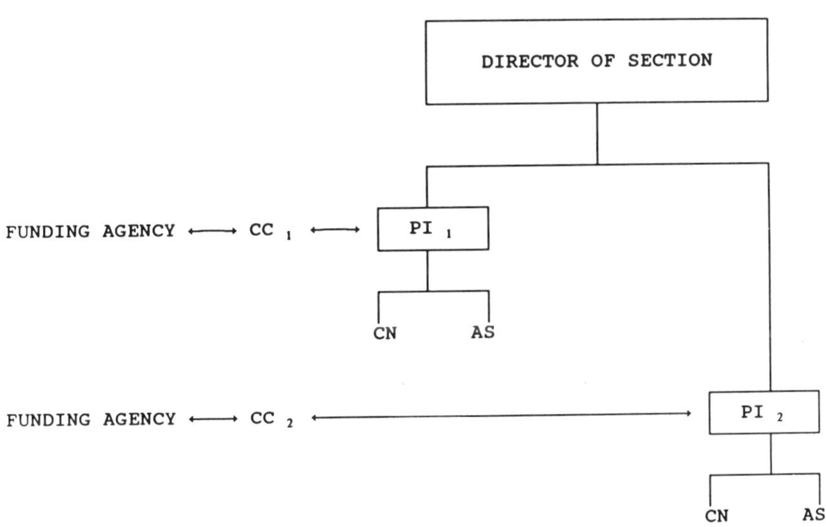

Figure 2. Simplest organizational structure for the conduct of a clinical trial within a single institution. The coordinating center for each trial (CC) answers to the funding agency, and the principal investigator (PI) answers both to the CC and to his immediate superior within the institution. Clinical nurses (CN) and allied scientists (AS) are responsible to the PI. In this model each trial within the institution acts independently.

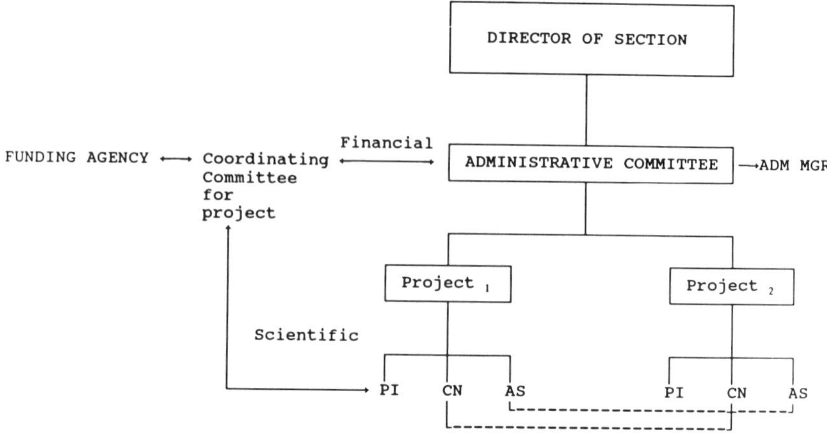

Figure 3. Complex model of research organization within an institution. This model allows for multiple trials to operate independently but optimizes resource utilization by allowing for cross-coverage between study personnel. An institutional administrative committee exists to coordinate resources and to establish institutional priorities. Larger operations may require an administrative manager. Coordinating committees or centers interact with the administrative committee about fiscal matters and with the institutional PI for the scientific conduct of the project.

may be a need for off-hour coverage. In this scenario (Figure 3), research associates may work on more than one project and are not accountable to a single investigator. Because of the complexities of these arrangements, it is often useful to have an internal administrative committee oversee priorities and to interact with either the funding agency or coordinating committee on financial matters. The principal investigator is still responsible for the actual execution of the trial and providing necessary periodical reports to the institutional review body, funding agency, or a multicenter trial administrative committee.

In between these two models various organizational structures may exist. Research staff may be largely responsible for a single project but provide coverage for vacation time and after hours studies. Advisory or administrative committees may have varying degrees of strictness over control of priorities and resources depending on the experience and style of the institution.

In single center studies, in-house statistical consultation and data analysis is necessary.

The Role of the Study Coordinator

The study or trial coordinator handles most administrative tasks on a day to day basis. The coordinator's responsibilities range from patient scheduling, ensuring accurate and complete data recording, conducting the protocol, and acting as a major contact person. The coordinator plays the most important role of ensuring the most efficient conduct of the trial.

The Role of Institutional Review Board

Institutional approval for a research project or clinical trial is now mandated by the federal government for federally funded projects to assure: (1) that the conduct of a clinical trial is ethical and will do no harm; (2) that informed consent is obtained; (3) potential conflicts of interest is eliminated; (4) patient confidentiality is maintained; and (4) confidentiality of the data is maintained.

An institutional review board must have at least five members, one of whom is not affiliated with the institution. It may not be composed entirely of men or women or from a single profession.

The principal investigator for a research project is responsible not only for obtaining initial approval but also for filing periodic reports, advising the IRB of any change in the protocol, and advising of any serious adverse reactions.

Funding Sources

Funding for research can be acquired by contracting with third parties or by grant application to public funding agencies such as the National Institute of Health, private endowments, and foundations.[24] Pharmaceutical based contracts are a very common source of funding and present some specific issues (see conflict of interest below) that are troublesome.

Various types of foundations exist and include: special interest foundations, corporate foundations, and family or community foundations. In general, funding from public agencies, endowments, and foundation are competitive and subject to peer review.

Estimating Costs of Research

The budget represents a major portion of a grant application. All costs must be identified.[24] In general, these costs can be categorized as follows:

1. personnel
2. consultant fees
3. equipment costs and maintenance
4. supplies
5. travel to either organizational meeting or to present the data
6. patient care costs
7. alteration or renovation to physical plant
8. contractural costs
9. miscellaneous costs

Grant agencies permit many of these costs although certain equipment items or physical plant renovations are often borne by the institution.

The budget requires careful scrutiny and integrity. Many funding agencies require multiple quotations on major equipment items and detailed explanations.

Conflict of Interest in Critical Care Research

There is a special need for the organization of research affairs within an institution to protect investigators against conflicts of interest.[25] The potential for conflict of interest is most obvious in the relationship between investigators and pharmaceutical manufacturers, especially where the latter act as the funding agency. To emphasize the implication of potential conflicts of interest, one study has found a correlation between the outcome of a study and its funding.[26]

Another ethical issue that arises when investigators receive reimbursement for drug testing is informed consent. This issue arises because patients are rarely told that their physician will be paid for doing the study and that this financial incentive may influence the type of therapy that the patient receives. Recent court decisions have affirmed that a higher standard of disclosure is necessary for research studies. In this context it may be advisable that patients be informed about the source of funding and the investigator's potential conflict of interest in receiving remuneration for enrolling patients.

A few simple measures may help alleviate concerns about potential conflict of interest in addition to the patient being told the source and mechanism of funding. This identifies to the patient the investigator's potential sources of bias.

The direct financial incentive to investigators can be diminished if not eliminated by the institution taking control of the money through a process that pays direct costs of the project first, indirect costs of the institution second, and remaining funds allocated throughout the institution to investigators or projects on the basis of need and merit. Patients should be informed of the arrangement. This represents a mechanism analogous to the external peer review funding agency.

Problems of Conducting Research in the Intensive Care Unit

Critically ill patients face the irony that, although they can benefit significantly from research activities, the emotion filled ICU remains a complex arena for effective research endeavors. The reasons for this complexity are numerous. First, the patients usually suffer from multiple system organ dysfunction, in greater frequency, complicating the patients physiological derangement and complicating therapy. Patients are generally receiving many drugs and often undergoing multiple procedures. There are often compelling reasons for these multiple therapies but they provide many confounding variables, making it a challenge for investigators to isolate the effects of a given investigational intervention.

Second, in view of the obvious discomfort the patient is suffering and frequently poor prognosis, any evaluation of therapy is often debated in ethical terms. Other health care providers and families alike need to be reassured that the trial is in the patient's best interest and that the study is important. Investigators must go out of their way to communicate the necessity of the study and address concerns regarding safety, patient distress, and importance. These concerns are justified and require careful and detailed discussions.

Third, it is important that staff performing the research are familiar with caring for such critically ill patients so that ongoing care is not compromised and other patient care issues are not neglected. This is often facilitated by having research staff who have already worked with the critically ill.

Fourth, the timing of study protocols has to be worked into the patients schedule for other treatments and tests. This requires excellent communication and significant effort but it carries the highest priority.

Fifth, the issue of obtaining informed consent has been a major handicap. Many institutional review boards have refused permission for research on acute care patients because of the difficulty satisfying the patient's legal capacity to voluntarily consent. Other alternatives to informed consent have been explored, such as using surrogates,[27,28] deferring consent,[29] and using established waivers for informed consent[30] (so long as the IRB oversees these waivers in a stringent and ethical manner).[31] These alternatives continue to be discussed widely, but until real consensus emerges, this troubling issue will continue to be a barrier.

Finally, it is important for the investigator to provide feedback to the staff on trial results. These activities are pointless unless they improve patient care. Future staff support is fostered both by demonstrating evidence of improved patient care and recognizing the contribution of involved health care workers.

Organizational Mission Statement and Goals

Much of the discussion in this chapter is an outline of how one prepares, initiates, and executes a single study. In this context, the discussion has been aimed at specific research requirements (the single investigator or team) as well as at an executive or administrative level. The administrative level needs control mechanisms to accomplish institutional goals. Investigators need to know what these institutional goals are and what support they can expect. To satisfy both needs and to optimize success, strong leadership is necessary to provide direction for the research effort and enhance teamwork especially in multidisciplinary areas.

The form of this leadership can be quite varied (Table 2), ranging from a very authoritarian to a consultative leadership to ad hoc planning and decision making.

Whatever the management style, mission statements are extremely useful tools for institutional leaders to clarify the institution's commitment to research, to determine what areas are felt to be of strategic importance, and to outline within what boundaries the research enterprise must operate. Early on in the development of a research enterprise, this statement is often written by the institutional leaders. If the need to write a statement occurs later in the process when multiple teams have been assembled who are looking for direction, a mutual process is helpful.

Table 2
Management Styles of a Research Organization

Type	Description
1) Rigid and authoritative	No delegation of responsibility nor decision making
2) Participative leadership	Responsibility and decision making is delegated appropriately
3) Consultative leadership	One individual consults with other and decides
4) Committee structure	Makes important decisions, reviews processes and progress of projects; structure and flexibility varies
5) No formal system	Ad hoc decision making

Specific goals for the institution's research enterprise as well as goals for each team of investigators or areas of investigation need to be set to provide a "compass" for research and to set "a priori" some measures with which to judge effectiveness. Again, this requires strong commitment to the research process throughout the institution.

Summary

More emphasis needs to be placed on critical care research if we are to achieve the goals of improving the prognosis of the critically ill and making this care more cost efficient. The areas of necessary research activity have been identified, the types of research studies reviewed with special attention paid to the clinical trial. Organization of clinical trials inside and outside the institution are discussed with emphasis on the interrelationships that exist.

References

1. Parrillo JE: Research in critical care medicine: Present status of critical care investigation. Crit Care Med 1991;19(4):569.
2. Knaus WA, Zimmerman JE, Wagner DP, et al: APACHE—Acute physiology and chronic health evaluation: A physiologically based classification system. Crit Care Med 1981;9:591.
3. Knaus WA, Draper EA, Wagner DP, et al: APACHE II: A severity of disease classification system. Crit Care Med 1985;13:818.

4. Teskey RJ, Calvin JE, McPhail I: Disease severity in the coronary care unit. Chest 1991;100:1637.
5. Sibbald WJ, Escaf M, Calvin JE: How can new technology be introduced, evaluated, and financed in critical care? Clin Chem 1990;8(B):1604.
6. Guyatt G, Drummond M, Feeny D, et al: Guidelines for the clinical and economic evaluation of health care technologies. Soc Sci Med 1986;22:393.
7. Bone RC, Slotman G, Maunder R: Randomized double blind multi-centre study of prostaglandin E1 in patients with the adult respiratory. Chest 1989; 96:114.
8. Holcroft JW, Vossar MJ, Weber CJ: Prostaglandin E1 and survival in patients with the adult distress syndrome. Ann Surg 1986;203:371.
9. Calvin JE and the Technology Subcommittee of the Working Group in Critical Care: Hemodynamic monitoring: A technology assessment. Can Med Assoc J 1991;145:114.
10. Pfeffer MA, Braunwald E, Moye LA, et al: Effect of captopril on mortality and morbidity in patients with left ventricular dysfunction after myocardial infarction. Results of the survival and ventricular enlargement trial. N Engl J Med 1992;327:669.
11. GISSI: Long-term effects of intravenous thrombolysis in acute myocardial infarction: Final report of the GISSI study. Lancet 2 1987;(2):871.
12. Lau J, Antman EM, Jimenez-Silva J, et al: Cumulative meta-analysis of therapeutic trials for myocardial infarction. N Engl J Med 1992;327:248.
13. Pocock SJ: Clinical Trials: A Practical Approach. Toronto, John Wiley & Sons, 1983, pp. 28–49.
14. Spilker B: Controls used in clinical studies. In Guide to Clinical Studies and Developing Protocols. New York, NY, Raven Press, 1984, pp. 18–20.
15. Spilker B: Types of blinds. In Guide to Clinical Studies and Developing Protocols. New York, NY, Raven Press, 1984, pp. 14–17.
16. Spilker B: Standardized information across protocols (polishing the boilerplate). In Guide to Clinical Studies and Developing Protocols. New York, NY, Raven Press, 1984, pp. 154–184.
17. DeAngelis C: Types of research models and methods. In Wissow L, Pascoe J (eds): An Introduction to Clinical Research. Oxford, Oxford University Press, 1990, pp. 38–74.
18. DeAngelis C: Data Collection Management and Analysis. In McCormick M, Wasserman RC (eds): An Introduction to Clinical Research. Oxford, Oxford University Press, 1990, pp. 75–110.
19. Spilker B: Comments on multicenter studies. In Guide to Clinical Studies and Developing Protocols. New York, NY, Raven Press, 1984, pp. 208–211.
20. Spilker B: Interview and selection of investigators. In Guide to Clinical Studies and Developing Protocols. New York, NY, Raven Press, 1984, pp. 217–225.
21. Spilker B: Monitoring and troubleshooting a study. In Guide to Clinical Studies and Developing Protocols. New York, NY, Raven Press, 1984, pp. 241–245.
22. Inmann KJ, Martin CM, Sibbald WJ: Design and conduct of clinical trials in critical care. J Crit Care 1992;7:118.
23. Spilker B: Management Styles, Staff and Systems. In Guide to Clinical Trials. New York, NY, Raven Press, 1991, pp. 953–960.
24. DeAngelis, Pragnatics C: In Duggan AK (ed): An Introduction to Clinical Research. Oxford, Oxford University Press, 1990, pp. 111–132.

25. Shimm DS, Spece RG: Industry reimbursement for entering patients into clinical trials: Legal and ethical issues. Ann Intern Med 1991;115:148.
26. Davidson RA: Source of funding and outcome of clinical trials. J Gen Intern Med 1986;1:155.
27. Buchanan AE, Brock DW: The Ethics of Surrogate Decision Making. Cambridge, Cambridge University Press, 1989.
28. Fost NC: A surrogate system for informed consent. JAMA 1975;233(7):800.
29. Miller BL: Philosophical, ethical, and legal aspects of resuscitation medicine. I. Deferred consent and justification of resuscitation research. Crit Care Med 1988;16:1059.
30. National Commission for the Protection of Human Subjects of Biomedical and Behavioral Research, The Belmont Report, OPPR. U.S. Government Printing Office, 1983.
31. Iserson KV, Mahowald MB: Acute care research: Is it ethical? Crit Care Med 1992;20:1032.

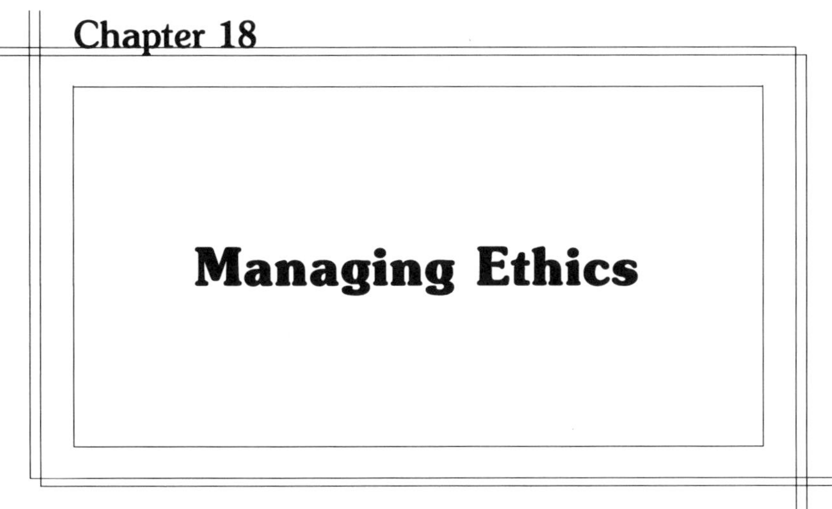

Chapter 18

Managing Ethics

Deborah J. Nyman, M.B., B.S.,
Charles L. Sprung, M.D., J.D.

Ethical Principles

Critical care medicine is an area in which health care professionals make life and death decisions on a daily basis. The laws concerning these decisions are fixed by the courts of the land and are constantly changing as courts in different jurisdictions reach differing conclusions and as legislators in various countries alter the law by new statutes.[1] Physicians must act within legal boundaries but must not be influenced entirely by the law. Physicians must also be guided by their ethical values. Medical ethics are "the principles of proper professional conduct concerning the rights and duties of the physician himself, his patients, and his fellow practitioners, as well as his actions in the care of patients and in relations with their families".[2] The major medical ethi-

From: Sibbald WJ, Massaro T (eds.): The Business of Critical Care: A Textbook for Clinicians Who Manage Special Care Units. © Futura Publishing Co., Inc., Armonk, NY, 1996.

cal issues in critical care, which include informed consent, triage of intensive care unit (ICU) beds, and foregoing life-sustaining treatments, will be discussed in this chapter.

The problem with individual physicians making decisions on the basis of their personal ethical thinking, of course, is that there may not be agreement between individuals, cultures, or religions. An example is the giving of blood to a Jehovah's Witness. It may seem abundantly clear to the treating physician that a bleeding patient requires a blood transfusion—the patient in this case, however, will clearly disagree. In the Netherlands, active euthanasia, although remaining a criminal offense, is a relatively common occurrence and the Dutch Medical Association even issued guidelines pertaining to its practice as far back as 1984.[3] In the US, a proposal to place a new law for active euthanasia in terminally ill patients on the November 1988 ballot in California was unsuccessful.[4] In 1989, however, a physician knowingly gave a 20-year-old terminal ovarian cancer patient a massive overdose of morphine that killed her.[5] This was clearly an illegal act, but whether it was an ethical one or not may be debated. When making decisions to carry out such interventions (or for that matter far less drastic ones) a physician must take into consideration the major ethical principles including autonomy, nonmaleficence, beneficence, and justice.

Autonomy is a basic premise of personal liberty establishing an individual's right to determine his own course of action in accordance with his own life plans.[6] For example, the patient's right to refuse intubation even though it may be a beneficial treatment is an act of self-determinism. Nonmaleficence is the duty of the physician not to inflict evil or harm whereas beneficence is the duty of a physician to promote good and to remove and prevent evil or harm.[7] Justice is the concept that a person receives what that person deserves.[7] At times it may be very difficult to realize all these principles simultaneously. For example, to give or not to give morphine to a patient in pain, but who may be in danger of respiratory arrest may present a moral dilemma. It may be that a patient will refuse a treatment recommended by the physician who knows, with as much certainty as possible, that it will be of benefit. Most of the time the difficulties of realizing all the ethical principles can be overcome by discussion and joint decision making by the health care team and the patient. On rare occasions one may have to go to court for, hopefully, a "just" decision.

Informed Consent

Informed consent is the process through which a patient decides to undergo a selected procedure or therapy based on information given by the health care provider.[8] Under normal circumstances there are five essential components of informed consent: disclosure of information, competency, understanding, voluntariness, and decision making. In a critical care setting many patients are unable to make important, rational health care decisions, however, and medical realities often make it difficult or impossible to obtain informed consent.

What defines a patient competent to make decisions? In most circumstances, persons are presumed to have the capacity to make decisions for themselves, unless they have been formally judged incompetent.[9] Competent persons comprehend and process information and are capable of understanding the consequences of their actions. Because competency is a legal term, medical determinations typically evaluate a patient's decision making capacity rather than competency.

Incompetency may be general or specific.[10] General incompetency refers to those patients who are unconscious, intoxicated, grossly psychotic, or senile. The term "specific incompetency" is applied to those patients who are incompetent to make certain decisions but competent to make others. Persons may be incompetent as a matter of law because they are minors, or incompetent as a matter of fact because they have been adjudicated to be incompetent by the courts. Some persons, however, who have been found by the courts to be incompetent may be quite able to make a specific medical decision. Although the law traditionally views persons younger than 18 years as incompetent to make decisions, some exceptions exist for emancipated minors, mature minors, and some children who have adequate capacity to make decisions.[11] It has been suggested that it may be more reasonable to ask of a person at any age, "is this person capable of making this decision?"[12]

In critical care medicine, a patient's lack of decision making capacity may be complete, limited, or intermittent. Medications given for sedation, anxiety, or analgesia may impair a patient's mental functioning, as can a patient's fear, depression, or denial. Caution must prevail in judging competency, because commonly used modalities (such as intubation) can prevent a competent patient from voicing preferences or from contradicting the staff's belief that he is incompetent. Because the status of the critically ill patient may change abruptly, competency should be re-assessed frequently.[13] Table 1 lists the various tests that have been proposed to determine competency.[1] Sliding scale standards applied for competency have been proposed for informed consent. A relatively low standard of informed consent and minimal scrutiny are appropriate when there is a favorable risk/benefit ratio and the patient assents, or when the risk/benefit ratio is unfavorable and the patient objects, whereas a higher standard and more intense scrutiny are appropriate when a patient objects to a procedure with a favorable risk/benefit

Table 1
Tests for Determining Competency

1. Is the patient capable of understanding the given information regarding:
   A. The illness—its nature and implications
   B. The treatment—its risks and benefits and those of any possible alternatives?
2. Is the patient capable of making a choice based on "rational" reasons?
3. Is the patient capable of communicating his preferences to the care givers?
4. Is the patient capable of arriving at a decision?
5. Is the patient capable of arriving at the "right" decision?

ratio, or when he consents to a procedure with an unfavorable risk/benefit ratio.[1]

The mere fact that a patient lacks decision making capacity does not automatically remove from him the rights accorded to all patients undergoing medical treatment, those of autonomy and privacy. However, the manner in which these rights are exercised differs for this patient in that another person, a surrogate, exercises these rights for the patient. Although family members have no legal authority to make most medical decisions for incapacitated patients,[14] next of kin routinely make these decisions. In fact, family members are best suited to be surrogates because they are most concerned about the patient and are the most knowledgeable about the patient's goals, preferences, and values.[11] Furthermore, most people have a strong expectation that their family members will make decisions for them if they are incapacitated[15] and family members best predict patient preferences.[16] When a surrogate must be chosen, the patient's "family" should be interpreted broadly to include not only relatives but also close friends.[11]

Physicians also play a substantial role in surrogate decision making because families rely heavily on their medical expertise. Physician input also helps diffuse the responsibility for making painful decisions.[13] The presumption that the family of the patient lacking decision making capacity should be the primary decision maker for the patient may be challenged under certain circumstances. For example, the family member or members may be incapacitated, unable to agree on a course of action, have conflicts of interest, or may abuse or neglect the patient.[11] Even if family members are disqualified as surrogates, it may be appropriate to consult with them for decisions, much as one should consult with the patient even if he becomes incompletely or intermittently incapacitated. If the patient has no family or court-appointed guardian, some surrogate decision maker should be designated to ensure a clear assignment of authority, continuity, and a foundation for decision making.[11] Usually, physicians become the surrogate decision makers under these circumstances,[17] but it may be more appropriate for a hospital ethics committee to appoint a third party to act as a surrogate under these circumstances, since there may be a conflict of interest on the part of the physician. It may, therefore, be preferable for another person—a patient advocate—to be appointed in court or by the hospital ethics committee. This person is an authorized representative who purely represents the patients' interests. In an emergency situation involving a patient lacking decision making capacity, there may not be enough time to obtain consent from a surrogate without endangering the patient. It is recommended, however, that assent of the patient, his surrogate, or both be obtained if time permits.[13]

Once a surrogate has been identified decisions should be made with specific regard to two concerns: respect for the patient's autonomy and the promotion of the patient's health.[11] Although patient autonomy is respected through the surrogate, there are differences between what patients want and what their surrogates think they want.[15,18] When a surrogate decides for a patient, therefore, it is different from the patient deciding for himself, and certain decisions have such potentially severe adverse outcomes that they may be made only by a competent patient, not by a surrogate.[11]

The two main standards advocated for use by surrogate decision makers making decisions for patients who lack decision making capacity are substituted judgment and best interests. Substituted judgment occurs when a surrogate attempts to determine what the incompetent patient would have decided had the patient been able to choose. This can only be used if the patient was at one time capable of developing preferences and values, and left reliable evidence of those attitudes concerning the current medical situation.[11] Most people avoid discussing illness and death, do not communicate their preferences to others, and do not have advance directives. Under these circumstances of lack of knowledge, substituted judgment cannot be used, and the best interests standard is typically used. The best interests standard attempts to promote the good of the individual as viewed by the shared values of society. Such factors as the avoidance of death, relief of pain and suffering, preservation or restoration of functioning, and quality and extent of life, as well as the impact on the patient's family are usually taken into account.[13] The course that will offer the greatest net benefit to the patient, as would be determined by a reasonable person in the patient's circumstances, is followed. Quality of life decisions should be made based on the value of life to the individual patient and not to society.

Most ethical and legal authorities have recommended the use of substituted judgment first. If the patient's views are not known, the best interests standard is used.[11]

Allocation and Triage of Scarce Resources

In caring for critically ill patients, professionals may have major ethical dilemmas in making decisions for these patients. As financial pressures mount, the ability to follow a patient's wishes may not always be possible, and these dilemmas will increase even more. Society may not be able to afford what each autonomous patient might desire. Although cost effectiveness is important, critical care professionals must not lose sight of their primary duty to their patient. Foregoing care should be based on a patient's desires and medical possibilities rather than upon financial considerations, especially considering the great uncertainties in medicine.[17]

In order to help physicians make major ethical decisions and in order to help diffuse decision making responsibility many hospitals have set up an ethics committee. This committee is made up of a multidisciplinary group of people from outside the ICU and may include physicians, a lawyer, an administrator, and lay people. These committees provide the physician with advice, opinion, consultation, and recommendations, but the actual treatment decisions are usually left to the physician.

At present, most individuals in society expect that "everything" will be done for their loved ones who require medical and critical care. The medical profession must educate the public and explain that maximum efforts for certain subgroups of patients who have no likelihood of surviving are simply not appropriate. Doing "everything" in some patients should mean maximizing comfort measures and not aggressive efforts at an unobtainable goal of survival.[17]

Of late, as scarce resources decrease, physicians seem to be becoming more concerned with societal needs as opposed to the needs of individual patients. Some specific conditions are particularly problematic: the patient in a persistent vegetative state (PVS), individuals with the acquired immunodeficiency syndrome, and the elderly. These classes represent the groups of patients who some may view as having lives not worthy of living.[19] If a treatment is deemed futile, not because it will fail physiologically and technically, but rather because the life saved is deemed not worthy of being saved, a moral judgment and not a medical judgment has been made. Indeed, there are considerable problems and a good deal of debate regarding the concept of futility. Physicians often face difficult decisions regarding continuation of treatments, for example, ventilating a patient in a PVS or instituting cardiopulmonary resuscitation in terminally ill patients. Youngner[20] suggests that open and full discussion with the patient and/or his surrogate can solve many of these problems, and that a satisfactory decision may often be reached. Lantos et al.[21] suggest that the clinical determination of futility is ambiguous due to disagreements of language, statistical uncertainty, and social prejudices. The additional factor of difficulty in predicting medical outcomes with complete certainty makes futility an elusive concept. These authors conclude that futility determinations must include both clinical judgments about the chance of success of a therapy and consideration of the patient's goals for therapy. Truog et al.[22] suggest that the whole idea of futility should be replaced by the concept of making therapeutic decisions based on what is in the patient's best interest. This, of course, involves full and open discussion with the patient and/or his surrogates. Under some circumstances, "unreasonable treatments" are demanded by the patient and/or his surrogates and these authors suggest that two other values be brought into the picture: those of professional ideals (i.e., respect for patient wishes, compassionate action, and minimization of suffering) and social consensus. For instance, a patient in a PVS whose surrogates demand full intensive care may present the professional carers with a serious moral dilemma. In the US, the Task Force on Ethics of the Society of Critical Care Medicine (SCCM), for instance, recommended that these patients should be removed from the ICU unless it is not possible otherwise to meet the patient's nursing care needs.[23] The President's Commission[24] stated that PVS patients should be removed from life-support if such action is necessary to benefit another patient who is not in a PVS. The SCCM Task Force stated that such a patient should not be maintained in the ICU to the exclusion of a patient who can derive benefit from ICU care and also recommended that, except in situations of pregnancy or where organ donation or research use has been validly authorized, there is no medical justification for continuing medical support of a patient who is diagnosed as brain dead.[23] In this case the Task Force suggested that it is inappropriate to seek the agreement of the family or the surrogate for the withdrawal of medical support. Although critical care medicine professionals have stated that the quality of life as viewed by the patient, the patient's likelihood of surviving the hospitalization, and the reversibility of the patient's acute disorder are the important criteria for deciding which patient should receive the last ICU bed,[25] it is not clear whether only medical criteria are used for triage decisions. Marshall et al.[26] noted that political power, medical provincialism, and income maximization rather than medical suitability were the reasons for physicians providing critical care services.

Foregoing Life Sustaining Treatments

There are many situations in critical care medicine that require decision making about whether to continue or forego life sustaining treatments. Smedira[27] found that although these treatments are withheld or withdrawn relatively infrequently (1% and 5%, respectively) approximately half of all deaths in ICUs (in the two hospitals studied) occur when life-sustaining treatments are foregone. When the patient is incompetent to make his own decisions the critical care physicians and family members (or surrogates) try to preserve the patient's autonomy by making decisions that the patient would have wanted.[17] Advance directives are means for individuals to exert more control over the decisions that will have to be made when they become incapacitated. They allow patients the self-determination to decide how decisions will be made and by whom. Advance directives are acts of an individual's will and therefore carry more weight than a mere preference that might be used for substituted judgment.[11] Advance directives have been used primarily for foregoing care at the end of life to ensure a patient's death with dignity, but may obviously be used for many other important medical decisions.

An instructional advance directive is an instrument, executed by a competent individual, in which it is specified which treatments should be given or not given under certain circumstances should the individual become incompetent. Commonly used instructional advance directives are the living will and organ donation cards. A proxy advance directive is an instrument executed by a competent individual in which he designates some other person to serve as a surrogate should he become incompetent. The most commonly known proxy advance directive is the durable power of attorney. Occasionally, the two types of advance directives are combined such that one designates a surrogate with instructions.

The advance directive, however, is not without problems. The living will usually provides that no extraordinary or artificial life-support will be used to prolong life in the event of a terminal illness rendering the drafter incompetent. The terms "extraordinary", "artificial life-support", and "terminal illness" are vague and great latitude has been given to doctors in interpreting these terms. Most physicians, however, are uncomfortable not knowing exactly what is permissible, and not all states (in the US) have made the living will legally enforceable. Some states require the patient to revalidate the directive after becoming terminally ill, a time at which most patients are unable to do so.[28] Other problems with living wills include the following: (1) it is a document for the future and all possible medical situations cannot be anticipated and decided in advance; (2) many individuals do change their minds when the actual situation arises; (3) therapeutic options may change from the time the directive is signed until the time it has to be implemented; (4) a competent person's decision concerning future contingencies is weaker under circumstances that the patient may not have envisioned than is a competent patient's contemporaneous decision; and (5) the physician's ethical imperative to preserve life and not let the patient give up too soon occurs for imprudent, contemporaneous decisions by patients but not for advance directives.[11] Finally, there may be practical problems concerning directives. There may be a question of whether the patient was competent, whether the patient was adequately informed or if he voluntarily signed, and the exact intent of the patient may not be clear as many directives may be vague and ambiguous.[11] A durable power of attorney avoids only some of these problems. Under many circumstances, the surrogate may not spend an appropriate amount of time adequately discussing and understanding the patient's values and preferences.

To overcome the uncertain legal status of living wills and patients without advance directives, several US states have enacted Natural Death Acts.[11,12] These statutes allow family members to withdraw or withhold treatment from certain patients. Many of the statutes require that the patient be terminal and that death be imminent.[11] Therefore, patients in a PVS may not be included in such statutes unless they are considered "terminal".

In general, where a valid and clear directive is present, it should be followed. It takes precedence over the other principles of decision making, as it advances the patient's self-determinism.[11] There may be rare circumstances when it is appropriate to refuse to respect an advance directive, such as when doing so would result in the death of a patient who though impaired would, with proper care, lead a life that clearly contains more pleasure than pain and suffering.[11] Difference of opinions between surrogates, between surrogates and health care professionals, and between health care professionals should be resolved with repeated efforts at discussion and communication. If disputes cannot be resolved, institutional ethics committees can help. Courts should only be used as a last resort.[17]

When making decisions concerning foregoing life-sustaining treatments, both preservation of life and quality of life must be taken into account.[23] In some circumstances, a patient may judge that it is preferable to forego therapy than to receive it, or clinicians may judge that major goals of therapy are unachievable. In cases such as these, it is sometimes ethically appropriate to forego therapy. Here we again encounter the problem of medical futility. A treatment may be considered medically futile either because it does not achieve its physiological goal or its therapeutic goal.[24] For instance, a patient receiving mechanical ventilation in the presence of respiratory failure may receive adequate oxygenation and carbon dioxide clearance, but if lung function will never recover, despite all medical interventions, then the therapy is futile even though it is physiologically successful. Others consider treatment futile only if it is physiologically unsuccessful.[22] Another problem encountered is that of semantics. In the US, the President's Commission[11] stated that there is no difference between the terms "withhold" and "withdraw". Life sustaining treatments may be necessary to permit full evaluation of the patient's condition and these therapies should not be withheld during evaluation.[23] Therefore a decision to withdraw a treatment already initiated and shown not to be effective may be regarded as less ethically problematic than a decision not to initiate a treatment. In the Jewish religion, however, treatments already instituted usually cannot be withdrawn, whereas treatments not yet instituted may be withheld. Catholics are required to take good care of their bodies and to use "ordinary means" to ensure their health and preservation, but are not required to use "extraordinary means".[29] They may withdraw treatments that become excessively painful or burdensome.

Any treatment derives its medical justification from the benefits that the informed patient and the physician hope to achieve by using it. When the treatment has achieved those benefits or can no longer reasonably be expected to do so, the treatment loses its justification and may be foregone.[23] Foregoing therapy should be discussed in the following situations: (1) when the patient has a diagnosis with a grave prognosis; (2) when the burdens of therapy outweigh the benefits; and (3) when the quality of the patient's life is expected to be unacceptable to the patient.[23] A health care professional has no obligation to offer, begin, or maintain a treatment which, in his best judgment will be physiologically futile.[23]

In a decision to withhold or withdraw therapy, there are no intrinsic moral differences between categories of treatment such as cardiopulmonary resuscitation, ventilatory support, or medications such as vasopressors, antibiotics, and insulin. There is some disagreement, however, concerning the status of the provision of nutrition and hydration by artificial means.[23] Many physicians place artificial nutrition and hydration in the same category as the aforementioned interventions. Others, however, maintain that hydration and nutrition (other than high technology total parenteral nutrition) are key components of patient care and should not be equated with medical interventions.[23]

Each available medical treatment or procedure should be considered from the patient's perspective in the light of the overall benefit that it may offer and the burdens that it may entail, and the professional duties that are involved. Treatment decisions should be considered in the context of the goals of the total treatment plan for the patient rather than in isolation.[23] The continued efficacy and justification for any ongoing course of therapy should be re-evaluated at appropriate intervals in light of changing conditions. One of the most important factors is the likely success of the continued course of treatment in achieving its goals and anticipated benefits that justified its initial use.[23]

Unlike a decision to initiate life sustaining procedures, which must often be made in an emergency situation, a decision to withdraw a life sustaining treatment should be made only after a deliberate consideration of the ethical factors involved. The basis for such a decision should be discussed with the patient and/or his surrogate and a joint decision reached.[23] It is also recommended that a treatment offering a reasonable expectation of physiologic benefit may be withheld in the case of a patient suffering from terminal illness, and that treatments offering no benefit and which serve to prolong the dying process should not be used.[23]

In order to ensure that treatments are not "wrongly" withheld or withdrawn there are several "safety-nets" available to physicians. Each country's legal system defines its own laws by which treating physicians must abide. For instance, in Israel, physicians are only allowed to withdraw life sustaining treatments already initiated in those patients who are brain dead, whereas many states in the US have enacted Natural Death Acts,[11,12] which allow family members to withdraw life sustaining treatments from certain patients. Also patients who have previously defined their wishes by means of a living will help physicians make these difficult decisions. Problems arise if a patient who has no living will is in a situation where treatment may be withheld or withdrawn. In these cases patients may not receive the treatment they would wish. A treatment may be withheld in a patient who, if able to express himself, would wish to continue with all possible treatments, or treatment may be given to a patient who would have preferred not to have received it. Problems may also arise if the family of the patient appears to be making clearly inappropriate decisions regarding the treatment of a relative. Under any of these circumstances it is helpful for the physicians to have recourse to the local ethics committee for support and guidance, and if unavoidable to the courts.

In situations where a patient does not receive medical treatment because it is withheld, or receives a medical treatment that is later withdrawn the term "passive euthanasia" is used. "Active euthanasia" or "mercy killing" occurs when individuals take an active role in the actual demise of a patient. In the US giving large doses of morphine to patients being withdrawn from ventilators and the withdrawal itself are considered passive euthanasia. In Europe, these actions are considered active euthanasia. In its 1977 policy statement on the physician and the dying patient, the American Medical Association condemned mercy killing as "contrary to the most fundamental measures of human value and worth". Although active euthanasia remains a criminal offense in the Netherlands, as previously mentioned, the Dutch Medical Association advocated guidelines for the medical practice of euthanasia in 1984.[3] These guidelines call for three "necessary conditions" for a physician to participate: (1) the request for euthanasia must be made consistently and freely by the patient; (2) the patient's state of illness and prognosis must be unbearable and beyond recovery; and (3) the physician must consult a colleague "to confirm the correctness of diagnosis and prognosis, to support and verify the correct medical performance of euthanasia, and to check if all (legal) requirements are met".[3] A new law is currently being proposed in the Netherlands that notes when euthanasia can take place. In the US public opinion polls have shown that approximately 60% of the American public favor legalizing active euthanasia under certain circumstances,[30] but it still remains illegal.

Clinical Research Trials

It is generally accepted that the physician's primary responsibility is to provide the best possible treatment to his patient and that this obligation overrides other competing goals such as the promotion of scientific knowledge.[31] Many medical procedures and therapies given in the critical care unit on a daily basis have not been scientifically proven to be effective. Interventional trials of the greatest benefit demonstrate validity, generalizability, and efficiency, and since validity has become a non-negotiable demand,[32] the randomized trial has become the gold standard. If there are therapies that we use that may help or harm patients, can we use our patients in randomized trials to evaluate these treatments? In a randomized clinical trial, the various procedures performed are not all necessary for the treatment of the individual patient. As a subject in a clinical trial, the patient may be exposed to added hazards, discomforts, and inconveniences. Treatment may not be able to be tailored to the patient's specific needs. On the other hand, there may be benefits for the patient to become a research subject. The patient may have access to a new drug that would otherwise not be available. In addition, the patient may be positively affected by the Hawthorne effect because the patient is part of a research activity with more attention from specialists who would not be as involved if the patient were not in the trial.[33] Recruiting patients as research subjects into randomized clinical trials is believed to be morally permissible because at the time of the trial it is not clear what the best treatment is and the randomized clinical trial is not inconsistent with the physician's duty to provide the best possible treatment for his patient.[31] In fact, there are those who argue that it is more ethical to use patients as research subjects in a randomized clinical trial than to use treatments that are unproven. Most of the recent clinical trials for sepsis have compared a new therapeutic agent to a placebo and all other therapies could be specifically tailored to the patient by his primary care physician.

There are, however, other ethical problems in the performance of randomized clinical trials in the critically ill. One is the potential conflict of interest for the physician who is responsible for the medical treatment of the patient and who is also the principal investigator of the research study.[31] As the primary care physician, the doctor's commitment is exclusively to his patient whereas as the scientist's obligation is to the proper running of the study and scientific knowledge. Often these two roles coincide but occasionally they may conflict. Therefore, it is best if these two roles be separated.

There are safeguards built into the performance of clinical trials. Restrictions on the use of human subjects in clinical research studies are accepted internationally. They are explicitly spelled out in the Nuremberg Code of 1947 and the World Medical Association Declaration of Helsinki, revised in 1975.[34] The Declaration of Helsinki, states that "concern for the interests of the subject must always prevail over the interests of science and society".[34] These codes require informed consent prior to using a human subject in a study. In the US, federal regulations for informed consent for research are more stringent than informed consent for therapeutic indications. In general, studies are reviewed by an Investigational review board (IRB) or Helsinki committee before being approved.

Informed consent for research presents additional ethical problems. In general, the patient should be informed as to the nature of the medical problem, what the proposed study treatment is with its risks and benefits, the fact that he does not have to participate in the trial, and that he can withdraw from the trial at any time. Most critically ill patients will not have the decision making capacity to decide for themselves and, therefore, surrogates will typically sign for them. Some countries and some states in the US specify that the surrogate must be "an authorized legal representative", which usually means going to court to appoint an official guardian but under most circumstances a close family member is accepted. All of the problems noted earlier as to differences between patient and surrogate decisions are relevant. One of the major issues with informed consent to clinical trials is whether the consent is truly voluntary. The added burden of information and decisions as to a trial adds to the extreme stress and anxiousness of the patient or family. They probably wonder how the patient's care will be negatively affected if they refuse or how it will be positively affected because they have agreed. The investigator should explain that the patient will receive the best possible care by the treating physicians whether he participates in the trial or not. Although there may be certain problems with informed consent in these situations, it may not be that different from informed consent under clinical situations and there are certainly more protections for research subjects.

Perspectives for the Future

The critical care physician's responsibility, apart from knowing the law and respecting a patient's individual rights, is also to know his own ethical principles. His behavior should be guided by these principles and by the patient's best interests. The physician does not have to agree to withdraw life-sustaining therapy, for example, because the patient requests this of him, nor must he administer a treatment he considers futile in a patient who is prepared to try anything.

Certainly disagreements will occur among the health care team and between the health care providers and the patient and/or his family and surrogates. Disagreements in this context may either be due to differences in opinion on basic issues, or due to poor communication. It is of paramount importance that everyone involved be aware of the true diagnosis and prognosis, and that a minimum of medical jargon be used. All members of the health care team must work hard to help the patient and his family or surrogates perceive and understand all the implications of a specific decision.

Finally, but of tantamount importance, is the physician's duty to an individual patient. In critical care medicine, particularly, difficulties may arise as scarce resources decrease, as they certainly will in the future. The physician must, however, retain his list of priorities, his duty to each individual patient and make decisions based on what he believes is medically, ethically, and legally correct.

References

1. Sprung CL, Winick BJ: Informed consent in theory and practice: Legal and medical perspectives on the informed consent doctrine and a proposed reconceptualization. Crit Care Med 1989;17:1346–1354.
2. Stedman's Medical Dictionary 25th Edition, 1990. Baltimore, USA, Williams and Wilkins.
3. De Wachter MAM: Active euthanasia in the Netherlands. JAMA 1989;262: 3316–3319.
4. The humane and dignified death act. Calif. Civ Code 10.5.
5. A piece of my mind. It's over, Debbie. JAMA 1988;259:272.
6. Siegler M: Searching for moral certainty in medicine: A proposal for a new model of the doctor-patient encounter. Bull NY Acad Med 1981;57:56–69.
7. Beauchamp TL, Childress JE: Principles of Biomedical Ethics. New York, Oxford University Press, 1989.
8. Salgo v Leland Stanford Jr. University Board of Trustees, 154 Cap App 2d 560, 317 P2d 170, 1957.
9. Winick BJ: Restructuring competency to stand trial. UCLA Law Rev 1985; 32:921.
10. Lidz CW, Meisel A, Zerubavel E, et al: Informed Consent: A Study of Decision Making in Psychiatry. New York, The Guildford Press, 1984.
11. President's Commission for the Study of Ethical Problems in Medicine and Biomedical and Behavioural Research: Deciding to Forego Life Sustaining Treatment: Ethical, Medical and Legal Issues in Treatment Decisions. Patients Who Lack Decisionmaking Capacity. Washington, DC, Government Printing Office, 121170, 1983.
12. Capron AM: The competence of children as self-deciders in biomedical interventions. In Gaylin W, Mocklin R (eds): Who Speaks for the Child? New York, Plenum Publishing Corp., 1982, p. 57.
13. Nyman DJ, Sprung CL: Ensuring informed consent: Essentials and specific exceptions. J Crit Illness 1991;6:891–906.
14. In re Brooks' Estate, 32 Ill 2d 361, 205 NE 2d 435, 1965.
15. High DM: All in the family: Extended autonomy and expectations in surrogate health care decision making. Gerontologist 1988;28:46.

16. Ouslander JG, Tymchuk AJ, Rahbor B: Health care decisions among elderly longterm care residents and their potential proxies. Arch Intern Med 1989; 149:1367–1372.
17. Sprung CL: Surrogate decision making. In Lumb PD, Shoemaker WC (eds): Critical Care State of the Art. Fullerton, CA, Society of Critical Care Medicine, 1990, pp. 367–378.
18. Uhlmann RF, Pearlman RA, Cain KC: Physicians' and spouses' predictions of elderly patients' resuscitation preferences. J Gerontol 1988;43:M115-M121.
19. Sprung CL: Changing attitudes and practices in foregoing life-sustaining treatments. JAMA 1990;263:2211–2215.
20. Youngner SJ: Who defines futility? JAMA 1988;260:2094–2095.
21. Lantos JD, Singer PA, Walker RM, et al: The illusion of futility in clinical practice. Am J Med 1989;87:81–84.
22. Truog RD, Brett AS, Frader J: The problem with futility. N Engl J Med 1992; 326:1560–1564.
23. Task Force on Ethics of the Society of Critical Care Medicine: Concensus report on the ethics of foregoing life-sustaining treatments in the critically ill. Crit Care Med 1990;18:1435–1439.
24. President's Commission for the Study of Ethical Problems in Medicine and Biomedical and Behavioural Research: Deciding to Forego Life-Sustaining Treatment: Ethical, Medical and Legal Issues in Treatment. Washington, DC, Government Printing Office 17.S., 1983, pp. 188–189.
25. The Society of Critical Care Ethics Committee. Attitudes of critical care medicine professionals concerning distribution of intensive care resources. Crit Care Med 1994;22:358–362.
26. Marshall MF, Schwenzer KJ, Orsma M, et al: Influence of political power, medical provincialism and economic incentives on the rationing of surgical intensive care unit beds. Crit Care Med 1992;20:387–394.
27. Smedira NG, Evans BH, Grais LS, et al: Withholding and withdrawal of life support from the critically ill. N Engl J Med 1990;322:309–315.
28. Martyn SR, Jacobs LB: Legislating advance directives for the terminally ill: The living will and durable power of attorney. Nebraska Law Rev 1984;63: 779.
29. Misbin RI: Physicians' aid in dying. N Engl J Med 1991;325:1307–1311.
30. Roper Organization of New York City: The 1988 Roper Poll on Attitudes Toward Active Voluntary Euthanasia. Los Angeles, CA, National Hemlock Society, 1988.
31. Schafer A: The ethics of the randomized clinical. N Engl J Med 1982;307: 719–724.
32. Sackett DL: The competing objectives of randomized trials. N Engl J Med 1982;303:1059–1060.
33. Murray M, Swan AV, Kiryluk S, et al: The Hawthorne effect in the measurement of adolescent smoking. J Epidemiol Comm Health 1988;42:304–306.
34. Angell M: Ethical imperialism? Ethics in international collaborative clinical research. N Engl J Med 1988;319:1081–1108.

Chapter 19

The Legal System: A Background for Clinicians

Walter Wadlington, A.B., L.L.B.

Background

Many physicians think of law almost entirely in the context of medical malpractice actions. Even in this context their views often are shaped by anecdote or horror story or perceptions about the legal system that are erroneous at worst or confused at best. Granted that concern about professional liability has become a factor in medical decision making—perhaps to a much greater degree than desirable—but it is important to recognize that because of the breadth, fragmentation, and intricacy of our health care delivery system, many more legal issues are implicated. This chapter seeks to provide a basic understanding of the legal system for physicians so that they can better understand these legal issues and the framework in which they are resolved. It also explains the segment now used to provide financial compensation to persons sustaining injury through the health care system.

From: Sibbald WJ, Massaro T (eds.): The Business of Critical Care: A Textbook for Clinicians Who Manage Special Care Units. © Futura Publishing Co., Inc., Armonk, NY, 1996.

State and Federal Roles

Under the federal system of the US, most of the law governing compensation for injury or enforcement of contracts between individuals is established and administered by the states. There may be substantial variance between jurisdictions in some instances, though the need for consistency in others has led to development and adoption of similar provisions. There also is an overlay of federal regulation in many areas, particularly where there is impact on interstate commerce, though today federal regulatory power is considered very broad in many settings.

For several decades the health care field has been subject to increasing federal regulation, much of it stemming from the government's provider role. This has been accomplished by legislation and through administrative regulation by agencies to which rule making and enforcement authority have been delegated. State regulation to implement federal policy sometimes has been induced by conditioning federal financial contributions on state adoption of specific initiatives or legislative provisions. Although state and federal regulations dealing with a particular area may and often do coexist (for example, some states deal more stringently in certain consumer protection or public health matters), federal regulations can be drafted so as to preempt and thus "trump" inconsistent state or local provisions on the same subject.

Important categories of private law that remain largely within the ambit of individual state regulation include torts, contract, property, trusts and estates, and family law. But even in these fields, a state rule that violates a right guaranteed by the US Constitution can be invalidated through judicial action.[1] Judicial willingness to interpret and protect such rights in recent years has been an important catalyst for legislative reform during the past decade even in areas such as family law, where intervention on constitutional grounds once was rare.

The Common Law Process

Much of the private law of the early US states was based on English common law, as modified by Parliament through some date specified in the legislative or constitutional provisions adopting it.[2] Under a common law approach, legal principles and rules develop through judicial holdings that serve as precedents for deciding subsequent cases. It remains of major importance in development of the law in some fields such as torts.

Supporters of a common law approach contend that its dynamism can allow ongoing consideration of technological as well as societal changes without abrogating established legal principles. For example, a principle to be used in gauging whether a particular medical procedure was appropriate or was performed in accordance with reasonable or customary practice at a specific point in time allows consideration in later cases of knowledge and techniques not available previously. A disadvantage of the common law, however, is that precedents often evolve slowly, a matter of special concern in times of rapid change. Courts decide only those cases that are brought before them, and only resolve those issues necessary to a decision under the circumstances of each case; the precedential value of the decision is limited to those issues that were reached. It is important to understand also that determination of the issues to be raised or emphasized can rest heavily on counsel, who may be more concerned about the impact of any decision on their clients than about implications for future litigants. The following brief description of the judicial process is designed to illustrate how law develops through judicial precedents.

The initial or "trial court" level is where witnesses testify and disagreements about facts are resolved. Usually one judge presides over a trial, applying rules of evidence and procedure that control who can testify and what evidence is admissible. If there is a jury, the judge instructs them about matters such as the scope of their duty, any tests to be applied in evaluating the probative weight of various evidence admitted during the trial, and the applicable law. Jury instructions usually are based on established legal rules or principles, though they may call for innovation when these are unclear. An example of the latter might be a judge's instructions about whether or how to apply an emerging test such as "cortical death" to determine whether a person was alive at a particular moment, in the absence of either a statute or a judicial precedent about such a test.

Appeal from a trial court's decision ordinarily is based on some misconstruction or misapplication of law. If the trial court's findings of fact are to be disturbed, the case usually will be remanded to the trial level for a new hearing. A typical reason could be that certain evidence was improperly admitted or excluded through an incorrect interpretation or application of the rules of evidence. Not all such mistakes will result in remand for a new trial; if an error is considered "harmless," in that it had no effect on the legal outcome, it may be disregarded by the appellate court.

In most jurisdictions appellate courts deal with issues of law rather than fact. Such questions can range from whether a particular witness should have been allowed to testify on a specific topic to matters of whether the facts that were proven can form the basis of a recognizable legal action. A good example of this is the so-called action for "wrongful conception", in which the issue is whether damages can be awarded to parents of an unwanted child who was conceived after an ineffective sterilization procedure.[3]

Appellate courts (and some at the trial level, such as federal district courts) produce written opinions that are published in official state reporters and/or an elaborate series of reports known as the National Reporter System. The latter includes published opinions of appellate courts from every jurisdiction, state and federal. Under the long-standing common law doctrine of *stare decisis*, holdings of an appellate court are binding on courts below them in the judicial hierarchy of that jurisdiction. Sometimes a lower court will interpret a higher court's arguably "binding" decision as distinguishable and from the case before it, perhaps leading to an appeal on that question. A court may overrule one of its own prior decisions or restrict its future application. Sometimes the precedential meaning of a decision may be difficult or impossible to determine because appellate courts at the highest levels often sit in large panels and their decision may be based on a plurality rather than a majority of those sitting. In such cases some judges may write separate dissenting opinions while others may concur in the result on the basis on a different theory.

Appellate opinions may include speculation about other situations or even discussion of hypothetical cases that might seem to suggest how they would decide issues not reached in the case before the court. Such statements are considered *obiter dictum*, or simply *dictum*. They are neither "holdings" nor "precedents" that courts lower in the judicial hierarchy must follow but they may have practical impact on how lawyers advise their clients, particularly if authored by a highly respected jurist or seemingly having wide acceptance among the judges. Such language may reflects a court's desire to articulate guidelines for conduct in related problem areas in order to obviate future judicial challenges.

An elaborate cross-indexing system permits locating each instance in which a reported opinion was cited by another appellate court anywhere in the US. Computerized data retrieval systems also facilitate locating opinions in which particular terminology has been used or interpreted.

Law schools in the US have long emphasized the use of appellate decisions to develop analytical skills. This "case method" of study is as much a key to how lawyers are socialized to respond to problems as is the clinical approach to training physicians. Law students are conditioned to question, analyze, and draw viable distinctions that will be important in coping with the enormous and continually growing body of legal precedent. Deemphasis of the case method is taking place as more law schools and authors of teaching materials expand their focus to include ideas and approaches from other disciplines, exploring how economic analysis and social science methodology can be integrated effectively into the legal process. Indeed some law schools today are in the forefront of interdisciplinary research and thought, with law and medicine one field for this.

The Increasing Importance of Legislation

The scope and significance of legislation have increased greatly in the US during this century. Some fields (e.g., antitrust and labor law) are based on statutory frameworks rather than judicial precedent, though even in such instances courts continue to play an important role through interpretation or determining issues of constitutionality.

When the common law in an area has matured into rules of general application, legislatures sometimes choose to codify them. Legislation may be enacted to overrule specific judicial holdings or to create new causes of action. Occasionally a court will decline to create a new cause of action, or to abolish an action or defense that has evolved through judicial development, when it is perceived that such a decision calls for investigating and evaluating the broader effects and policy implications that such a step may have. This may be accompanied by express judicial suggestion that legislative consideration of the problem would be appropriate. But even though courts may prefer to have legislatures address certain issues, failure or delay by the latter in doing so does not mean that the judiciary will not seek to resolve problems in the interim. Modern illustrations of this include such issues as whether life-support systems might be removed even in the absence of passage of a natural death or durable power of attorney law.

Locating and comparing the different states' legislative approaches to the same or similar problems can require tedious examination of inconsistently indexed state codes. And unlike the situation with regard to the US Congress, there is usually little legislative history of state legislative debates that might provide clues useful for subsequent interpretation.

Steps Toward Uniformity Among the States

Even under a federal system, there is obvious need for uniformity in many private law areas. Facilitating commercial transactions across state lines provides a key example. Recently there has been increased willingness to seek greater compatibility (and, on occasions, uniformity) in areas where this formerly was the exception. Family law, which can include decision making about children's medical care as well as issues of child support, neglect and abuse, and family breakdown, presents such an example. Some of the impetus has been economic, as in the case of enforcing support obligations across state lines; in other instances, such as interstate child custody, change sometimes has reflected popular concern abetted by media coverage.

When states wish to achieve uniformity, availability of model statutes can be important. Their use can be influenced by whether they were drafted by respected groups who weighed the alternatives and reviewed the language for nuances, or whether they have been adopted in some jurisdictions and are working effectively. A model that initially may have seemed *avant garde* or unnecessary may later achieve popular acceptance as the problems it was designed to confront become acute.

Best known among nongovernmental groups who develop legislative models is the National Conference of Commissioners on Uniform State Laws, founded in 1892. The term "Uniform Law" is considered a term of art for a model developed by the Commissioners rather than a generic label for legislative models.

The Expanding Role of Administrative Law

Administrative law has seen extraordinary growth in the US during the past 3 decades. It is of major importance in regulation of the health industry because of extensive involvement of the Department of Health and Human Services and corresponding state agencies. Under power legislatively delegated to them, administrative agencies engage in a variety of regulatory functions. In health care this has ranged from determining whether new hospital facilities can be built (or old ones expanded) to establishing limitations on physicians' assistants' practices and hospital reimbursement under Medicare. Important to the system are special administrative law tribunals that remove much burden from the judiciary. Procedures that must be followed by various agencies in a given jurisdiction usually are set forth in laws of general application known as administrative procedure acts. There are usually procedures for invoking limited judicial review of administrative actions, and questions also can reach courts regarding whether an agency exceeded its authority or adequately followed required rule making procedures.[4]

It is through the administrative process that much of the regulation of credentialing and licensure takes place in the US.

Criminal Law

Criminal law deals with conduct regarded as an offense against the state. An act may constitute both a tort and a crime; in such instances tort law can provide compensation to the injured party while criminal law is invoked to punish or deter such conduct in the future. For example, violation of a prohibition against unlicensed medical practice may result in a fine or jail sentence imposed by a criminal court because of the danger posed to the general public. But an individual harmed by the unlicensed practitioner must bring a separate action in tort to recover damages for injuries sustained through substandard conduct. In some legal systems both tort and criminal law issues would be adjudicated in the same proceeding. In the US they are separate, and a criminal prosecution typically requires a higher level of proof.

Fear of criminal prosecution now seems greater than ever among physicians. This reflects both the litigious disposition of our time and fundamental differences of opinion within society about matters such as abortion, treatment of defective neonates, and withdrawal of life-support from terminally ill incompetents, as well as slowness in coordinating modern technology and long-standing legal rules adopted at a time when it would have been near heresy even to predict such developments.

Law Reform Commissions

The "commission" approach to promoting law reform is used frequently in Commonwealth countries to assess either broad or specific issues of social and technological change with an eye to stimulating appropriate legal responses. Products of this approach include the 1984 Report of the Committee of Inquiry into Human Fertilisation and Embryology, known as the Warnock Committee Report, in Great Britain. Officially appointed committees have dealt with similar issues elsewhere, such as in the Australian states of Victoria and Queensland and the Canadian Province of Ontario. Some governments have established law reform commissions that remain in continuous operation, prepared to accept instructions to examine and make proposals about specific issues or practices.

Resort to commissions has been less frequent in the US, though this may be changing. During the past decade the Presidential Commission for the Study of Ethical Problems in Medicine and Biomedical and Behavioral Research published a series of influential volumes dealing with issues that included genetic screening and counseling, access to health care, making health care decisions, deciding to forego life-sustaining treatment, splicing life, defining death, and implementing human research regulations. The readable, extensively annotated volumes of the Report include findings and conclusions of the Committee, and they have been cited extensively in judicial opinions. Though broad in scope, the specific congressional mandate to the Commission did not encompass all areas in which major ethical and legal issues are emerging as the result of biomedical progress. Among those not dealt with were artificial conception and new reproductive techniques, aside from the role of heterologous artificial insemination in genetic counseling.

Since the Report of the President's Commission, several state governments have appointed special committees or commissions to focus on problems of biomedical technology and medical decision making with regard to specific areas such as reproductive techniques and death and dying. Such an approach is likely to become increasingly important in light of recent US Supreme Court decisions making it more important for states to develop their own rules to govern practices in these and other areas including abortion.

The Framework for Medical Professional Liability

As noted earlier, some physicians seem to view "law" as almost synonymous with "malpractice suit". Though undeniably narrow and perhaps overstated, this depicts the intensity of the concern of many medical practitioners that they may be sued after an untoward outcome even if they followed an accepted medical standard. Some such fears may be justified, though many stem from lack of knowledge or misconceptions about the legal system and the incidence of successful actions for medical injury. Because it is widely believed that fear of liability often influences medical decision making and encourages medical procedures to protect against liability more than promote patient well being, examination of the framework governing professional liability seems appropriate. Important questions are: (1) do legal rules about liability of physicians, hospitals, and allied health care personnel vary significantly from those governing other professionals or business entities?; (2) are there valid reasons for a distinct approach for health care providers?; and (3) are current legal rules for compensation workable in the medical milieu, and have they been articulated with sufficient clarity that physicians and other health care practitioners can understand when and why their conduct may be actionable?

Contractual Liability and Waiver

An action for breach of contract is based on failure to comply with an obligation created by personal agreement rather than a duty imposed independently by law. Physicians may expressly or impliedly agree to use a particular level of care or skill, but it is unusual (and foolhardy) to guarantee a result or cure. The contract action thus has not been used extensively to recover damages suffered through medical treatment, even though it could provide a tenable basis for legal action based on the specific terms of an agreement. Sterilization and elective, cosmetic surgery are examples of cases in which patients have been more likely to contend that a specified result was promised but not effected. Because statutes of limitation may differ according to whether an action is framed in contract or tort, contract actions sometimes have been used when the time has expired for a tort suit. Contract actions also have been initiated in attempts to circumvent procedural obstacles such as sovereign or charitable immunity barring tort actions against certain institutions.[5]

Courts have long frowned on contractual agreements waiving liability for hospital or physician negligence, even in cases involving nonpaying patients. In concluding this they have applied a general rule against exculpatory clauses in contracts affecting the public interest to a high degree. In rejecting such an exculpatory clause in a medical context, the California Supreme Court[6] described the situation in which a contract would be "affected by the public interest":

> [T]he attempted but invalid exemption involves a transaction which exhibits some or all of the following characteristics. It concerns a business of a type gener-

> ally thought suitable for public regulation. The party seeking exculpation is engaged in performing a service of great importance to the public, which is often a matter of practical necessity for some members of the public. The party holds himself out as willing to perform this service for any member of the public who seeks it, or at least for any member coming within established standards. As a result of the essential nature of the service, in the economic setting of the transaction, the party invoking exculpation possesses a decisive advantage of bargaining strength against any member of the public who seeks his services. In exercising a superior bargaining power the party confronts the public with a standardized adhesion contract of exculpation, and makes no provision whereby a purchaser may pay additional reasonable fees and obtain protection against negligence. Finally, as a result of the transaction, the person or property of the purchaser is placed under the control of the seller, subject to the risk of carelessness by the seller or his agent.

Regarding it as unrealistic to expect patients to bargain over such clauses or seek to find another hospital instead, the court noted that "The admission room of a hospital contains no bargaining table where, as in a private business transaction, the parties can debate the content of their contract."

The language of the 1963 opinion provides interesting judicial insights about the place of health care in our society. However, today there is significant support for at least a modified "market" approach that would allow patients and providers more latitude in fixing their respective rights and duties regarding compensation for harmful or unsatisfactory results in advance through private ordering. Current cost control concerns and increased emphasis on shopping for price among competitive providers in other fields may well lead to relaxation of the historic restrictions against contractual limitation of liability in connection with medical treatment. Indeed, it is probable that the limitation of the cases on exculpatory contracts has been considerably overstated: Generally the cases arose in the context of total waiver of liability, a far cry from negotiating either a different scheme for determining liability or a different regime for providing compensation. One reform approach now being urged is to permit greater contracting between patients and providers with regard to liability coverage and procedures for fixing liability.[7]

The Framework of Tort Liability

Theories of Recovery

Tort law provides financial compensation in the form of money damages for injury caused by conduct violating a duty imposed by law independent of a contract. Although its basic purpose is injury compensation, the tort system also is regarded as serving a quality control function through its deterrent effect. In limited instances it also may serve a role more analogous to the criminal law through punitive damage awards. Substantive tort law is governed by each state through rules and principles that have evolved largely through common law development, though an increasing body of legislative regulation, some of it focusing specifically on medical malpractice litigation, has been added in recent years.

The three basic theories on which recovery can be grounded are classified as intentional tort, negligence, and strict liability. Negligence is the most widely used in medical injury cases, though concern about intentional tort has led to widespread establishment of protocols for obtaining consent. Strict liability, also known as liability without fault, has developed most significantly in the context of products liability and extrahazardous activities. Some reformers have suggested formal extension of strict liability to some untoward results of medical care as an efficient method of risk distribution. And some physicians contend that negligence rules are being twisted into something akin to strict liability in the medical malpractice context.

Intentional Torts. An intentional tort is an intentional, unauthorized, and unprivileged invasion of a legally protected interest of some person. Courts have named and defined the elements of a number of specific intentional torts. Battery, perhaps the best known of them, is the violation of a protected interest in bodily integrity. Assault involves placing someone in apprehension of such harmful contact. Other examples of "nominate" torts include defamation (encroaching on a protected dignitary interest), and intentional infliction of emotional harm.

Among intentional torts, battery probably is most relevant to physician conduct because many routine medical procedures could be actionable without either express or implied authorization by a patient. The Restatement of Torts (2d) includes the following hypothetical example of actionably "offensive conduct": "A, a surgeon, while B is under anesthesia, makes an examination of her person to which she has not given her consent. A is subject to liability to B."[8]

Desire to avoid a battery action provides the basis for obtaining patient consent before performing risky or seriously invasive procedures. In many lesser "invasions," consent will be implied from patient conduct, and an emergency exception has been developed by courts to allow medical personnel to take immediate steps to preserve the life or health of an ill or injured person who is incapable of consenting.

Special problems can arise when a person is legally incompetent either because of minority or mental incapacity. In non-emergency situations consent generally must be obtained from a person legally authorized to do so, usually a parent or legal guardian. A large number of the states have enacted specific statutes dealing with the special situation of minors nearing adulthood. Typically the latter have been authorized to consent to certain procedures such as crisis care for mental health, communicable disease, alcoholism of drug abuse therapy, and family planning (other than abortion or sterilization).[9] A few states have gone further and adopted "mature minor" provisions that allow a minor "of sufficient intelligence to understand and appreciate the consequences of the proposed surgical or medical procedure" to consent.[10]

Because invasion of a protected interest is the basis for an intentional tort, proof of actual physical harm is unnecessary. Without consequential damages, a recovery may be low, but it is in the context of intentional torts that the potential for an award of punitive damages is most likely to exist. Punitive damages sometimes are based also on reckless or outrageous conduct, and are awarded to deter the wrongdoer rather than simply to provide compensation for injury.

Negligence. Negligence, to use another Restatement of Torts (2d) definition, is "conduct which falls below the standard established by law for the protection of others against unreasonable risk of harm. It does not include conduct recklessly disregardful of an interest of others." To be actionable, any breach of the standard must cause actual damage to a person to whom a duty was owed. The duty is generally based on existence of a physician-patient or hospital-patient relationship. Proving that the breach of duty was the "legal" or "proximate" cause of the injury can be complex, particularly when there has been some intervening agency subsequent to the original act or omission that forms the basis of the complaint. A special concern in case of medical negligence is the manner for determining the applicable standard of care. It is not enough to show that there was a mistake in diagnosis, an untoward result, or an unnecessary procedure unless there was injury resulting from failure to exercise the minimum degree of skill and care required under circumstances.

1. The standard of care: Determining the standard of care for negligence is an example of the common law's potential for reflecting ongoing technological and social change rather than embedding past practices in inflexible rules. Whether conduct was unreasonable under the specific circumstances will be determined by a judge or jury as a matter of fact. In deciding about reasonable-

ness of particular conduct, a jury is instructed by the court as to what factors may be considered and what weight they may be accorded. In nonmedical cases, the standard often is described as that of a reasonable person under the circumstances. Custom in a particular industry or profession can be important but in determining what conduct is reasonable, courts often use what is described as a "calculus of risk" test to balance severity of foreseeable harm against the onerousness of requiring additional precautionary burdens. The watchword is "reasonable" conduct under the particular circumstances.

In medical malpractice actions, physicians are accorded special advantage because the standard applicable to them usually must be established by expert (physician) testimony, thus emphasizing the role of custom much more than in other cases involving professional conduct. The generally accepted rationale is that lay persons could not gauge appropriate conduct for medical procedures. The practical result is that as to distinctly medical issues unless a plaintiff produces testimony from a medical expert to establish the standard, the suit can be dismissed on the motion of the defendant. That requirement once produced accusations that physicians (and their insurers) engaged in a "conspiracy of silence" that made it virtually impossible to obtain expert witnesses in malpractice actions.[11] This concern has largely dissipated in recent years, replaced in part by physician concern about whether some expert witnesses are "hired guns" rather than adequate evaluators of good medical practice standards.

Not long ago the standard of care applied in medical malpractice cases was that exercised by physicians of ordinary skill and care in the defendant's locality or a similar community.[12] This "strict locality" rue permitted recognition of practice standards that varied according to geographical location and exacerbated then existing problems of obtaining expert testimony; by statute or judicial decision, it generally has been replaced by a broader standard of what a reasonable and prudent physician (or "a reasonably competent practitioner in the same class" would do under the same or similar circumstances.[13] An additional "expert" standard has been developed in some jurisdictions for physicians with special training and qualification. However, the language in which standards are articulated remains subject to significant variation among the states, some of which retain vestiges of the older "locality" rule.[14]

An expert testimony requirement accords great weight to

customary medical practice in determining acceptable physician conduct. Professional views may differ as to what is customary, and the trier of fact must resolve disparities between conflicting expert testimony regarding both the customary standard and the reasonableness of the conduct at issue. There also can be instances when courts decide as a matter of law (without jury involvement) that a customary standard is too low. Washington's Supreme Court in 1974 reached such a conclusion about the general practice among ophthalmologists of administering glaucoma tests to patients under age 40 only in unusual cases. The court found that the simplicity of the test and the magnitude of the risk made it unreasonable to apply such a rule without exception.[15] Though criticized by some in the medical world, the court's action applied an established principle used in tort actions other than for medical malpractice.

Treatment in an Emergency: Both courts and legislatures have responded to the problem of what standard of care should be applied for medical care rendered in emergency situations. An "emergency exception" has been developed in many states to allow physicians to proceed when a patient is incompetent. Many states also have adopted what are dubbed "Good Samaritan" or "rescuer" statutes. The usual approach of the latter is to lower the legal standard of care owed by a physician (and often a lay person as well) who renders emergency assistance gratuitously outside of a medical facility. Generally speaking, physicians have a moral rather than a legal duty to persons other than those with whom they have established a physician-patient relationship. Thus the purpose of the statutes is to assure that physicians will render emergency care, through what might be described as positive reinforcement. Some statutes provide that the actor can be held liable only for gross negligence. Others afford near blanket immunity rather than simply lower the standard. Whether the statutes were legally needed is subject to debate because the customary standard of physician care could consider emergency circumstances and settings. Adoption of the statutes has generally been deemed desirable, however, if only for their symbolic quality.

2. Burden of proof: A plaintiff must prove each element of the particular action, though in some circumstances a court or jury may be permitted to draw an inference that a particular result would not have occurred without negligence. The latter approach, known as *res ipsa loquitur*, developed outside the ambit

of medical care. In its most common form it is considered appropriate where expert testimony is unnecessary to determine whether proper skill was used (e.g., medical testimony is not necessary to establish that a scalding water bottle will cause burns). "Foreign body" cases, in which a sponge, instrument, or other object is left inside a patient after the close of surgery, are typical examples for invocation of *res ipsa loquitur*. The doctrine also may be used in highly technical cases that require expert testimony to establish that the particular harm usually does not result if reasonable care is given.[16]

Courts differ on the procedural effect of *res ipsa loquitur*. The majority treat it as a form of circumstantial evidence that permits, but does not require, a jury to draw an inference of negligence. However, some in the medical community fear that the doctrine will be misused by invoking it even if adverse results can stem from a particular procedure in a significant number of instances of even high level care.

Another controversial use of *res ipsa loquitur* involves its use in dealing with multiple defendants when it is uncertain which one caused the harm. In a famous California case, a patient who suffered shoulder trauma while undergoing an appendectomy under anesthesia subsequently sued all parties connected with the operation.[17] The court invoked *res ipsa loquitur*, which had the practical effect of requiring each party to come forward and explain what happened as far as (s)he was involved. New Jersey's Supreme Court has used a similar approach in a case involving a rongeur that broke during orthopedic surgery while embedded in a patient's spine. It was unsuccessfully argued that not all the parties who might appropriately have been held liable were before the court.[18] Critics of such an approach worry that it reflects a judicial orientation toward assuring a recovery against someone for every undesirable result.

3. Defenses: The most obvious defense to a malpractice action is to refute the evidence. And once there has been final judgment on the merits of a particular claim it is said to be *res judicata*, which bars relitigation of the same issues. Other defenses based on general negligence law principles may be available, including those discussed below.

   Contributory and Comparative Negligence: Under a "pure" contributory negligence rule, proof that a plaintiff's negligence was a contributing factor will bar recovery even though the defendant's negligence was significantly greater. Contributory negligence has not had substantial impact in medical malpractice cases, though it has been asserted in instances of patient noncooperation or refusal to undergo tests or follow-up treatment. In the latter cases, however, some courts consider that the plaintiff alone may have been negligent under the circumstances. Some jurisdictions have adopted comparative negligence schemes in which a plaintiff's negligence does not bar recovery but may diminish an award.

Statutes of Limitation: Statutes of limitation set forth the maximum time period during which a legal action can be commenced. Special statutes of limitation for medical malpractice exist in many states, with substantial variation between them. Of special importance is the time when the limitation period commences. It was long common to begin when the negligent act occurred, whether or not the injured party was aware of it. A more modern approach, known as the "discovery" rule, does not start the limitation period until the injured patient knew or should have discovered that there was injury. A further variation based on the physician-patient relationship can preclude commencement of the statutory limitation period until continuing treatment for the particular condition has ended.

Special statutes of limitation can apply when the plaintiff is a minor. Some provide that the limitation period does not commence until the plaintiff reaches adulthood (usually age 18). Because this can present special problems for pediatricians and pediatric surgeons, some states have adopted statutes suspending commencement of the filing time only until some age well below majority; others have allowed only a moderately longer period for filing children's claims compared with that for adults. The courts that have reviewed such statutes have reached conflicting results about their validity, usually applying the constitutional law of their own states.

4. Informed consent—The negligence framework: State courts early in this century recognized that competent persons have the right to decide whether to submit to a particular medical procedure,[19] though these statements were made within the framework of concern about intentional torts such as battery. Recognizing a physician's duty to "inform" a patient in the context of negligence is a much later development.[20] Under the latter doctrine a physician should disclose to a patient those risks of serious harm that may be reasonably expected to stem from a given procedure, as well as feasible alternatives. The

underlying concept is that patients should be partners in the treatment decision process.

Using the negligence formula, the appropriate standard of disclosure must be determined once it is decided that there is a duty to disclose. To meet the causation it also must be established that the patient would not have consented to the procedure had there been adequate disclosure. Some courts use an "expert" standard to define the disclosure standard (what physicians normally disclose),[21] while others use a "lay" test (what a reasonable patient would expectably want to know).[22] It is widely accepted, however, that causation should not be determined on the basis of what the particular patient would have decided, but on what a reasonable person would have done under the circumstances.

The distinction between consent to avoid a battery action and consent to comply with the standard of care for a negligence action still may be widely misunderstood by physicians. The confusion is not helped by use of the same terminology in the context of human experimentation with a special set of administratively promulgated federal rules and standards. Because of this uncertainty the informed consent doctrine, which developed as a response to a perception of physician paternalism,[23] has been viewed as a major threat by many clinicians even though relatively few plaintiffs recover solely on the basis of negligent failure to disclose.

Strict Liability. The term "strict liability" can be an overly broad label. It is used here to denote imposition of liability without proof of negligence or other culpable conduct. In the US, the doctrine has been developed most prominently in cases involving ultrahazardous activities and, more recently, defective products placed in commerce. In addition, various compensation schemes that minimize or replace the use of fault as the criterion for fixing responsibility have been introduced. Best known is worker's compensation. Others include "no fault" automobile compensation schemes, and most recently, compensation schemes for birth related neurological injuries.

1. The product liability background: Strict liability to deal with dangerously defective products has been effected through either legislation or judicial action, and through either commercial law or tort law. The latter is illustrated by Restatement of Torts (2d) § 402 A, which has been effectively "adopted" by some courts

and has served as a model in others: "One who sells any product in a defective condition unreasonably dangerous to the user or consumer or to his property is subject to liability for physical harm thereby caused to the ultimate user or consumer, or to his property, if (a) the seller is engaged in the business of selling such a product, and (b) it is expected to and does reach the user or consumer without substantial change in the condition in which it is sold." The rule applies even though the seller has exercised "all possible care" in preparing and selling the product, and there is no contractual relation between user and seller.

The reporter's commentary to § 402 A describes an exception for "unavoidably unsafe products", referring specifically to ethical drugs. Recognizing that they may have harmful side effects that are outweighed by benefits justifying a high degree of risk, the commentary suggests that such a product, if "property prepared, and accompanied proper directions and warning, is not defective, nor is it *unreasonably dangerous.*" While this can insulate the manufacturer of an ethical drug from tort liability, it can produce special problems for physicians who do not heed the manufacturer's warnings and instructions in the "package stuffer" or elsewhere. The physician may be negligent for prescribing when it is not the appropriate drug of choice and an efficacious and significantly less dangerous alternative is available, or for failure to maintain adequate monitoring for side effects in accordance with the manufacturer's instructions.[24] Thus the manufacturer's directions may be important to the standard of care of the prescribing physician. Widespread over prescription of chloromycetin more than a decade ago provided such a problem for physicians.

A widespread legislative exception to strict liability in the hospital field developed in response to judicial opinions fixing liability on hospitals for hepatitis acquired through blood transfusions when there was no effective scientific test to detect presence of the virus in whole blood. Numerous state courts followed the lead of a 1970 Illinois Supreme Court decision that blood was a "product" within the meaning of § 402 A, that it was "sold" by the hospital, and that if it contained hepatitis virus it was "in a defective condition unreasonably to the user." In a subsequent legislative movement, however, such decisions lost future precedential effect when special statutes removed blood (and other transplantable tissue) from coverage under strict liability provisions in tort, warranty, or the Uniform Commercial Code.

The Action for Violation of Civil Rights. Although not generally thought of as part of the tort system, the federal action for violation of civil rights under 42 U.S.C.A. § 1983 deserves mention in any broad appraisal of professional and hospital liability because it can result in a damage award as well as declaratory or injunctive relief. The action is based on deprivation of some right, privilege, or immunity secured by the Federal Constitution. It can only be invoked if the defendant acted "under color of state law", a requirement not ordinarily satisfied simply by acceptance of Medicare or Medicaid reimbursement or Hill-Burton funds.

Damages

The term "damages" describes a monetary award to compensate for injury received through tortious conduct or breach of contract. In the medical malpractice setting, concern has been expressed both about specific items that are deemed compensable and the high level of some awards. Fear that dramatic publicity about large recoveries for malpractice might promote filing of claims has led some insurers to seek agreements maintaining confidentiality of settlement amounts.

Some critics argue that it is difficult, if not impossible, to translate "pain and suffering" into a monetary award without undue reliance on emotional responses. They argue that this element of damages is unduly susceptible to manipulation based on subjective views rather than objective proof. Also criticized is the "collateral source rule", which provides that amounts received by the injured party from a source other than the defendant (e.g., the injured person's own accident insurance or social security) will not lessen an award. It is often suggested, however, that the collateral source rule is retained to make up for the portion of a damage award that a plaintiff's attorney receives as a contingent fee in typical US practice in which each party bears the costs of litigation.

One damage law reform proposal would modify the traditional practice of reducing an award to a fixed amount that cannot be modified either up or down based on changing needs. Such awards take into account actuarial projections of life span and predictions about the need for future treatment. Alternatives could be structuring awards in future installments terminable on a payee's death, or using annuities or insurance to cover certain expenses. Many states already allow or require consideration of periodic payment of awards in some medical malpractice cases.

In countries with broad national health schemes, damages that are legally recoverable by a patient will be lower if future medical care is to be covered under the government scheme. This presents an interesting question for contemporary health care planners. For example, should the national health plan be subrogated to actions of patients for medical care paid by the state based on substandard care? Thus far such an approach has not been considered appropriate, and thus it is easily conceivable that a universal access health care system could lower the overall size of damage awards in the US.

The 1970s and 1980s "Malpractice Crises" and Its Impact

The 1970s Experience The mid-1970s saw considerable publicity about an avowed medical malpractice "crisis". Usually it was defined only sketchily, and its causes and extent were unclear though there was no shortage of anecdotal information. Major concern centered on the rapid cost increase and diminishing availability of professional liability insurance in many states. As late as 1973 a special Commission on Medical Malpractice appointed by the then Secretary of HEW to investigate the problems reported that malpractice insurance was available to health-care practitioners and that the market for it was competitive. Within a year that statement was considered almost ludicrous as premiums began climbing and some underwriters began to withdraw selectively from some markets.

Although the ostensible crisis was triggered by availability and cost of insurance, it is important to understand that professional liability insurance merely indemnifies an insured physician for claims based on legal liability. In theory at least, the system thus mirrors contemporary tort law. Despite the lack of hard data, many reasons were offered about why the underwriting changes took place. Among the most popular were: (1) an increased number of lawyers and a perception of their willingness to bring marginal suits under the lure of contingent fees; (2) substantive and procedural tort law changes, including a shift to "discovery" timing in statutes of limitation and expansion of the doctrine of *res ipsa loquitur*; (3) casualty insurers' poor investment results; (4) the characteristically long period between filing and settlement of medical malpractice claims, producing what is described as a "long tail" phenomenon; (5) lower standards of medical practice; (6) greater likelihood of iatrogenic injury because of increased technological complexity in medicine; (7) changes in the traditional physician-patient relationship; (8) costly administration of liability claims under the existing system; and (9) a growing public view that persons should receive at least some compensation for injuries from "diseases of medical progress" or untoward results of medical care.

Demoralizing, costly, and harmful results were attributed to the crisis, most of them difficult to verify or quantify from existing evidence. Some probably resulted less from the "insurance crisis" itself than from physician anxiety in the face of uncertainty about claims. Some of the effects attributed to the crisis at the time are described below.

Defensive Medical Practice. "Defensive medicine" can be defined in several ways, some of them connoting desirable practice from a consumer standpoint. In its most objectionable sense, it refers to undertaking or prescribing diagnostic or other procedures more to protect the physician from tort liability than to promote patient health. Concerns about defensive medicine range from potential physical danger through excessive x-rays or other tests carrying inherent risks, to imposition of medically unnecessary costs that must be absorbed at some level of the health care system. The volume of "defensive medicine" of this genre is unclear, but the term has become common in the health care lexicon.

A more subtle form of defensive medicine is reluctance to publish suggestions for change or results of studies indicating that existing or prior procedures may be incorrect or even harmful, for fear that this will provide an avenue for tort suits based on repudiation or criticism of previously accepted practices.

Lowering Standards of Medical Practice. A frequently voiced concern was that fear of malpractice actions could lead to physician reluctance to perform procedures with greater potential benefit but substantially higher risk. The thesis is that physicians will conform to a standard of the least risky alternative, creating greater exposure to the more imaginative and conscientious practitioners. Implicit in such an assumption is that concern about tort liability on physicians in their day to day practice is highly significant.

"Going Bare." This refers to practicing without professional liability insurance. Problems can arise regarding exposure to bankruptcy and the possibility that injured patients with legitimate claims will go uncompensated. An important feature of professional liability policies is their provision for defending insureds as well as indemnifying them against judgments within the policy limits. The uninsured physician must bear the cost of legal counsel even if the defense is successful. Another important consideration is the requirement by some hospitals that all physicians with staff privileges maintain a minimum level of liability insurance.

"Dropping Out." Though suggested as a concern, information about how many physicians actually leave practice because of the malpractice action fears is largely anecdotal. Generally regarded as a more serious concern is physician withdrawal from certain procedures, such as delivering babies. Also relevant are considerations of whether a physician is influenced to join a large group practice or an HMO to assure liability coverage.

Responses to the Crises

During the 1970s, many state legislatures adopted legislative responses to the perceived crisis. Legislative responses ranged from extensively publicized malpractice "packages" to subtle (and not so subtle) provisions lobbied through without careful scrutiny or consideration of how (or whether) they might affect existing medical practice. Even when enacted, some were considered as likely to have little impact, or even to be of questionable constitutionality. The latter concern was justified by subsequent court decisions in some states. Examples of the most popular legislative responses of the day were:

1. Ceilings or "caps" on damages: These provisions varied according to whether they "capped" all damages or merely those for pain and suffering (the more typical approach). While subsequent studies have shown that damage caps can have an effect on insurance rates, the approach nevertheless has been criticized because their practical effect can be to require only the most seriously injured persons to participate in the process of keeping insurance rates down. Although the US Supreme Court declined to review a decision by one state supreme court consti-

tutionally upholding such a law,[25] the highest courts of several states have invalidated such provisions based on their state constitutions.

2. Eliminating *ad damnum* clauses: The ad damnum clause in a claimant's petition sets forth the amount of damages requested. Critics argue that eliminating it is largely cosmetic because there is little evidence that it significantly influences the ultimate recovery amount; some also assert that it infringes on the right of free speech. Supporters disagree, and also contend that it helps keep down spectacular publicity that might foment malpractice claims.
3. Pretrial screening and review panels: Many states enacted provisions for pretrial review of medical malpractice claims by special screening panels. Such panels usually are a precondition rather than a substitute for court trial and their conclusions typically are not binding. Provisions vary on such aspects as panel membership, whether findings will be admissible in subsequent litigation, and whether suit should be filed before or after requesting panel. Critics argue that such panels unreasonably restrict access to the courts and cause further delays.
4. Arbitration: Arbitration of medical malpractice claims has seen limited use for many years in some jurisdictions, but in others there have been questions about its feasibility and reluctance from lawyers and physicians to use it extensively. The latter reflected factors including concern about enforceability of agreements to arbitrate executed before delivery of health care; fear that arbitration might lead to a larger number of recoveries, albeit of smaller dimensions; possible limitations on agreements for binding arbitration; and a limited number of arbitrators with medical backgrounds. Responsive legislation in many states was designed to clarify the use of arbitration specifically in the health care context.
5. Changing the collateral sources rule: Many states adopted provisions modifying or largely eliminating the collateral source rule. They vary in approach, with some allowing evidence of such payments to be received, with the trier of fact left to determine the weight to be ascribed, and others requiring an offset. Under the latter approach, the deduction may be made by the court after a jury award.
6. Regulating contingent fees: Contingent fee agreements, under which a plaintiff's attorney is compensated by receiving a portion (typically one-third) of any recovery, is feature of malprac-

tice litigation specially maligned by health care providers. In some areas of law, such as domestic relations, contingent fees have been limited by opinions of legal ethics committees or courts that regulate practice standards. However in personal injury cases of all types the approach is widely used.

Some critics of contingent fees argue that they produce excessive attorneys' fees and encourage filing of marginal claims for nuisance or settlement value. Others question whether an attorney should be a joint venturer with a defined economic stake in a claim that (s)he is asserting for someone else. Defenders of the practice contend that it provides effective representation for worthy claimants who otherwise could not afford it because of the cost of legal services. They also contend that market factors will discourage bringing untenable claims, and that there are other and better ways of policing frivolous actions.

The 1972 Report of the HEW Secretary's Malpractice Committee found that through averaging plaintiff lawyers' contingent fees to an hourly basis for comparison with the charges of defense lawyers there did not appear to be any gross discrepancy between them in medical practice cases. They made the additional interesting and little noted finding that "the contingent fee arrangement discourages the acceptance of meritorious low-recovery cases" but that "on a fee-for-service basis, potential clients would be similarly discouraged from pursuing these same meritorious low-recovery cases, since the average citizen cannot financially support the required lawyer's services."

Regulation can take several forms, including the establishment of a maximum percentage or a series of maximums varying according to recovery amounts, or the requirement of judicial approval of fee agreements for fairness.

7. Modifying *res ipsa loquitur* and informed consent: Concerns about possibly burring the distinction between negligence and strict liability through aggressive use of the doctrine of *res ipsa loquitur* led some states to modify or limit use of the doctrine in medical malpractice cases. Similarly, some states elected to codify the doctrine of informed consent purportedly to clarify the duty to disclose.[26] Some statutes permit a physician to rely on a patient's written acknowledgment as conclusive that consent was "informed", though one state's highest court has construed such a statute as creating a rebuttable rather than a conclusive presumption that informed consent was obtained, noting that the state's right of privacy doctrine assures that pa-

tients can determine whether to accept or reject medical treatment.[27]

Changes in Insurance Underwriting Practices

There were also changes in insurance practices, though many of these had no specific legislative impetus. One key example was the movement toward "claims made" rather than occurrence based policies. Under the latter, long-standing approach, a physician or hospital would purchase an annually renewable liability policy that would cover the insured (within policy limits) against claims based on conduct taking place during the policy year, even though such claims might not be filed until afterward. Under many statutes of limitation, an action might be filed considerably longer than a year after the date of the conduct giving rise to it occurred. Under the "discovery" rule, for example, or under a statute that does not start to run against a minor until (s)he reaches majority, potential exposure of an underwriter might continue for a considerable period of time. This was reflected in what actuaries referred to as the "long tail phenomenon". From the insurer's standpoint, it was argued that this makes it difficult to establish a fair annual premium rate on an experience basis except over a considerable period of time.

A "claims made" policy indemnifies the insured only against claims filed during the policy year, regardless of when the actionable conduct took place. The underwriter thus can better define exposure by knowing the number of outstanding claims at the end of each policy year. But this advantage is achieved by increasing exposure to the insured. To be covered against unfiled claims for conduct during the period, (s)he must maintain future coverage. A retiring physician who wishes to be protected must, therefore, purchase a special policy covering this unprotected "tail".

The "claims made" policy is now typical for physicians as well as many other professionals.

Physician Mutuals. Another popular approach was the establishment of mutual insurers owned and controlled by physicians. They responded both to fear that commercial insurance might become unavailable and to belief that administrative costs could be contained better through such organizations, as well as to the perception that they might better reflect and protect physician's views and interests. The idea behind such groups was not new. Physicians and dentists in the British Commonwealth long were defended and indemnified chiefly by medical defense unions. Although in England, it has been held that these organizations are not "insurers" in the strict legal sense; it is clear that they performed such a function for physicians whether or not they fell within the ambit of formal insurance regulation. They also actively sought to educate their members about conducting themselves to avoid malpractice claims—a practice continued today even though the government has taken over the defense of medical injury claims for that part of a practitioners work under the National Health Service.

At one time there was concern that some physician owned companies, often known as "bedpan mutuals", might be insufficiently capitalized to survive major unfavorable underwriting experience. Although some start-ups experienced such financial difficult, on balance, many physician mutuals have survived and grown and today they are writing a significant amount of professional coverage.

The "Crisis" of the 1980s

Before there had been time for the legislative measures adopted in the 1970s to have any identifiable effect, claims incidence and insurance rates tapered off. Some observers saw this as an illustration of the clearly cyclical nature of insurance underwriting. They were not surprised, therefore, when another insurance-driven crisis surfaced in the 1980s. At that time some of the earlier measures were adopted in states that had not done so earlier, and attempts at fine tuning were made. Though little new in the legal sense was initiated, at this stage it became more widely recognized that the problems did not rest simply with the tort and insurance systems. New approaches to risk management and quality control were implemented, and there were finally some initiatives to undertake serious studies regarding the etiology and dimensions of the problems involved.

Among the most important findings dealt with were the extent of medical injury sustained in hospitals. A 1970 study in California, undertaken to evaluate feasibility of a no-fault compensation system surprised many with the finding that 4.65% of inpatient stays produced injuries that might be compensable under a no-fault scheme. Even more surprisingly, 17% of those seemingly provided the legal basis for negligence awards.[28] However, only ten from the last group actually filed a claim.[29] These findings were largely confirmed in 1990 by the Harvard

Medical Practice Study. In the latter, which uses cases drawn from a probability sample of 31,000 hospital patients in New York State, the incidence of adverse events for hospitalization there in 1984 was estimated as 3.7%; of that number 27.6% (1% of all hospital discharges) were considered due to negligence.

These findings obviously hold special significance for any new compensation not based on fault because they permit more realistic estimates of the cost savings necessary through administrative efficiencies, damage ceilings, or other means. Alarmingly to some, they also suggest that the present tort system is not working very efficiently and that there is a sizeable "overhang" of cases that might reach the courts if there were a change in claiming behavior for any reason.[30]

Tort Law In a Qualitatively Multitiered Health System

Federal and state regulations can affect health care practice standards in many ways. Since government is a major third party provider, its efforts to monitor quality should be expected. In today's economy, escalating health care costs have led to imposition of new regulations aimed almost exclusively at cost control. But uncoordinated measures directed toward the separate goals of establishing standards for quality control and fixing procedures to minimize cost can produce not only confusion but the possibility of serious tort liability problems for health care providers by introducing conflicts of interest to provider-patient relationships and what may be perceived as dual standards of care according to who is paying. For example, a third party provider's approaches of providing fixed amounts for reimbursing health care providers based on a formula such as average projected cost, or of setting specific goals for decreasing certain types of operations or conditions, may have the desired effect of cutting costs through promoting efficient use of hospital facilities. However, its overly rigid application could also result in lowering the quality of care for some patients. Whether this occurs may depend on what numbers are placed in the formula. Use of such an approach thus has the potential for altering care standards in order to reach specific economic goals. If the lowered compensation formula is designed to cover all costs rather than introduce greater cost sharing by the patient, the state is set for a qualitatively multitiered system. However tort law does not recognize different standards of care for patients whose care is being reimbursed through Medicare or other third party providers.

An interesting dimension with regard to federal involvement in treatment standards is added when one examines the provision for physician tort immunity for acting in compliance with or in reliance on professional norms developed by PROs for their geographical areas. While the statute did not exempt physicians from liability for failure to exercise due professional care, it provided strong incentive to follow the "established" norm if one were concerned about malpractice. Although encouraging more standardization of medical care may be a desirable goal in some or even many instances, there are some costs that should be considered in accomplishing it through this means. What impact will reinforcement of the standard through an offer of tort immunity have on quality in cases where the standard offers the legally safer but medically less efficacious alternative? The PRO exception on its face might be regarded as possibly negating or denying a key quality control aspect of the malpractice action by its assurance that the quality standard it sets will not be affected by tort action.

It is in the context of a major shift in the process for delivering health care that some major new approaches are being drafted and discussed. These range from substitution of a new system of no-fault coverage to retaining fault as the basis for liability but removing adjudication from the courts and replacing it with a more administrative law type of model (a proposal by the American Medical Association) would introduce a variation of this approach. Another less drastic approach would allow greater use of contract, as discussed previously. Reflecting the changes in practice that already have occurred, a proposal for enterprise liability has achieved support in some quarters. The last would provide that actions for medical enterprise would be brought against a hospital or other entity rather than the individual physicians involved. Advantages include the fact that it could be used regardless of the underlying basis of the system for compensation, it could achieve significant operating efficiencies, and it would encourage greater quality control through the entity with liability.

The incidence of claims has remained fairly stable or even declined in some locations during the past several years, although the severity factor has continued to rise. In this environment, however, there has been less widespread concern about a "crisis". Additionally, some in the health care system seem to question whether further legal reforms are likely to accomplish this. Several of the new schemes are reaching a stage of development at which large scale demonstrations could test their effectiveness. If such demonstrations are carried out and one or more of the new proposals proves to be better than the present system gauged in terms of both fairness and efficiency, a shift in the present system could well occur when the next crisis appears.

Some Comparisons with Other Systems

The preceding discussion has placed special emphasis on the legal system in the US. In the health care world this is the approach that is being watched most widely and which has produced special concern. It is important to recognize that in most other common law jurisdictions such as Great Britain, most of Canada, and Australia, differences from the US system are for the most part not major. In some, such as Canada and Australia, similar problems of federalism can arise though the role of courts in the constitutional sphere may not be so great. And it is only in the US that jury trials are widespread in civil actions for medical injury.

Civil law jurisdictions such as France, Germany, and the Canadian Province of Quebec differ significantly from the common law jurisdictions because of the latter's emphasis on judicial precedent. Their typical starting point is a code that is comprehensive and internally integrated to provide the basis principles for legal reasoning in decision making by the courts. Such codes are much different from collections of statutes that are described as codes in the US and which are regularly annotated with judicial decisions that provide a highly important gloss. While one state in the US, Louisiana, still maintains some of its French and Spanish civil law heritage and has a civil code, the emphasis on judicial precedent in some areas such as torts has moved it closer to the common law group.

References

1. See, e.g., Loving v. Virginia, 328 U.S. 438(1972).
2. See, e.g., 1 Va. Code Ann. §§ 1–10, 1–11 (1995 Repl. Vol).
3. See Procanik by Procanik v. Cillo, 97 N.J. 339, 478 A.2d 755 (1984).
4. See, e.g., American Academy of Pediatrics v. Heckler, 561 F. Supp. 395 (D.D.C. 1983).
5. See, e.g., Berry v. Druid City Hospital Bd., 333 So.2d 796 (Ala. 1976).
6. Tunkl v. Regents of Univ. of California, 60 Cal.2d 92, 32 Cal. Rptr. 33, 383 P/2d 441 (1963).
7. See, e.g., Clark Havighurst, Reforming Malpractice Through Consumer Choice, Health Affairs 63, (Winter 1984).
8. 1 Restatement of Torts 2d 32 (1965).

9. See, e.e., 7A Va. Code § 54.1–2929 (1994 Repl. Vol.).
10. See Arkansas Code 20-9-602 (1991 Repl. Vol.).
11. See, e.g., L'Orange v. Medical Protective Co., 394 F.2d 57 (6th Cir. 1968).
12. See Shilkret v. Annapolis Emergency Hospital Ass'n, 276 Md. 187, 349 A.2d 245 (1975).
13. See Shilkret v. Annapolis Emergency Hospital Ass'n, 276 Md. 187, 349 A.2d 245 (1975).
14. See, e.g., 7A Va. Code § 8.01-581.20 (1992 Repl. Vol.).
15. Helling v. Carey, 83 Wash.2d 514, 519 P.2d 981 (1974).
16. See, e.g., ZeBarth v. Swedish Hospital Medical Center, 81 Wash.2d 12, 499 P.2d 1 (1972).
17. Ybarra v. Spangard, 25 Cal.2d 486, 154 P.2d 687 (1945).
18. Anderson v. Somberg, 67 N.J. 1, A.2d 1 (1975).
19. See, e.g., Pratt v. Davis, 118 Ill.App. 161 (1905). *aff'd* 224 Ill. 300, 79 N.E. 562 (1906); Schloendorff v. Society of New York Hosp., 211 N.Y. 125, 105 N.E. 92(1914).
20. See Salgo v. Leland Stanford, Jr. Bd. of Trustees, 154 Cal.App.2d 560, 317 P.2d 170); Canterbury v. Spence, 464 F.2d 772 (D.C. Cir.), *cert. denied*, 409 U.S. 1064 (1972).
21. See, e.g., Bly v. Rhoads, 216 Va. 645, 222 S.E.2d 783 (1976).
22. See, e.g., Cobbs v. Grant, 8 Cal.2d 229, 502 P.2d 1, 104 Cal. Rptr. 505 (1972).
23. See Jay Katz, The Silent World of Doctor and Patient, The Free Press 1984); and Walter Wadlington, Breaking the Silence of Doctor and Patient, 93 Yale L.J. 1640 (1984).
24. See, e.g., Mulder v. Parke Davis & Co., 288 Minn. 332, 181 N.W.2d 883 (1970).
25. Fein v. Permanente Group, 47 U.S. 892 (1985).
26. See, e.g., N.Y. Public Health Law §2805-d (McKinney 1993).
27. Hondroulis v. Schuhmacher, 553 So.2d 398 (La. 1989).
28. See D.H. Mills, Report on the Medical Insurance Feasibility Study (1977) for a review of further findings.
29. See P. Danzon, Medical Malpractice Theory, Evidence, and Public Policy, at 19–29 (Harvard 1985).
30. See Walter Wadlington, A Medical Malpractice Crisis in 1995?: Some Conceivable Scenarios, 36 St. Louis U.L.J. 903 (1992).

Chapter 20

Management of the Neonatal Intensive Care Unit and Neonatal Service

Morris Cohen, M.D., M.B.Bch

Up until 1950, the nursery was essentially an adjunct to the obstetric service. During the late 1960s, hospitals that delivered more than 2,000–3,000 newborns began to develop neonatal intensive care units (NICUs) (Figure 1). Over the last 2 decades with advances in therapy and technology, the provision of neonatal services has become increasingly complex. The demand for these tertiary services continues to increase.

The need for tertiary care services became the impetus for regionalization of neonatal care. This began in the 1970s and peaked during the 1980s. Neonatology became the leading discipline in the regionalization effort. While most other specialties have moved in the direction of regionalization, only a few, such as trauma, have been quite as successful.

The rapidly enlarging patient population creates excessive demands on personnel and the high expectations for good neonatal care have made the job of managing neonatal/perinatal systems increasingly difficult and complex. The rapid growth of tertiary facilities in the face

From: Sibbald WJ, Massaro T (eds.): The Business of Critical Care: A Textbook for Clinicians Who Manage Special Care Units. © Futura Publishing Co., Inc., Armonk, NY, 1996.

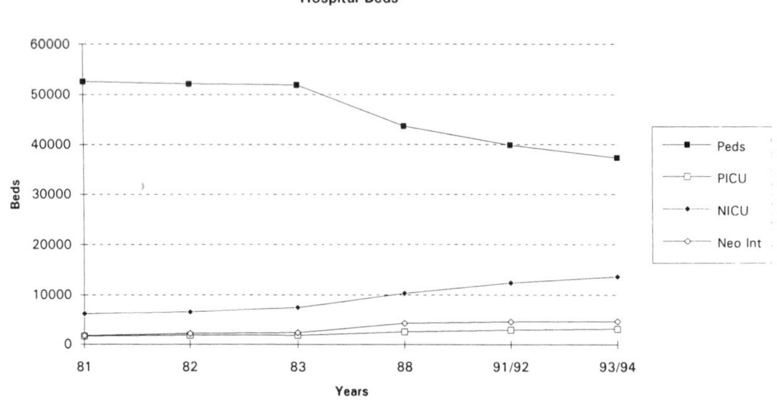

Figure 1.

of a shrinking "health care dollar" has created difficult problems in various aspects of neonatal health care.

In order to address the management of neonatal services, we need to look at those factors implicit in the management of the patient as well as the various factors that impinge upon this inner nucleus.

Neonatal Services and Facilities

Neonatal units are generally categorized into four levels of care, levels I-III and regional perinatal centers (RPC). The classification used in assigning levels of care to neonatal units, designates the most basic unit as level I, unlike some other disciplines including, pediatric intensive care and trauma units in which level I is the most intensive.

Level I (Community Perinatal Center-Basic)

The level I facilities provide for the management of uncomplicated newborn patients. They are generally located in community hospitals with a very low-risk population or in geographically isolated communities that cannot support a higher level of care. The primary goals of this service, in addition to providing care to healthy term babies, are directed toward education in parenting and caring for the newborn, and early detection of existing or potential problems. Since some of the pregnancies will present with unanticipated complications, these units must be capable of providing emergency medical services to both mother and baby, efficiently and competently in order to stabilize the patient until help arrives!

Level II Intermediate Care (Community Perinatal Center-Intermediate)

The level II facility is described by various terms including intermediate care nursery, special care nursery, and community perinatal center-intermediate.

Level II facilities provide a full range of services for uncomplicated mothers and newborns and for neonates with intermediate level of illness or prematurity. They are located in suburban or smaller urban hospital with a delivery rate of 1,500–2,500 births per annum. The range of services in these facilities vary quite widely. At the lower end of the spectrum, these facilities provide basic intravenous therapy and oxygen supplementation. At the high end they have the capabilities for short-term assisted ventilation. The size of these units is quite variable, ranging from 4–6 beds to 12 beds.

Level III Intensive Care Nursery/Neonatal ICU

These units provide the full range of services, providing care for normal uncomplicated well newborns and mothers on the one hand and for all types of materno-fetal and neonatal illness and abnormality on the other. They must, therefore, provide full range of resources and expertise required for the management of any complication of pregnancy or complication of the newborn. Neonates who require maximal care, generally require constant observation with highly specialized supportive services and frequent medical intervention. The NICUs are generally large ranging from 20–40 beds with a high level of acuity.

The number of patients and ventilator-patients is generally more than that of any other intensive care unit (ICU) in the hospital. Ventilator patients often account for a third to half of the patients in the unit. The needed equipment and supplies are often unique to the patient population and not available elsewhere in the hospital.

Regional Perinatal Center

RPCs provide services from basic to intensive care and in addition provide specialized services. They are generally located in larger urban areas and have a delivery service of > 2,500–3,000 infants per annum. The RPC has formal or informal transfer agreements with surrounding urban and suburban community perinatal centers. In addition to providing transfer and transport of mothers and newborns they often provide perinatal and neonatal consultation and education. Other specialized services, include extracorporeal membrane oxygenation (ECMO), and surgical services such as cardiac surgery, neurosurgery, urology, and general surgery.

Special Services

High-Risk Follow-Up Clinic

The majority of larger NICUs have established high-risk follow-up (HRFU) clinics. The goals and objectives of these vary quite broadly. Some provide comprehensive primary and preventive pediatric care. The majority, however, track these high-risk infants with the major goal of identifying developmental and other delays. Screening for cognitive and physical abnormalities are performed at regular intervals during the first 1–2 years of life. Some follow the children to school age and beyond. Included among the clinic personnel are the following: neonatologists, psychologists, developmentalists, social workers, and physical therapists. In our clinic we have, in addition, opthalmology and neurology.

Regionalization

In almost all regions of the US and Canada, neonatal/perinatal health services are organized into "regionalized networks" or consortia. Hospital supporting facilities of various levels of neonatal care within a geographic area, develop a voluntary cooperative relationship with the goal of coordinating care, in order to ensure access to optimum care for each mother and newborn within the region. The "Committee on

Perinatal Health" promoted this concept in the monograph *Towards Improving the Outcome of Pregnancy.*[1]

The need for neonatal services provided by a hospital must take into account the size and specifics of the population served by that hospital, but taken in the context of the region. In addition to the absolute number of deliveries, the needs assessment must account for the high-risk nature of the population. Most problems of the newborn, except for prematurity and low birth weight (LBW), occur at a relatively constant rate in all population groups. The number of beds recommended by the American Acadamy of Pediatrics (AAP) and the American College of Obstetrics and Gynecologists per 1,000 deliveries is one intensive, three to four intermediate, and one convalescent care bed.[2] The total number of seven beds per 1,000 is similar to that recommended by the British Paediatric Association.[3] These calculations appear best suited for a low-risk population of 60 LBW babies per 1,000. As the number of LBW and very LBW babies increases the number of intensive care beds should be increased by a factor of two to three.

The Newark Beth Israel Regional Perinatal Network consists of eight hospitals: one RPC, five level II nurseries (Community Perinatal Center [CPC]-intermediate), two level I nurseries (CPC-basic), and one birthing center. It provides care to over 10,000 newborns annually. The overall LBW rate is almost 10 per 1,000 live births. The five level IIs have 35 intermediate/convalescent beds (average seven beds per unit) with the RPC having 17. In addition, the RPC has 30 intensive care beds. This represents three intensive and four intermediate care beds per 1,000 deliveries.

Regional programs also provide a variety of other services to the region that they serve, including transport, education, administration, and professional consultation.

Central to the regional operations is the neonatal transport team. This is generally run by the RPC, which provides the professional staff. The team usually consists of a physician and a nurse, and or neonatal nurse practitioners or clinicians. Some will additionally use a respiratory therapist. In our system attending neonatologists and specially trained transport nurses participate on transports. The ambulance is either owned or leased by the hospital, and is specifically designed and outfitted for newborn transport and generally dedicated for this one purpose. The RPC thus provides a highly skilled team to its referral hospitals. This arrangement ensures that competent personnel with a high level of expertise are sent to site in need of assistance. Over a period of time the RPC team learns the capabilities of each referral nursery, which helps in determining the level of urgency of any given transport. It also establishes personal rapport and a level of trust between the referral hospital personnel and those of the transport team from the RPC, which is seldom duplicated by other medical services.

Outreach education is an important aspect of the approach to regionalization. The primary goals are continuing education and education of the staffs to upgrade the level of care provided at a particular nursery. Most referral nurseries are too small to have their own neonatal/perinatal educators. The RPC at Newark Beth Israel Medical Center has two nurse educators dedicated to outreach education and all of the attending faculty are involved. Our educational program is quite extensive and includes a variety of programs and formats as listed in Table 1. Approximately 125 nursing and medical continuing education programs were presented in 1993. Professional continuing eduation credits were offered for 90% of these programs. Nearly 1,100 perinatal health care professionals attended the programs offered.

Perinatal advisory commitees have been established at each network hospital. These committees are represented by medicine, nursing, and administration from the referral center and the neonatologist, perinatologist, and outreach educators from the RPC. Meetings are held regularly, generally every other month. Issues discussed range across the spectrum of perinatal-neonatal care from planning to patient-care, education to equipment needs.

Role of the Director of Neonatal Services

The neonatologist and/or director of the unit plays a pivotal role in establishing the level and quality of care provided. He/she must work with the hospital administration to function at a level that is economically feasible. This entails an evaluation of the patient population and referral sources. After an in-depth needs assessment has established the size of the unit (number of beds), an appropriate determination of the professional staffing and equipment needs can be established. This will require close collaboration with various departments including at a minimum nursing, respiratory therapy, and social work. The director must ensure appropriate hospital supportive services, nursery support staff, and pediatric and surgical consultation. Finally, he/she must establish and maintain good relations with referral hospitals and clinics, including if necessary, the RPC, while at the same time cultivating relationships with the referral private practitioners, both pediatricians and obstetricians, midwives, and family practice physicians.

Table 1
Sample List of Annual Educational Programs: The Regional Perinatal Center–Newark Beth Israel Medical Center

Program	Description	Length	Frequency
Perinatal Advisory Committees	Meetings at each network hospital.	1–2 hours	Monthly
Educational Planning Meetings	Meetings with RPC Educators and hospital nurse managers at each referral hospital.	As needed	Bi-annually
Perinatal Nurses Advisory Board Meeting	Group meetings with RPC Educators and nurse managers from all referral hospitals.	2 hours	Bi-annually
*Annual Fall Perinatal Symposium	Directed towards physicians, nurses and other health care providers. Held at central location	8 hours	Annually
*Issues in Perinatal Nursing	Day long nursing program held at RPC.	8 hours	Bi-annually
*Nursing Seminar Days	Offered at individual hospitals. Select 1–6 topics from 32.	1–6 hours	As requested
*Nursing Inservices	Offered at each individual hospital. Topic selected by hospital.	1 hour	Monthly
*Neonatal Nursing Care Course	Held at the RPC. Clinical time also available.	6 days	Annually
*Perinatal Post Anesthesia Care Course	Held at the RPC. Meets State standards for Perinatal Post Anesthesia Care.	2–3 days	Bi-annually
*Perinatal Post Anesthesia Care Update	Held at the RPC. Provides update for those who have taken the full course.	1 day	Annually
*Basic Electronic Fetal Monitoring Course	Rotated at network hospitals.	4 hours	Quarterly
*Advanced Principles in Electronic Fetal Monitoring	Rotated at network hospitals.	5 hours	Bi-annually
*Breastfeeding Program: The Nurse as Lactation Consultant	Rotated at network hospitals.	4 hours	Bi-annually
Physician Programs	Presented at network hospitals. Topics as requested.	1–2 hours	Monthly to quarterly as requested
Neonatal Resuscitation Program (NRP)—Instuctor Course	Offered at each hospital. Trains physician and nurse instructors for the NRP Program.	2 days	As needed
*NRP Provider Course	Offered at each hospital.	8 hours	As needed
Consumer Programs	Held at a central regional location in the evening.	2–3 hours	Bi-annually

* Continuing Education Units (CEUs) and/or Continuing Medical Education Credits (CMEs) offered.

Table 2
New Jersey Neonatal DRGS 1991

DRG	Description	Number of Patients	Average Length of Stay	Charges/ Patients
600	Died Within One Day of Birth	441	1	1,350
601	Transferred <5 Days Old	1,312	1.34	1,041
602	Birth Wt <750g, Disch Alive	349	42.44	40,151
603	Birth Wt <750g, Died	78	16.76	22,748
604	Birth Wt 750–999g, Disch Alive	261	68.28	62,990
605	Birth Wt 750–999g, Died	39	39.18	43,418
606	Birth Wt 1000–1499g, With Signif O.R. Proc, Disch Alive	21	88.95	87,165
607	Birth Wt 1000–1499g, Without Signif O.R. Proc, Disch Alive	873	43.03	34,593
608	Birth Wt 1000–1499g, Died	30	50.17	56,432
609	Birth Wt 1500–1499g, With Signif O.R. Proc, With Mult Major Problem	15	69.13	74,232
610	Birth Wt 1500–1999g, With Signif O.R. Proc, Without Mult Major Problem	3	19.33	19,118
611	Birth Wt 1500–1999g, Without Signif O.R. Proc, With Mult Major Problem	325	29.74	23,897
612	Birth Wt 1500–1999g, Without Signif O.R. Proc, With Major Problem	395	21.28	13,769
613	Birth Wt 1500–1999g, Without Signif O.R. Proc, With Minor Problem	295	20.98	12,223
614	Birth Wt 1500–1999g, Without Signif O.R. Proc, With Other Problem	679	14.32	6,880
615	Birth Wt 2000–2499g, With Signif O.R. Proc, With Mult Major Problem	22	41.86	38,293
616	Birth Wt 2000–2499g, With Signif O.R. Proc, Without Mult Major Problem	9	15.44	9,674
617	Birth Wt 2000–2499g, Without Signif O.R. Proc, With Mult Major Problem	331	21.61	18,833
618	Birth Wt 2000–2499g, Without Signif O.R. Proc, With Major Problem	634	11.1	6,732
619	Birth Wt 2000–2499g, Without Signif O.R. Proc, With Minor Problem	458	8.72	4,966
620	Birth Wt 2000–2499g, Without Signif O.R. Proc, With Only Normal Newborn	3,335	4.25	1,478
621	Birth Wt 2000–2499g, Without Signif O.R. Proc With Other Problem	523	7.71	3,546
622	Birth Wt. >2499g, With Signif O.R. Proc, With Mult Major Problem	61	40.9	43,205
623	Birth Wt >2499g, With Signif O.R. Proc, Without Mult Major Problem	119	7.19	5,633
624	Birth Wt >2499g, With Minor Abd. Procedure	59	4.14	4,037
626	Birth Wt >2499g, Without Signif O.R. Proc, With Mult Major Problem	1,038	12.8	10,751

(continued)

Table 2 *(continued)*

DRG	Description	Number of Patients	Average Length of Stay	Charges/ Patients
627	Birth Wt >2499g, Without Signif O.R. Proc, With Major Problem	3,855	6.2	3,196
628	Birth Wt >2499g, Without Signif O.R. Proc, With Minor Problem	3,363	5.09	2,449
629	Birth Wt >2499g, Without Signif O.R. Proc, With Only Normal NB Diag.	103,861	3.05	889
630	Birth Wt >2499g, Without Signif O.R. Proc, With Other Prob	986	5.08	1,924
635	Aftercare for Weight Gain	167	12.16	5,136
	Totals	123,937		

DRG = diagnostic related group; WT = weight.

Patient Population

The newborn population represents a microcosm of society and is, indeed, a unique hospital population. There are two major groups of newborns: healthy and sick. Each have very specific but very different needs during their stay in the hospital during the first day of life.

Healthy Newborns

The majority are full-term or near-term, healthy newborns. Based on the New Jersey Diagnosis-Related Groups (DRGs) for the calender year 1990, these two groups, DRG 629 and 620, respectively, accounted for almost 87% of the population. The majority of these normal newborns are of normal birth weight of at least 2,500 g (DRG 629) and have an average length of hospital stay of 3 days, but a range from < 1 day to several weeks (Tables 2 and 3).

Those that remain for only a day or less generally come from two patient pools. The first is from the small proportion of parents who choose to deliver in a more "natural" environment with minimal medical intervention. Some deliver in birthing centers, others in hospital settings geared towards natural childbirth. More recently and in recognition of these desires many hospitals have moved towards Labor, Delivery, and Recovery and Labor, Delivery, Recovery, and Postpartum

Table 3
Admissions to the NICU at NBIMC—Inborn Deliveries Only, 1993

BW	<10 Days	10–60 Days	>60 Days	Totals	%
<1500g	31	65	57	153	30%
1500–2500g	44	132	8	184	36%
>2500g	135	33	2	170	34%
Total	210	230	67	507	100%
	41%	45%	13%	100%	

departments. The second pool has been created from the new managed health care programs that encourage the practice of very short stays and strongly advocate for hospital stays of 1 day.

When cesarean is the mode of delivery, the normal newborn's hospital stay will be prolonged until the mother is ready for discharge. Almost a quarter of births in the US and a fifth in Canada are by cesarean. While the rate of cesarean is high in almost all industrialized countries, the rate of repeat cesarean without any complication of the fetus or mother remains significantly higher in the US.[4] The length of stay (LOS) of these babies will generally be from 3–5 days. Finally, a small but growing population is the "boarder baby".[5] These healthy newborns must remain in the hospital after discharge of the mother, for weeks to months because of unfavorable social situations, including maternal drug abuse and homelessness, or in those cases where mothers, often teenagers, choose to give up their babies for adoption.

The neonatal service must be flexible to accommodate these needs. Protocols and screening procedures must be established for early discharge, in order to identify apparently healthy newborns who are at risk of problems such as jaundice, non-obvious congenital malformations, etc., prior to early discharge. Appropriate plans for follow-up must be in place. At the other end of the spectrum the service must accommodate the long-term custodial care of newborns awaiting placement. This includes volunteer "baby sitters", active social service involvement, and interaction with city and state child protective agencies and adoption agencies.

Sick Newborns

Sick newborns account for 10%–15% of the newborn population. The mortality rate during the newborn period (0–28 days) is higher than at any other time, with a rate of 5.5 per 1,000 live births.[6] The majority of deaths occur within the first week and most of these at < 24 hours of age. About 10% of all newborns are delivered prematurely at < 37 weeks of gestation. Seven percent of babies are of LBW, weighing < 2,500 g. The mortality rate among these infants is 10–12 per 1000 or four times greater than the full-term infant.

This ill newborn population can be divided into three broad categories based on the severity of their illnesses: acute short-term illnesses (30%–40%); intermediate illnesses (40%–60%); and critically ill newborns (10%–20%). Babies with acute short-term illnesses tend to be larger term or near-term newborns who require oxygen therapy, intravenous fluids, and antibiotic therapy. Included among these, are infants who experience difficulty in making the pulmonary transition to extrauterine life and present with pulmonary mal-adaption diseases, including transient tachypnea, and infants of diabetic mothers with hypoglycemia. Their course is short and they require NICU for 3–7 days and hospitalization for 5–10 days.

The majority of NICU admissions (40–60) represent the larger preterm newborns of birth weight 1,500–2,500 g (32–36 weeks gestation) and term babies with severe diseases such as sepsis and meningitis, severe respiratory diseases including meconium aspiration and pulmonary hypertension, and isolated congenital anomalies especially of the GI tract that require surgical management. The vast majority of these newborns recover completely, generally have an uncomplicated course, but remain in the NICU setting for 2 weeks to 2 months (average 20–30 days).

At the other end of the spectrum are the critically ill newborns who require hospitalization for 2–6 months and account for 10%–20% of NICU admissions. Most of those babies are either extremely small having birth weight of < 1,000 g (DRGs 602, 604, and 606), larger preterms with major problems (DRG 609), and the near-term and term newborns with severe diseases (DRGs 615 and 622). This latter group often require surgical procedures and frequently have congenital malformations. While the babies from the eight DRG groups accounted for only 9.9% of admissions, they utilized 39% of sick-newborn hospital days. Their courses are quite complicated and they present a multitude of acute complications and disorders along with their primary disease process. In addition to the acute medical and nursing problems, they have the additional problems of long LOS, uncertain outcome, and fluctuating (roller coaster) condition. The psycho-social challenge that they often present impacts heavily on the parents and family, as well as the professional staff of the NICU. They often present difficult ethical dilemmas to further complicate their stay.

Personnel

The role of the director is to coordinate a broad scope of health professions into a smooth running team in order to ensure optimum care of the patient. In addition to delivering the most appropriate skills and technologies effectively, a secondary management objective is to provide these services at the least cost.

Because of the complex nature of the illnesses that many of these newborns have, such as prematurity and congenital malformations, the patients require care from numerous personnel. Included among these are the following: neonatologist; neonatal fellow; pediatric resident; pediatric subspecialists; neonatal nurse; neonatal nurse practitioner; social worker; respiratory therapist; physical therapist; developmentalist; and perfusionist.

Caring for the neonatal patient requires the cooperation and integration of the skills of these varied professions. One of the difficulties for the manager is to deal with the roles, ambiguities, and conflicts of such specialized expertise. Each discipline brings its own values and intellectual assessment of patient problems and recommended interventions. It is necessary to obtain the observations and evaluations of the different disciplines involved, in order to make the best decisions regarding the patient's care. While each discipline demands autonomy to practice its own skills, independence is limited in this very obvious group setting.

In the traditional medical model the physician makes the patient diagnostic and treatment decisions unilaterally. The physician, who is clearly in charge, orders services from the other disciplines, which carry them out. While this works quite well in many settings, it poses some problems in the NICU.

The complexity of the illness and treatments and the proliferation of the other health professionals, as well as the long LOS has made this structure somewhat burdensome. Management of neonatal patients has, therefore, become a hybrid of the traditional medical model and the team model. Each of the professional personnel function as a member of the team with the physician assuming the role of the team leader. This is further complicated by having the parent integrated as an active member of the team.

A further obstacle in the management of this team of health professionals is the rather ambiguous hierarchical structure. The team caring for the neonatal patient develops a close rapport and working relationship. While the team members in a practical sense are responsible to the neonatologist as team leader, within the hierarchical structure of the hospital they report to another individual often in another department. For example, the nurse reports to the unit head nurse who in turn reports to the Director of Nursing. This ambiguity can create problems because the nurse does not report to the person issuing the instruction.

Staffing

Staffing by the various disciplines is primarily the responsibility of that discipline. None-the-less, it is incumbent on the Director of Service to be involved and participate in ensuring appropriate staffing of the neonatal service, particularly the NICU.

Nurse staffing needs are rather intense. Nurse:patient ratios for the well baby nurseries (WBNs) run from 1:6 to 1:8. The nurse:patient ratio for intermediate is 1:3 to 1:4. For NICUs, the ratio is 1:2 to 1:2.5. These staffing ratios are similar in countries outside of North America.[7] For an average 30-bed NICU this would require some 85–100 RNs and for a similar size WBN, this would require some 30 RNs. Much of the difficulty in staffing is due to the daily fluctuations in the number of patients. Since there are no elective admissions to these services, there is very little control on the number of patients being admitted. Consequently, it is quite difficult to maintain appropriate nursing numbers for the number of patients on any one day.

Respiratory therapy staffing is generally somewhat easier to regulate provided there is an adequate pool of therapists, specifically allocated to the neonatal services. Fortunately, some of the respiratory functions can be assumed by the neonatologists or nursing staff during critical crisis periods. Our unit, which has 44 beds, has three respiratory therapists at all times in the unit.

Medical staffing of the NICU is generally accomplished by neonatologists together with residents and/or nurse practitioners. As with nursing it would seem that a moderately large patient population is conducive to better neonatal coverage. For the most part it would seem that a minimum of three to four neonatologists is necessary in order to provide adequate neonatal coverage. Preferably, most busy neonatal units have over four and up to ten or more neonatal faculty.

There are several mechanisms that the successful manager uses in order to accommodate the daily fluctuations in patient census. The first is to build in some flexibility in the ability to shift patients within the system. Many neonatal services have a unit for long-term "boarders" and "room-air" growing prematures attached to the WBN and/or a similar "step-down" unit on the pediatric floor. Thus, with the use of these three services, NICU, WBN, and Pediatrics, each with its own nursing staff, it is possible to decompress into one of the units in accordance with the fluctuating census. An effective regional system offers a similar deflating mechanism through the referral hospitals. Patients are transferred back to the level IIs for convalescence in order to accommodate new admissions to the NICU at the RPC.

The second mechanism is to accommodate an increased census by increasing nurse staffing. In order to be able to recruit nurses to work overtime during busy periods, it is necessary to have a relatively large staff. This tends to work more successfully in those units that run over 25–30 beds, and therefore, have a staff of over 70–80 nurses, thereby having a larger pool from which to recruit nurses for overtime.

An alternate means of increasing nurse staffing is to use nurses from a hospital pool or per diems. The former is less desirable in that often the nurses who are sent to the NICU are inexperienced in neonatal care. The latter poses problems of unreliability and variable experience and, in addition, per diem staff from agencies tend to be very expensive. Furthermore, nurses from both sources are often not familiar with the NICU and the specific practices of a particular NICU.

To regulate the amount of staffing requires considerable planning and communication between the various caregivers. It requires cooperation of physicians and nurses to move patients to a lower level of care in a timely but appropriate fashion in order to admit new patients. This should include the involvement of social workers as well. Establishing an appropriate rapport with the parents is essential in order to allow for such accommodations to occur.

Stress and Burnout

The acuity of neonatal intensive care results in a significant amount of stress and consequent burnout among the personnel of these units. Critical care stresses include: caring for critically ill and dying patients; and the ethical dilemmas of terminal conditions and difficult work loads.[8] The NICU in addition has the stresses of the chronically ill newborn,[9] as smaller prematures survive but require ventilation for weeks and months while they recouperate and gain weight. There are also the issues relating to newborns with severe non-lethal congenital malformations and anomalies and others particularly the premature, with devastating complications, such as severe intracranial hemorrhage and short gut syndromes.

Burnout is a psychologic process that has been described by Maslach as having three components: emotional exhaustion, depersonalization, and low personal accomplishment.[10] Emotional exhaustion is an early sign of burnout. The neonatal faculty, nursing staff, and other professionals are exposed to the same high stresses of work overload and emotional drain. It is important to pay particular attention to provider:patient ratios, acuity, and intensity of the patient load.

Attending Neonatologists

It is essential to limit attending months in the NICU, as well as night and weekend call. In addition, it is important to ensure adequate time free of clinical responsibilities and vacation time. Adequate numbers of attending faculty for the patient volume and acuity and on-call coverage is essential.

Staff Nurses

Burnout among neonatal nurses, which is probably similar to other ICU personnel, is not well documented in the existing literature. Neonatal units will run about a 10% nursing turnover rate per annum. Some of this is due to the usual issues of people moving and changing jobs. Since many in neonatal nursing are younger and of child-bearing age, family needs may supersede. However, some of this turn-over is probably related to burnout, particularly in the younger and less experienced nurse.[11] Nursing overtime and excessive working hours must be monitored. Job dissatisfaction is a very important variable in the development of stress and burnout.[12] Interactions with co-workers has been sited as one of the most important sources of emotional exhaustion.[13] The support systems are important particularly for younger and less experienced personnel. Of special importance is the support from supervisors and superiors. Oehler et al.[11] concluded that less experienced nurses may need more support from the head nurse to feel a sense of accomplishment.

The "team" concept prevailing in the NICU environment may play an important role in providing much needed support to all disciplines. In our unit family meetings with the neonatologist, social workers, and nurses are held periodically (at least monthly in non-acute situations) with the parents, to discuss the babies' progress and problems. "Psychosocial rounds" are held weekly with the same group of professionals together with the developmentalists and discharge planners. While intended to discuss patient related issues, including their families, these rounds help foster a sense of group professional involvement and support.

In a setting where babies are transferred out as soon as they are well, it is often difficult for the personnel to maintain a sense of accomplishment. The HRFU clinic fulfills some of this role. When families return periodically for evaluation of their babies' development and progress they are encouraged to visit the NICU. We also hold two annual events when parents are invited back to visit with the staff; the annual NICU picnic held at an outside venue and the annual Halloween Party held in the NICU and environs.

The responsibility of the Neonatal Director of Service in supporting all the staff of the NICU is bound to increase in this new era of health care reform. At a time when the needs are increasing, the resources available to the director are decreasing as cost containment, efficiency and resources allocation become the terminology of the era. As hospital administrations and insurance companies heed the bottom line, the Director of service must identify new means to justify appropriate staffing, maintain a pleasant and rewarding work environment, and protect the personnel from the prevailing depersonalization invading our units.

Education and Research

The rapid increase in the number of neonatal units, the advances in the available technology and the increased expectations of neonatal intensive care, demand a high level of continuing education for the professionals involved in these units.

Physicians

Education of physicians in neonatal care is targeted at four major levels; residents, fellows, pediatricians, and neonatologists. During the

1970s training programs in neonatal care blossomed. Residents generally spent 6–10 months of their 3-year pediatric residency programs in neonatal care. In the 1980s the AAP and the Residency Review Committee began to place increasing emphasis on primary care. As of July 1992 the requirements for subspecialty training in pediatrics limited the number of months allocated to any one specialty to a maximum of 6 months.[14] In neonatal medicine this allocation includes both intensive and intermediate care. The result of this is that most residents currently spend no more than 4 months of the 3-year pediatric residency in the NICU. It seems probable that pediatric residents will be limited to a total of 4 months in neonatology as of early 1996. The obvious consequence of this is a short fall in the medical coverage for the service needs. The less obvious, but possibly more important consequence in view of this, is the challenge of educating the pediatrician with a significantly reduced time allocation on an increasingly demanding service. To achieve this, major changes in the approach to education will be necessary.

First, the emphasis of current activities will have to be altered. The service will need to be structured so that residents spend a greater proportion of their time focused on activities such as delivery room resuscitation, stabilization on admission to the NICU, and discharge evaluation and planning, while much of the time-consuming routine daily care will be assumed by others. Although more resident time will be free to engage in other educational activities, some of this time will be allocated to continuity care in the pediatric outpatient department. The remainder, should be geared towards education in areas of neonatal medicine important to the pediatrician. Hopefully, included among these will be ethical and psycho-social issues that the pediatrician, as the primary care provider, will become involved in with families. The other major challenge for the attending staff will be to ensure the resident "students" continue to be engaged in the activities of the NICU, at the same time that they are being focused away from intensive care; to establish a role and function for them while others, such as nurse practitioners and clinicians are assuming a predominant role in the care of patients. The danger for the pediatric residents is that they are destined to become passive observers and bystanders, who are no longer essential members of the neonatal team. As their exposure and experience becomes more limited, they may graduate without many of the skills of past years, into a world where others exclude them from previous pediatric domains, especially the delivery room where they can interact with the referring obstetrician and have their first contact with new parents.

Fellowship training in neonatal medicine has gone through its own transitions over the past years. The training program was expanded to 3 years in 1989. At the same time that 1 year was added for research activities, more demands were placed on fellowships to ensure that less of the remaining 2 years be allocated to service delivery. As these future neonatal fellows come out of pediatric residencies with less exposure and knowledge in neonatal care, the demands on the service to address the deficiencies in their clinical skills will be greater. As with residency programs, fellowship programs will need to adapt, accommodate, and become more focused and efficient in teaching these clinical aspects of neonatal care.

Neonatal faculty across the country have increasingly assumed more and more direct hand-on clinical involvement. The number of neonatologists who provide in-house coverage appears to have increased significantly over the last decade. As the hours of direct clinical service increase, especially night and weekend coverage, the ability to participate in continuing educational activities becomes less. This affects personal education in the form of reading journals and text, group activities such as in-house conference, patient review, and external conferences.

There are a variety of approaches to ensure adequate continuing education. A regular schedule of weekly and monthly in-house conferences is essential. There should be an expectation of attendance by the majority of faculty. While residents may often present a case and even lead the discussion, the assigned attending should be expected to have reviewed the literature and direct the discussion. A reasonable monthly schedule might include a perinatal morbidity/mortality conference, a perinatal case review, and a surgical conference. On our service we hold, in addition, a weekly patient review conference. Furthermore, the neonatologists participate in similar conferences at our affiliated level I and II hospitals on a monthly, quarterly, or semi-annual basis.

The observant director will identify areas of interest among the attending neonatologist. They should be encouraged to pursue these interests by attending outside conferences, visiting centers with special expertise in the particular area, and be encouraged to be guest lecturers in these areas. This is especially valuable for units that do not pursue active research and might be a mechanism to initiate a measure of research effort.

Nursing Education

Nursing education for the most part comes under the pervue of the Department of Nursing. Much of the educational activity is directed at new graduates or new recruits to the service. The result is that ongoing in-service education is neglected to a greater or lesser degree. A minimum of education is generally mandated by some outside state or regulatory body.

Cross-disciplinary education is also a neglected area. In our experience this has worked well when there is a specific focus such as in cases with a major ethical dimension or in initiating a new program that involves the education and training of all the disciplines, for example the introduction of ECMO. In order to achieve maximum efficiency in a unit, particularly in the new cost-containment era of the 1990s, integration of education will be seen as more necessary.

The Neonatologist as Generalist

Neonatal medicine is almost universally a division within the department of pediatrics. Its early beginnings, however were in the department of obstetrics-gynecology. Prior to the 1950s, obstetricians and midwives provided care to the newborn after delivery. In fact, even today the obstetrician has the primary responsibility for the newborn at birth, until the pediatrician or neonatologist formally assumes care of the newborn.

Neonatal intensive care developed during the 1960s and gained impetus during the 1970s. The 1980s saw an expansive growth, particularly in the number of level II units. This rapid growth is punctuated by the increase in the number of neonatal beds during a period in which the number of pediatric beds, nationally, has declined. Over the last decade the number of NICU and intermediate beds has increased such that neonatal beds, excluding the regular or WBN, now account for 24% of all pediatric beds as compared to 14% in 1980 (Table 4).

As the discipline grew it assumed a greater role within the department of pediatrics. In larger centers it is often one of the larger divisions

Table 4
Pediatric and Neonatal Beds—USA

	1981	1982	1983	1988	1991/1992	1993/1994
PEDS	52,601	52,143	51,866	43,659	39,859	37,292
PICU	1,635	1,839	1,788	2,502	2,881	3,110
NICU	6,187	6,538	7,432	10,279	12,364	13,595
NEO INT	1,743	2,169	2,336	4,237	4,537	4,610

within the department. This growth brought with it a financial reward. Many pediatric departments find themselves depending on the income from neonatology to support the less financially productive divisions. It is important for the division director to recognize the issue and to deal with the conflict that this may bring with it. On the one hand, the division must continue to support the department, while on the other hand, the director has an obligation to protect the neonatologists and to ensure appropriate remuneration for the neonatal faculty while appreciating the need to retain some financial symmetry within the department.

There is a co-dependency in the relationship between neonatology and all the other subspecialties. A high proportion of the major chronic problems of childhood present in the newborn period. These patients require the service of the neonatologist during their initial hospitalization, but ultimately will be followed by the general pediatrician. A high percentage of admissions to the pediatric inpatient service, especially to the PICU are graduates of NICU. Thus the relationship of the neonatal faculty and the other sub-specialties extends far beyond the neonatal period and has implications for the department of pediatrics and indeed the hospital.

Neonatologists generally retain primary responsibility for all patients in the NICU. All the other physicians involved in the newborns care, including the pediatrician, remain as "consultants". During the ill newborns course in the NICU, a variety of consultants will be requested to assist in the care of the newborn. These include cardiology and neurology, infectious disease, gastrointestinal and hematology, and all the other pediatric specialties. Often their involvement is limited to several brief consultations. In many cases these sub-specialties will be involved in the aftercare of the baby. In either circumstance and almost without exception, these babies remain under the care of the neonatal faculty, who remain the primary and major care provider. Similarly, while the surgical consultants play a major role in the pre-operative and diagnostic phases of the "surgical newborn's" care, during the post-operative and recouperative phases the neonatologist remains primarily in charge. Perhaps the only exception, is for some post-operative cardiacs, where in some centers they are transferred to the cardio-thoracic service. In fact, in these circumstances the patient is generally transferred to the PICU post-operatively. The obvious advantage is that a single individual (or service) will provide continuity and coordination of the care. This arrangement has clear advantages to the family, nursing staff, and social workers and to the pediatric residency staff. The major challenge for the neonatal service is to ensure that the consultants, particularly the pediatrician and the surgical specialties, remain involved.

The relationship with obstetrics is, similarly, a symbiotic one. Obstetrics needs neonatal services when newborns are in trouble; the neonatologist is dependent on the obstetricians to deliver the "high-risk" mother in that center and to involve neonatology in the decision making process, prior to the delivery. Of particular importance is the involvement of the neonatologist in helping to determine the most appropriate time and location for the delivery. Obstetric involvement with the family after delivery is an extremely valuable and often under-used resource for families struggling with the dilemmas and anxiety of a sick newborn. Finally, on the busy services of regional centers, consultation regarding available beds for transfer of high-risk mothers requires a coordinated effort of both services. This type of collaborative involvement is hard to achieve. This is further complicated on those services with residency programs, when the resident is often the first physician to interact with the patient or the outside referring physician.

Economics

The soaring cost of health care and the attempt to contain this have initiated a deluge of efforts to scrutinize and review medical practices. NICUs are seen by many as a very expensive service. In fact, there are some who are beginning to question whether the expense is justified. Up until recently the Director of Service had little more to do than stay within the hospital budget for the department, ensure adequate salaries for faculty, and run the neonatal office. As hospital administrators, insurance companies, state and federal government, and planners get more involved, the director's role must focus increasingly on the economics and financial aspects of the service. The alternative, is to abdicate these responsibilities and with it lose much of the control of the unit as well as the level and quality of the service provided.

Costs of newborns requiring NICU is often reported as extraordinarily high. Extremely LBW babies with multiple complications or term babies with multiple major congenital malformations can exceed "$125,000". The average reimbursement for the 280 ELBWs newborns weighing 750–999 g who survived in New Jersey during 1991 (DRG 604) was $87,360. Their average LOS was 82 days. The 129 term newborns with multiple major problems, who required a significant operating room procedure (DRG 622), had an average LOS of 37 days and the average reimbursement was $44,656. The vast majority of these very LBW babies and this group of term newborns who require significant NICU resources survive and have an excellent future outcome. Thus, while a very small number of newborns who have a predictably costly NICU course but a very uncertain outcome, may engender much discussion and present difficult ethical questions and decisions, they represent significantly < 5% of the NICU population and < 5 per 1,000 of the total newborn population.

In reviewing the newborn DRG rates for New Jersey, it's interesting that the inlyer rate for vastly different groups of babies varies very little when justified for LOS. The daily reimbursement, calculated from the total charges and the total LOS in 1991, for similar babies who survived and did not need an operating room procedure but of vastly different birth weights (BWs) were: for a BW 1,000–1,499 g the charges were $905; for a BW of 1,500–1,999 g $890; for a BW of 2,000–2,499 g $806; and BW > 2,499 g they were $805. The LOS for each was 42 days, 30 days, 20 days, and 13 days.

The most effective way of achieving economy of patient cost is to shorten LOS. The effect of this was clearly seen in New Jersey with introduction of DRGs in 1980. With a fixed reimbursement per admission, LOS decreased from in 1981 to 1991. The discharge weight for newborns has consistently dropped over the past two decades. In 1986 Brooten et al. reported on the successful early discharge of very LBW infants at an average weight of 2,072 g ± 131 (range 1,880–2,500) when the routine weight for discharge was 2,200 g.[15] In 1990 many units discharge babies at 1,900 g and at even below this weight. Each 100 g saves as much as 3–5 hospital days. Another problem which constantly plagues the neonatologist in planning for discharge is the newborn who has occasional brief apneic episodes without significant bradycardia or cyanosis. This can often require an additional 2–3 weeks of hospitalization. In our unit we have been sending these babies home on an apnea monitor for the past 3 years, with extraordinary success.

That vastly different babies cost similar amounts might seem improbable until one recognizes that most of the expenses incurred are for personnel. Much of the personnel expense is for nursing. Most NICUs utilize an average nurse to patient ratio of 1:2 to 1:2.5. By using some of the strategies noted in the section under personnel, the patient census can be maintained at > 90% (many NICUs run a census close to 100%), and thus optimize the use of nursing, as well as respiratory therapy, social work, and physicians.

The costs of NICU in addition to personnel include all those encountered by other inpatient services, including laboratory, blood bank, pharmacy, and radiology. To date, few hospitals have use micro-costing and thus, have few specifics as to where the costs for a specific patient are expended. Neonatologists have generally tried to use few medications and generally have not embraced newer more expensive medications for fear of side-effects. The pharmacy expenses may thus be lower than other areas of the hospital. The same philosophy of limiting x-ray exposure has been adopted. It is my impression that less x-rays were taken than a decade ago, our success is less obvious. In order to limit exposure to transfusions some efforts have been made to reduce blood tests.

The new age of cost-containment and total quality improvement will require the neonatologist to evaluate these areas in a much more critical fashion. If the service does not want to be more controlled by those external to the unit, the director and staff will have to become involved in this process much more intimately.

Many hospitals, like insurance companies and HMOs recognize the long-term investment of attracting young families. Marketing the obstetric and neonatal services ensures a steady flow of patients to all the other services of the hospital. This is even more true when one understands that decisions regarding health care are overwhelmingly made by the female spouse.

A disproportionate number of newborns at risk for problems requiring care in an NICU come from low-income families. The rate of LBW babies among low-income urban populations (14%–18%) is double the national average. Low-income families also have a three times greater rate of teenage pregnancies with an associated 1.5 times increase in prematurity. Despite these abhorrently high rates, it is important to recognize that the majority of preterm newborns are not born to the inner city low-income families. Review of New Jersey DOH date for 1991 shows that of the 1,496 babies weighing < 1,000 g, 771 (52%) had insurance, 541 (36%) medicaid, and 184 (12%) self-pay.

The majority of term newborns requiring intensive care have conditions that are not the result of poor socio-economic conditions (Table 5). They together with the majority of preterms, however, come from a financially disadvantaged group of society in that their parents are young, early in their jobs and careers, and thus at the lower end of the salary scale. In addition, 30% of children come from single parent families.

As hospitals begin to look more closely at costs and reimbursements, the high cost of NICU may not appear as advantageous when compared with the relatively low-cost, high-volume well baby service. Physicians, nurses, and other providers will need to ensure that a bal-

Table 5
Admissions to NICU-NBIMC 1993—Diagnosis of Term Newborn

Resp		Medical	Surgical	Total	(%)
	TTN	97			
	MAS/PPHN	47			
	Total			171	52%
Metabolic	Hypoglycemia/IDM			36	11%
Anomalies	Cong Anomalies			35	11%
Asphyxial	Low Apgar/HIE			11	3%
Infectious	Sepsis/Meningitis			13	4%
Hematologic	Jaundice/Incompatibility			11	3%
Other Surgical			25		0%
Other Medical	Other		51	51	16%
Total			76	328	

anced approach is taken and due consideration given before NICUs are closed down under the onslaught of the mighty dollar.

Summary

Neonatology had its birth in the 1940s and 1950s. Neonatal intensive care developed during the 1960s. Regionalization gained impetus during the 1970s. The 1980s saw a consolidation of these systems. Over a few decades, the development of NICUs and regionalized systems resulted in a marked reduction of neonatal-perinatal mortality and morbidity.

The shrinking "health-care dollar" of the 1990s in the face of a stagnant system is now placing increasing demands on both the neonatal-perinatal system and those dedicated to providing this care. The challenge of the 1990s will be to further reduce neonatal-perinatal mortality and morbidity by integrating the well established high-tech tertiary services with a rather neglected but all important primary and preventive perinatal-system. It will be important to maintain the high levels of care in the NICU for the acutely ill newborn, while resources are increasingly redirected towards prevention programs.

The physician director will need to increasingly become involved in the political and economic environment far beyond the walls of the NICU, if we hope to continue to play a central role in the provisions of health-care services to newborns.

References

1. Committee on Perinatal Health. Towards Improving the Outcome of Pregnancy: Recommendations for the Regional Development of Maternal and Perinatal Health Services. White Plains, NY, The National Foundation-March of Dimes, 1976.
2. Guidelines for Perinatal Care, Third Edition. Elk Grove Village, Illinois, and Washington, DC. American Academy of Pediatrics and American College of Obstetricians and Gynecologists, 1993.
3. Walker CH. Special and intensive care baby units and nurse staffing in the UK. Arch Dis Child 1983;58:387–392.
4. Notzon FC, Cnattingius S, Bergsjo P, et al. Cesarean section delivery in the 1980s: International comparison by indication. Am J Obstet Gynecol 1994; 170:495–504.
5. Dahl-Regis MM, Oyefara BI. Boarder Babies: Children with special health needs. J Natl Med Assoc 1990;82:473–477.
6. Wegman ME. Annual Summary of Vital Statistics—1992. Pediatrics 1993; 92:743–754.
7. Williams S, Whelan A, Weindling AM, et al. Nursing staff requirements for neonatal intensive care. Arch Dis Child 1993;68:534–538.
8. Stechmiller JK, Yaranndi HN. Predictors of burnout in critical care nurses. Heart and Lung 1993;22:534–541.
9. Marshall RE, Kasmen C. Burnout in the neonatal intensive care unit. Pediatrics 1980;65:1161–1165.
10. Maslach Paine WS, ed: Job stress and burnout. Beverly Hills, CA, Sage Publications Inc., 1982, pp. 29–40.
11. Oehler JM, Davidson MG, Starr LE, et al. Burnout, job stress, anxiety, and perceived social support in neonatal nurses. Heart Lung 1991;20:500–505.
12. Stechmiller 1993; Paredes 1982; Hackman 1978; Jayaratne 1983; Stone 1984.
13. Leiter and Maslach. The impact of interpersonal environment on burnout and organizational commitment. J Org Behavior 1988;9:297–308.
14. American Academy of Peditrics. Special reqirements for training in Pediatrics. Graduate Medical Education Directory AGME 1991;95–101.
15. Brooten D, Kumar S, Brown L, et al. A Randomized clinical trial of early discharge and home follow-up of very-low-birth-weight infants. N Engl J Med 1986;315:15:934–939.
16. Hospital statistics. American Hospital Association—1993 edition, p. 235.

Chapter 21

Managing Respiratory Intensive Care and Respiratory Therapists

Charles G. Durbin Jr, M.D.

A frequent reason for intensive care unit (ICU) admission is potential or actual failure of the respiratory system. One of the first respiratory ICUs was established in Copenhagen, Denmark during the poliomyelitis epidemics in 1952–1953. Since mechanical ventilators were not yet invented, medical students provided artificial ventilation to paralyzed patients by ventilating them by hand.[1] The mortality in patients with bulbar symptoms was dramatically reduced with this simple supportive intervention. Soon after, simple pressure-cycled ventilators were built and widely used in newly organized, specialized respiratory care units. Individuals with interest and skill in using and maintaining mechanical devices, often nurses, thrived in these units and the profession of "oxygen therapy" was born. Physicians skilled in diagnosis and treatment of lung diseases also found the respiratory care unit as a place to provide specialized treatments to a wide range of critically ill patients. Pulmonary medicine had its birth in this environment. Today, almost all pul-

From: Sibbald WJ, Massaro T (eds.): The Business of Critical Care: A Textbook for Clinicians Who Manage Special Care Units. © Futura Publishing Co., Inc., Armonk, NY, 1996.

monary medicine training programs in the US include extensive intensive care experience and the potential for physician certification in critical care medicine.

Although specialized areas devoted only to the treatment of acute respiratory failure are rare today, chronic respiratory care units (or "weaning units") are becoming more common. Artificial airways and mechanical ventilators are common in all ICUs and many critically ill patients will undergo a period of artificial ventilation. Mechanical support of respiratory function is often necessary even when the primary disorder or injury is non-respiratory. Often during the course of recovery from prolonged treatment of critical illness, survivors require an extended period of mechanical ventilation. Respiratory support and weaning units are an economical, efficient way to reduce the cost of prolonged ICU care of these patients.[2] At some point in the disease process the patient has only a single organ failure and can be efficiently cared for in this less intensive (less expensive) environment. Equipment needs are simpler and staff-to-patient ratios can be reduced.[3]

The respiratory therapist is an important contributor to improved outcome and less expensive care in both the acute and chronic setting. This chapter describes the roles that these skilled non-physicians can play in delivery of respiratory care to critically ill patients in and out of traditional ICUs. Educational background, personnel management and deployment strategies, and innovations in practice will be presented. The principles outlined that have been learned from these service providers can be generalized to other areas of critical care practice.

Respiratory Care Service Characteristics

Attention to the needs of patients and life-support devices must be provided continuously to patients in respiratory failure. These patients may be within a specific area, such as an ICU or a wider geographic location. The structure of a respiratory care service reflects the geography of the patient care areas and the hospital support systems. In general the service consists of centralized and decentralized components. Some of these functions and components are listed in Table 1. Direct patient care is provided in slightly different ways in various units by individual respiratory care practitioners (RPCs), thus it is a decentralized service. All areas need almost identical support systems to process and provide equipment and recruit staff. Some functions are provided in both a centralized and a decentralized manner. Inservice

Table 1
Centralized and Decentralized Activities of a Respiratory Care Service

Activity	Typical Location
Patient activities	
Patient assessment	Decentralized
Patient education	Decentralized
Mechanical ventilation	Decentralized
Bronchodilator treatments	Decentralized
Pulmonary function testing	Centralized
Lung hyperinflation	Decentralized
Equipment management	
Purchasing	Centralized
Inservice instruction	Decentralized
Repair	Centralized
Evaluation	May be decentralized
Cleaning	Centralized
Personnel	
Recruitment	Centralized/decentralized
Deployment	Decentralized/centralized
Staff size (FTEs)	Centralized
Salaries	Centralized
Staff coverage	Centralized/decentralized
External relations	
Physicians	Decentralized
Other departments	Centralized
Regulatory agencies	Centralized

education about a ventilator only used in a single area may be confined to those individuals who are likely to use it. These organizational divisions are arbitrary and individual institutions will solve their unique organization and structural issues differently. All functions, however, are necessary for adequate respiratory care services.

Continuous Availability of Service

Since the support of respiration is a full time job, individuals with needed skill and experience must be available throughout the day and night. Some investigators have suggested that the night hours pose an exceptional risk in hospitalized patients.[4,5] The same level of attention and quality of care must be available to the critically ill at all times. When all ventilator dependent patients are collected in a common area, consistent and uniform care can be provided efficiently. When patients receiving mechanical ventilation are widely dispersed throughout the hospital in multiple ICUs, there is a need for centralized management of respiratory care services. Departments of respiratory care have been organized to deal with issues of equipment maintenance and standardization, hiring of personnel, orientation of new employees, consistency in performance of practitioners, distribution of staff, and evaluation of quality and cost.

One of the most basic functions of any hospital respiratory care department is to ensure that enough appropriately trained individuals are available and deployed to provide adequate, safe, and quality care in every area throughout the day and night. These staffing and scheduling functions requires competent and creative management and support from the hospital administration. Trust and negotiation on both sides are essential to ensure cost effective and medically sound staffing decisions. By having competent individuals providing around the clock assessment and management services, length of stay and respiratory complication rates should be improved.

Many institutions have diverse patient populations and critical care may be provided in smaller, highly specialized units. Examples of these are neonatal, pediatric, neurologic, cardiovascular, and transplant ICUs. The respiratory care provided in these areas has unit-specific aspects. These areas need as well the centralized support systems listed above. RCPs providing direct patient care are often assigned to one specific area (or a few similar areas) for an extended period of time. This allows development of higher level skills and more consistent service. Some cross coverage of different areas is desirable to increase flexibility of staffing and to maintain the RCP's skills in different areas. This is also an employee satisfier and reduces staff turn over.[6,7]

Centralized activities often include equipment support and processing, purchasing, recruiting, hiring (with local unit input), cost accounting (inventory), vacation scheduling (with consideration of local needs), long-term planning, dispute resolution, office functions, and administrative relations with the other areas of the hospital. These activities can be roughly divided into equipment issues, personnel issues, and external relations.

The needed department size, requirements for specific individual RCP competencies, distribution of staff, hiring and supervision of support staff, and relations with other departments and the hospital are other centralized functions. The volume of these activities and the number of full time equivalent employees (FTEs) needed to provide them should be in proportion to the department activity loads and service demands. These employees (or non-clinical time) must be seen as supporting the bedside caregivers. If a department is to improve, adequate energy must be available for these activities as well as planning for and implementation of new, state-of-the-art services.

Respiratory Support Equipment

Equipment support (acquisition and service) is a centralized function in most hospitals. This allows cost reduction by increasing purchasing power. Also, by limiting the number of different kinds of ventilators in use, the chances of improper operator use causing harm to individual patients is reduced. Physicians often want the latest technologies, failing to appreciate the need to educate a large group of providers in its appropriate and safe use. The cost of the equipment is often inconsequential compared to these training costs. A centralized empowered management allows rational evaluation of new technology and prudent acquisition and implementation. Physician input to these purchase decisions is essential. This is often provided by a formal medical director or a user group of interested physicians.

Supervision and Clinical Support

Because the need for respiratory care service is patient-driven, the ability to respond to changing demands is essential. To ensure efficient use of all personnel, oversight of the entire service is needed on a 24-hour basis. In specialty areas such as neonatal or pediatric critical care units, service line or specific areas may need to provide internal mechanisms for staffing flexibility, but there must be an empowered decision maker or a set of explicit rules to guarantee adequate staff deployment for the entire hospital system.

Medical Direction

Unlike nurses and other medical professionals who have an independent scope of practice, respiratory therapists are physician extenders. In the organizational structure their activities are always overseen by a physician and are entirely guided by physicians' orders at the bedside. The scope of their practice is set by a physician medical director with input from other involved physicians or the general medical staff. In most states in the US and all provinces in Canada, respiratory therapists are not licensed for independent practice, they cannot bill patients directly for professional services and can only treat patients by physician prescription. The Medical Director of Respiratory Care (MDRC), a hospital appointed physician, is responsible for the overall medical quality of respiratory care provided in the institution. By having an organized, centralized department structure within the hospital, caring out of this responsibility is possible. A MDRC is mandated by regulatory agencies and is important to guarantee that the safety and adequacy of life-support systems are addressed. In some institutions this responsibility rests with a committee of the medical staff, however, an individual physician active in the care of patients with respiratory compromise must be available to assist the respiratory care department on a continuous basis. If respiratory care is provided by persons other than hospital staff therapists, active medical direction is essential to ensure quality and consistence of this contractual service.

Education of the Respiratory Care Practitioner

In the early 1950s and 1960s, respiratory therapists received their education on the job. Individuals with manual skills and interest in very sick patients found respiratory care as a satisfying career available to them. Now there is an organized, didactic route to the practice of respiratory care. Students are selected for good mechanical skills, compassion, dedication, and the ability to work as a member of a team. The entrance requirements to most programs include a high school diploma (or equivalent) and satisfactory performance in math and science courses.

There are several recognized levels of educational preparation of RCPs. The entrance level practitioner, officially designated "Certified Respiratory Therapy Technician" or CRTT, receives instruction in assembling and using respiratory equipment and is exposed to machine cleaning and management in a 9-month to 1-year training program. These programs often were established within a hospital rather than an institution of higher learning. The content and quality of the individual training program is evaluated and accredited by a national certification body. The trend is to use an educational institution as a base for RCP training programs, often within the community college system. Completion of such a program allows the individual to sit for a national examination administered by the National Board of Respiratory Care. The examination is technology oriented and includes patient safety questions. If the candidate is successful in passing this written examination, he or she is granted the title "CRTT". Most candidates enrolled in 2- or more year respiratory therapy programs succeed on this examination after the first year. Only about 70% of 1-year program candidates are initially successful.

The designation of "Registered Respiratory Therapist" or RRT is reserved for individuals who have completed at least 2 years (and up to 4 years) of an accredited didactic program, obtained the CRTT certification, and successfully completed a two-part "registry" examination. The examination consists of a cognitive multiple choice part taken after finishing the 2-year didactic program, and the "clinical simulations" examination following successful completion of the first examination. This examination consists of patient assessment and management scenarios. The examinees must request additional relevant data and formulate treatment plans. Requesting unnecessary information or not requesting appropriate tests decrease the candidate's score.

The success rate on the multiple choice examination is approximately 75% and repeated attempts to pass are allowed. The first time pass rate for the "clinical sims" is only about 65%, most individuals eventually being successful after repeated attempts.[8] Since the basis of this examination is patient management, the RCP increases his knowledge and chances of success with additional patient care experience. This examination includes all types of patients and employment that includes an ongoing broad didactic program can help employees achieve registry. This educational opportunity can be used as a recruitment tool.

Four-year baccalaureate degree programs are becoming more common routes for RCP preparation. Graduates from these programs have a broad based general liberal arts education, more in depth science, exposure to management theory, and several additional years to acquire practical skills prior to entering the work force. Masters and doctorate degree programs are also available. Advanced training in specialty areas such as pulmonary function testing and neonatal intensive care are other routes to advanced education. Special examinations are offered or being developed in these areas.

Respiratory therapy education is now standardized, organized, and subjected to a rigorous accreditation process. Accreditation of individual education programs requires a detailed self-study and a site visit including a therapist educator and a physician. The Joint Review Committee for Respiratory Therapy Education is the certifying arm of the Council for Allied Health Education Association, an advisory group to the American Medical Association. These bodies have physicians, therapists, and lay members. All educational programs must include an active physician medical director and an involved physician teaching staff. One educational goal of all programs is to establish in each student effective communication skills with physicians. Clinical affiliations with accredited hospitals are required for all respiratory care educational programs. Clinical competence and cognitive mastery of care is the goal of the educational and examination process.

Employers may not understand or recognize the different educational backgrounds of practitioners in RCPs. Entry level salary is often the same for 2- and 4-year graduates, usually higher than for 1-year, CRTT trainees. Many hospitals award therapists a higher salary once they have passed their registry exam. RRTs usually receive significantly less pay than equally prepared nurses. This is illustrated in the data presented in Table 2. Physical therapists also provide some respiratory care services to patients. They are much more expensive than either nurses or therapists and rarely have the depth of knowledge to treat patients requiring mechanical ventilation or inhalation treatments. Departments of respiratory care also have less administrative overhead than most nursing departments. These issues should be kept in mind when considering cross-utilization of these other groups to provide respiratory care services.

Table 2

Comparison of Salaries for Various Health Care Workers Capable of Providing Respiratory Care Services

Category	Salary	Source
Respiratory Care Technician (CRTT)	$21,002	1, p. 72
Registered Respiratory Therapist (RRT)	$24,934	1, p. 72
Physical Therapist	$30,705	1, p. 71
Licensed Practical Nurse (LPN)	$16,976–24,929	2
Registered Nurse (RN)	$26,410–41,789	2
Physician's Assistant	$37,500	1, p. 73

1. Opportunities for a lifetime. A Health Careers Reference Manual, 1993–1994, p 36. Virginia Health Council, Richmond, VA, 1994.

2. Nursing 94, Career Director. Springhouse Pub. Co., Major Scientific Books, Inc., 1851 Diplomat, Dallas, TX 75234, 1994.

The Science of Respiratory Care Practice

As with other professions, RCPs rely on scientific methods to validate the efficacy of therapy. A large body of knowledge related to equipment and techniques used for respiratory therapy has been developed and published. The main journals publishing peer reviewed literature related to respiratory care are: *Respiratory Care, Chest, Critical Care Medicine, Journal of Critical Care, Anesthesiology, Anesthesia and Analgesia, New England Journal of Medicine, Heart and Lung, British Journal of Anesthesiology*, and the *Canadian Medical Association Journal*. These should be available in the department or hospital medical library. Most of these journals are indexed in the National (American) Library of Medicine and available in abstract form through Medline®. In addition, the CINAHL (citation index of allied health literature) database includes specific references from allied health journals.

Respiratory Intensive Care Practice-Mechanical Ventilation Orders

Many patients residing in ICUs receive mechanical ventilation. Orders directing the delivery of this care can be in several forms. Several of these are listed in Table 3. Standing unit orders often specify the

Table 3
Techniques for Ordering Respiratory Care Services

Type of Physician Order	Authority	Examples
Standing Orders	Unit or department policy—Medical Director	Suction endotracheal tube, PRN secretions. Oxygen 2–4 L/min by nasal prongs PRN chest pain. Retape endotracheal tube daily.
Policies or Guidelines	Medical Director	Ventilator selection. Ventilator alarm settings. Inspiratory time limit.
Therapist-driven Protocols	Medical Staff	Mechanical ventilation weaning. Low-flow oxygen weaning. Chest hyperinflation. ABG sampling for clinical changes.
Explicit Orders	Attending Physician	Extubate now, ABG in 10 minutes.
Stop Orders	Medical Staff	Oxygen 2–4 L/min for 24 hours.

Table 4
Components of an Order for Mechanical Ventilation

Component	Examples	Who Decides?
Mode	Intermittent Mandatory Ventilation, Pressure Support Ventilation, Assist/control Ventilation	Physician
Manufacturer	Seimens 900c, Bear 1,000	Therapist
Rate	10 BBM	Physician*
Tidal Volume	500 ml	Physician
FiO_2	0.5	Physician*
Inspiratory Time	0.9 sec	Therapist
Alarm Settings	Low pressure, low volume, high pressure, high volume, FiO_2	Department Policy
Inspiratory Flow	Shape, rate	Therapist
Humidification system		Therapist

* Initial settings are usually followed by modifications to meet specific ABG endpoints.

usual routines for initiating therapy and monitoring of efficacy. These often include the frequency of endotracheal suctioning (usually left to the discretion of the caregiver or "PRN"), use of oxygenation monitoring, and routines for obtaining of arterial blood gases.

Initiation of mechanical ventilation or inhalation treatments usually requires a physician's signed (or verbal) order. As shown in Table 4, an order initiating mechanical ventilation should include at least the following: the mode of ventilation; the desired inspired oxygen concentration; level of end-expiratory pressure (PEEP) and the desired minute ventilation (or frequency and tidal volume); or the inspiratory pressure level (for pressure support ventilation). Other ventilatory parameters such as: the specific machine chosen; the inspiratory time; the wave form of delivered ventilation; and the pressure limits and other alarm settings are often left to the RCP to determine. Respiratory care departmental policies can be used to set boundaries for these additional functions. Quality improvement activities should include monitoring of appropriateness of actual settings employed by RCPs of these discretionary functions.

Using RCPs to Optimize Mechanical Ventilation

One of the most efficient ways to optimize ventilation management is to have the responsible RCP make independent routine modifications and report only significant changes to the physician. This takes advantage of the depth of the educational background and experience of the RCP. The management plan can be guided by the philosophy of the attending physician. This use of the RCP can be achieved in several ways. In an individual patient, the responsible physician can establish goals and parameters to be achieved and endpoints or deviations at which communication should occur. This is a frequently used method and allows for individual physician variation in approach and experience. The MDRC acts as a quality control officer available to the therapist to evaluate those individual plans that seem to deviate from usual acceptable practice. The medical director must take an active role in these cases to negotiate with the attending physician and therapist to resolve differences of opinion.

Therapist-Driven Protocols

A more formal and effective way to promote uniformity and high-quality respiratory care management is use of therapist-driven protocols. These are specific management plans that represent a consensus of the physicians' and RCP's opinions of good practice. They give the RCP autonomy in decision-making within specified limits. Physicians are guaranteed consistent, efficient care. Most protocols identify under what circumstances the physician should be called. Although not all therapy is easily "protocolized", the frequently performed procedures and management issues can be addressed using this technique. Therapist-driven protocols have been well accepted by both physicians and therapists and offer economy and improved care.

Calling these standardized algorithms "therapist-driven" does them a political disservice. They are really "patient-need driven." The RCP assesses the patient and makes adjustments within the specified parameters to meet the needs of the patient. As therapists are always present, therapeutic changes can be effected around the clock. This increases effectiveness, efficiency, and perhaps improves outcome.

Respiratory treatments besides mechanical ventilation and ventilator weaning also lend themselves to protocols. For instance, lung hyperinflation therapy used to treat (and prevent) atelectasis and pneumonia consists of several options: coughing and deep breathing; incentive spirometry; and intermittent positive pressure breathing (IPPB). Clinical criteria as illustrated in Figure 1 can be used to guide the appropriate choice. Therapists can gather the appropriate laboratory values (vital capacity), choose the appropriate therapy, institute it, and assess the

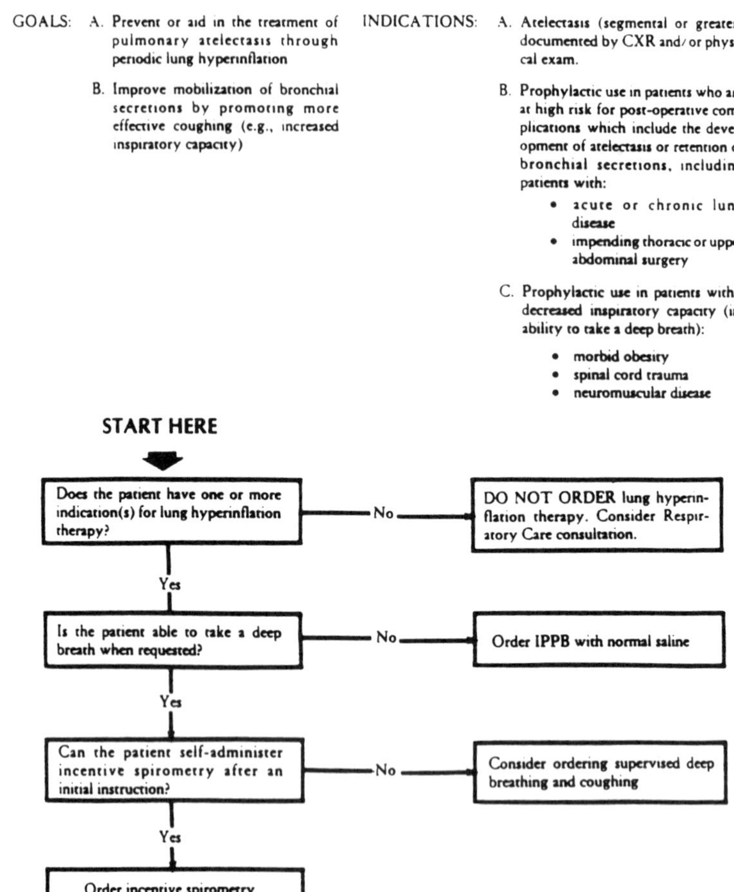

Figure 1. Guidelines for lung hyperinflation therapy. Reproduced with permission from Hart SK, Dubbs W, Gil A, et al: The effects of therapist-evaluation of orders and interaction with physicians on the appropriateness of respiratory care. Resp Care 1989;34:185–190.

success at meeting the therapeutic goals. This approach has been shown to decrease the frequency of unnecessary treatments and increase the number of patients receiving appropriate treatments.[9] This approach is accepted by physicians, patients, and therapists and saves the hospital money by standardizing care. These protocols or algorithms can also serve as an educational device for other caregivers including physicians and nurses.[10,11]

Stop Orders

Another method to limit provision of unnecessary respiratory care is to use "stop orders". Often used in pharmacy orders, these define specific lengths of time that an order will be carried out. At the end of the time period the therapy will be discontinued unless a new order is entered to continue therapy. These are often used with medicated aerosol and inhalation treatments. The time before automatic stopping is usually about 72 hours. Therapy is usually delivered by a technician-level person. This can decrease personnel costs, however, often the treatments could have been discontinued sooner if proper patient assessment were being carried out by a therapist-level individual and contact with the physician was made. In addition, at the end of the specified time period the patient may still require intensive treatment and the renewal order may be overlooked by the physician. Needed changes in therapy are poorly handled with stop orders.

One area where stop orders have proved safe and effective is in the area of low-flow oxygen. Often patients are begun on nasal oxygen or a face mask for minimal indications. Removal of the oxygen at a specified time after initiation is reasonable. Those patients needing oxygen continued will have been identified and the others will automatically have the oxygen stopped in a short period, usually 24 hours. The costs of evaluating all these patients by a therapist is probably excessive and few (if any) patients will be harm by low-flow oxygen discontinuation.

Stop orders are used to administratively control physician ordering behavior. Their use sometimes reflects the failure of the respiratory therapy department to establish physician confidence in the quality of respiratory assessment and services offered. Staffing make-up strategies and shortages may make the use of this method necessary. This is a particular problem when non-therapists are providing respiratory care.

The Costs and Cost Savings of Respiratory Care

Alluded to above, other allied health professionals can provide some aspects of respiratory care. In general they are more expensive and less effective than respiratory therapists. In a recent study of metered dose inhaler use, nurses were significantly less effective than therapists in administering this treatment modality.[12] Another advantage to the hospital of having RCPs available on a continuous basis, is that they may provide additional services efficiently and economically. Services such as blood sampling, starting intravenous lines, recording EKGs, obtaining EEG studies, providing metabolic cart services, assisting in invasive procedures, supporting the operating room, leading hospital cardiac arrest teams, staffing the cardiac catheterization laboratory, and other activities can easily be added to the respiratory therapy department's tasks. Because of concerns for patient safety and skills in patient assessment, therapists can become contributing members of the care team, filling multiple clinical roles. Nurse and therapist teams can provide safe and efficient transport of critically ill patients within and between hospitals.[13]

Therapists demand lower salaries than many other caregivers. Their flexibility, accountability to physicians, communication skills, and ability to make independent decisions, make them a bargain and an asset to most hospitals.

Management of the Respiratory ICU

Patients with isolated respiratory failure may be cared for in a separate physical area identified as a respiratory ICU. The importance of respiratory therapists in these units is obvious. Being at the bedside, they monitor both patient and mechanical ventilator. They can identify patients whose condition is deteriorating and institute needed changes in therapy. They can replace defective equipment and place the patient on the most appropriate ventilation device available to them. They keep the physician informed of important changes in the patient and suggest alternative treatment strategies.

Respiratory therapists are excellent teachers. They routinely instruct patients in proper methods of self-administrating bronchodilators and postural drainage. These same teaching skills can be used to increase the other professional staffs' knowledge and decision skills about respiratory management. House staff and general doctors (non-specialists) in particular can benefit from the knowledge and skills of these individuals. Their indepth knowledge and practical experience allow them to predict and explain the effects of mechanical ventilation and avoid preventable catastrophes. They are able to instruct physicians in a non-threatening way due to the fact that they derive their support from a respected, senior physician or physician group. Diplomacy is a requirement for successful practice as a respiratory therapist.

As a physician manager of a respiratory ICU, the respiratory therapists are important extenders of your skills and beliefs. They support the quality and consistency of care at the bedside and when you are not physically present. With various and different attending physicians, the therapists become the consistent factor in the unit. They will carry out the unit "policies" whether they are explicitly or custom written. Unlike other non-physician caregivers, these respiratory policies are developed and endorsed by the medical director and medical staff, rather than with other professions such as nursing that functions independently from physicians. Although they are required to carry out physician's orders, if the request is deviant from their concept of good care, they will contact their medical director for conflict resolution. It is essential to have such an individual readily available to the therapists at the bedside. This informal but mandatory consultation with a respiratory care expert provides consistency in critical care practice.

Quality assurance and care improvement is a natural part of the therapist's role. As a manager, the quality of respiratory support services is an essential component of your responsibility. Mechanical ventilation is a high-risk, expensive, and frequent service. It needs to be provided as safely and efficiently as possible. Respiratory care policies for ventilator checks, documentation, order writing requirements, and equipment servicing and repair are developed to deal with and reduce these risks. Monitoring of consistency of these activities and results of servicing of ventilators is an important indicator of quality and identification of areas needing attention. Reports of mechanical failures or undesired patient outcome resulting from respiratory misadventures should trigger detailed investigation into systematic problems that should be corrected. Therapists are in the appropriate position to identify and investigate these events.

Respiratory therapists can serve similar roles in all intensive care areas in which airway management and mechanical ventilation are performed. They can provide support and respiratory management assistance in transporting patients in the hospital, helicopter transfers, in the recovery room, in the emergency department, and during cardiopulmonary resuscitation activities.

Respiratory step-down or weaning units are intensive care areas designed for support of patients with the single problem of respiratory failure. They often admit patients who have secondary respiratory failure. These are patients who have survived multiple organ dysfunction and require a prolonged, gradual ventilatory course prior to hospital discharge without mechanical ventilation. Occasional patients with acute, primary respiratory failure are admitted to take advantage of the respiratory expertise and avoid a more expensive ICU course. These units should have the same ratio of respiratory therapists to patients as an ICU but may have fewer nurses and other support personnel. They are usually able to expand and contract staff and space to meet the needs of a changing population. Therapists often rotate from the ICU to staff these beds.

Summary

Respiratory failure is an important problem in critical illness. Specialized units providing mechanical ventilation and respiratory care improve hospital efficiency and patient outcome. Respiratory therapists provide quality mechanical support, patient assessment, and physician support continuously. Their training and practice are based on rational, scientific principals. They are able to extend the physician's care and function within narrow or wide limits. They can easily be cross-trained to meet many additional hospital needs. They are less expensive than other health care providers and more accountable to physician needs and concerns. To function well, a respiratory care department needs strong, efficient central administration, involved medical direction, and hospital support and respect. Appropriate numbers of educated practitioners and optimal deployment will ensure quality, efficient care. Respiratory care units are an economic alternative to keeping patients with isolated or persistent respiratory insufficiency out of the ICU.

References

1. Hilberman M: The evolution of intensive care units. Crit Care Med 1975; 3:159–165.
2. Nochomovitz ML, Montenegro HD, Parran S, et al: Placement alternatives for ventilator-dependent patients outside the intensive care unit. Respir Care 1991;36:199–204.
3. Bone RC, Balk RA: Noninvasive respiratory care unit: a cost-effective solution for the future. Chest 1988;93:390–394.
4. Gold DR, Rogacz S, Bock N, et al: Rotating shift work, sleep, and accidents related to sleepiness in hospital nurses. Am J Pub Health 1992;82: 1011–1014.
5. Alward RR, Monk TH: A comparison of rotating-shift and permanent night nurses. Int J Nursing Studies 1990;27:297–302.
6. Synder GM: Patient focused hospitals: an opportunity for respiratory care practitioners. Respir Care 1992;37:448–454.
7. Hmelo C, Axton K: Job satisfaction and task complexity among respiratory care practitioners. Respir Care 1989;34:1129–1134.
8. NBRC Horizons. National Board for Respiratory Care, Lenexa, KA, 1994; 20:7.

9. Hart SK, Dubbs W, Gil A, et al: The effects of therapist-evaluation of orders and interaction with physicians on the appropriateness of respiratory care. Respir Care 1989;34:185–190.
10. Browning JA, Kaiser DL, Durbin CG: The effect of guidelines on the appropriate use of arterial blood gas analysis in the intensive care unit. Respir Care 1989;34:269–276.
11. Beasley KE, Darin JM, Durbin CG: The effect of respiratory care department management of a blood gas analyzer on the appropriateness of arterial blood gas utilization. Resp Care 1992;37:343–347.
12. Guidry GG, Brown WD, Strogner SW et al: Incorrect use of metered dose inhalers by medical personnel. Chest 1992;101:31–33.
13. Beyer JA, Landn G, Zaritsky A: Nonphysician transport of intubated pediatric patients: A system evaluation. Crit Care Med 1992;20:961–966.

Chapter 22

Managing the Coronary Care Unit

James E. Calvin Jr, M.D.

The treatments of acute coronary ischemic syndromes such as myocardial infarction and unstable angina have undergone radical change in the last 25 years.[1] The activities of the coronary care unit that was first devised as a means to prevent arrhythmic death[2] after myocardial infarction, have escalated as a result and the efficient organization of these activities are pivotal to the success of such interventions as thrombolytic therapy[3,4] and percutaneous transluminal coronary angioplasty.[5,6] Early intervention, often initiated in the critical care unit (CCU) is a critical success factor, and adjunctive therapy such as heparin[7] and beta blockers,[8] now of proven utility, further emphasizes the important role of the coronary care unit organization for the best outcomes. Interestingly, in many locales, because of the economics involved and the level of care available, coronary and intensive care units (ICUs) are often combined into single units.

Beyond these exciting advances aimed at early restoration of coro-

---

From: Sibbald WJ, Massaro T (eds.): The Business of Critical Care: A Textbook for Clinicians Who Manage Special Care Units. © Futura Publishing Co., Inc., Armonk, NY, 1996.

nary blood flow in acute ischemic syndromes, the management of acute pump failure often necessitates the use of mechanical ventilation,[9] intra-aortic balloon pumping,[10,11] mechanical ventricular assist devices,[12–15] and heart transplantation[16] in addition to potent vasopressor and inotropic agents. The fact that these aggressive measures are conducted in the CCU underscores the importance of an efficient and effective unit organization.

Finally, acute coronary care is an integral part of any critical care system. The need of a patient with an uncomplicated myocardial infarction including thrombolytic therapy can be provided in smaller CCUs and combined CCU/ICU units. Recent studies suggesting better efficacy of primary angioplasty compared to thrombolytic therapy in acute myocardial infarction, improved survival of revascularization techniques for cardiogenic shock, and ventricular assist devices for severe heart failure place a major responsibility on a critical care system to provide the necessary access and availability of these resources to the critically ill cardiac patient. Regional CCUs that can provide this type of care coupled with transport and communication systems will need to be developed allowing better access for referring hospitals and their patients.

The purpose of this chapter is to review the organization, activities, and acuity of the coronary care unit and to provide an outline for reviewing and managing outcomes.

Patient Population

Although CCUs were devised for the management of acute myocardial infarction, the case mix is now quite broad. Currently at Rush-Presbyterian-St. Luke's Medical Center only 17.6% of admissions are for acute myocardial infarction. Patients with unstable angina comprise the largest group at 29.2% of admissions. Congestive heart failure comprise 9.4%. Patients with undiagnosed chest pain (the so-called "Rule out MI") comprise 11.4%, and patients with serious dysrhythmia also comprise 11.4%. Other assorted diagnoses comprise the remaining 21% (Figure 1). This case mix represents the experience of a US tertiary care center and may differ in other countries or smaller community hospitals. Nonetheless, it illustrates that much of the activity in the CCU is involved in working up suspected myocardial infarction, and treating other ischemic syndromes and other forms of severe heart disease.

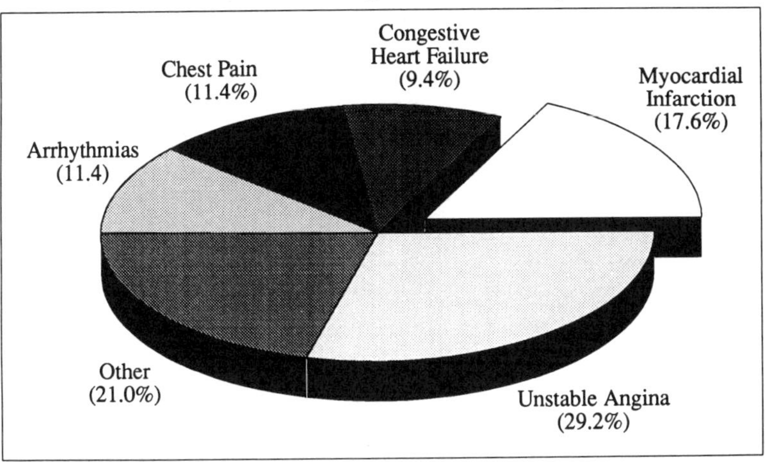

Figure 1. Distribution of admission diagnoses to Rush-Presbyterian-St. Luke's Medical Center.

Acuity of Patients in the Coronary Care Unit

Some of the earliest acuity scoring systems in critical care were for patients with myocardial infarction. Both the Killip classification[17] that is still commonly used and the Norris Prognostic Index[18] were introduced in the late 1960s and early 1970s. To some degree they were usurped by a hemodynamic classification first published in 1976.[19] Although this latter classification predicted mortality better, it necessitated the use of right heart catheterization (an invasive monitor) that has significant complications.

The Use of APACHE II to Assess Acuity in the Critical Care Unit

Recently Teskey et al.[20] published a retrospective review of the efficacy of APACHE to predict mortality in the broad range of diagnoses found in the CCU. The distribution of APACHE II scores for this study was compared to previously published data for ICU patients[21] and this comparison is shown in Figure 2. The distribution of APACHE II scores in coronary care is shifted to a lower range of values. The mortality of admitted CCU patients did correlate with APACHE II (Figure 3). However, comparison of the distribution of APACHE II scores in surviving and non-surviving patients revealed an interesting observation (Figure 4). The APACHE II scores for non-survivors was bimodal with peaks both at relatively low and high APACHE II scores. This reveals an important difference in the patterns of mortality of patients in CCUs. Although most patients are admitted to the CCU with little derangement in normal physiology, a significant proportion of CCU mortalities occur in this apparent low-risk group primarily of single organ failure. Patients are admitted also with high APACHE II scores reflecting multiple organ system dysfunction with the poorer prognosis that is more characteristically observed in the ICU.

In addition to comparing the worst APACHE II score in the first 24 hours between survivors and non-survivors for various diagnoses (Table 1), the utility of APACHE II was assessed by constructing a receiver operator characteristic curve for each diagnosis.[22] This type of analysis involves calculating the area beneath the relationship of sensitivity as a function of 1-specificity. A perfect test or scoring system would have a value of 1.0. A test with no predictive value (i.e., a coin toss) would have a value of 0.5 (represented by the diagonal). Using

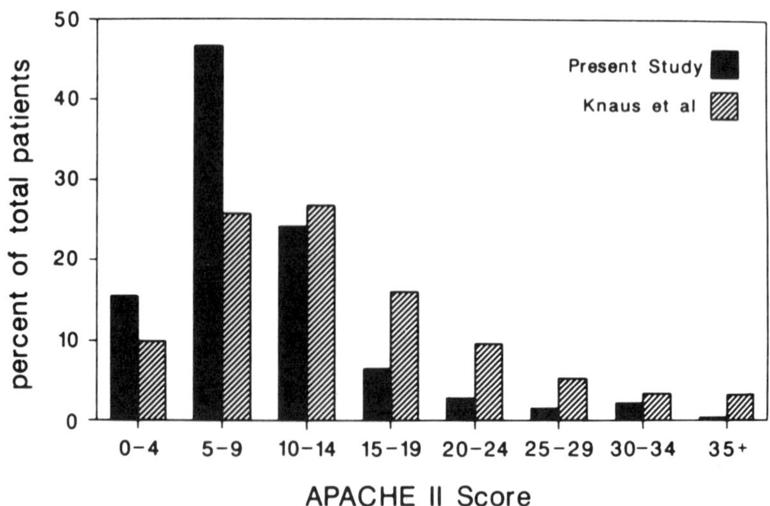

Figure 2. Distribution of APACHE II scores for CCU cohort (present study; solid bars) and a multidisciplinary ICU cohort.

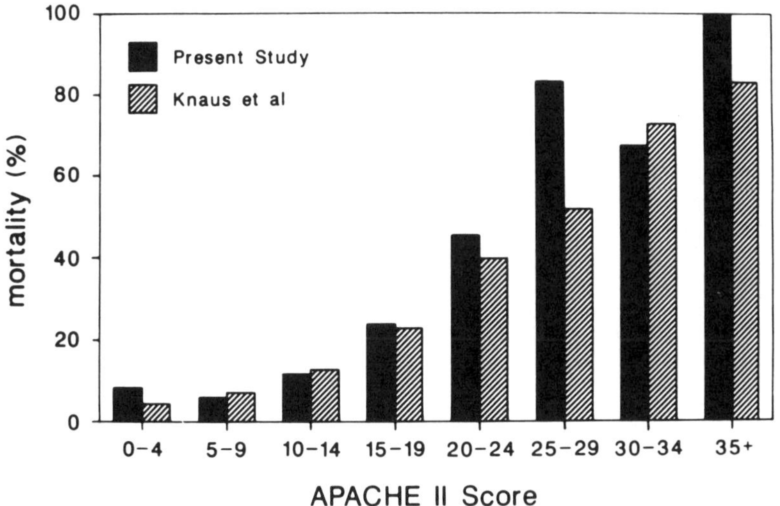

Figure 3. Coronary care unit in-hospital mortality by APACHE II score.

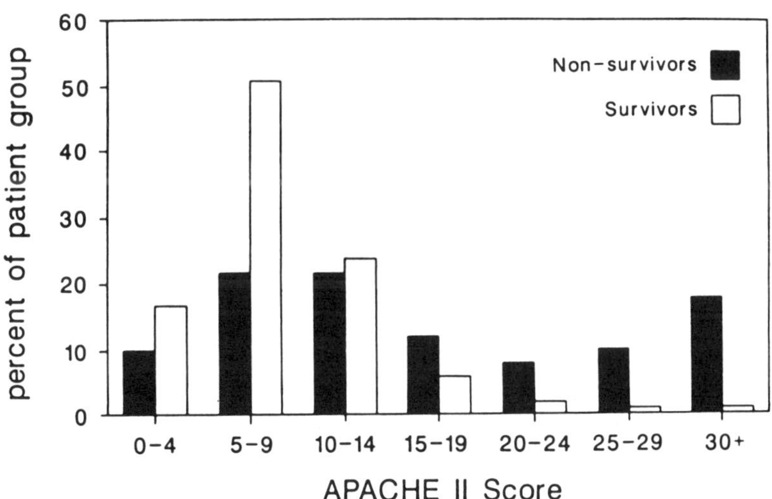

Figure 4. The APACHE II score distribution among survivors is unimodal, whereas that of nonsurvivors is bimodal, with a second peak at high APACHE II scores.

Table 1
Diagnostic Groups

Diagnosis	n	Mortality (%)	APACHE II Score*	
			Nonsurvivor	Survivor
Arrhythmia				
Out-of hospital cardiac arrest	10	70	31.1 ± 1.4	22.0 ± 6.1
Other	34	12	9.5 ± 1.0	8.4 ± 0.6
Total arrhythmias	44	23	23.3 ± 3.3	9.6 ± 1.0†
Congestive heart failure	20	15	23.3 ± 3.8	12.5 ± 1.9‡
Chest pain, not yet diagnosed	21	14	3.0 ± 0.6	7.6 ± 0.9‡
Myocardial infarction:				
non-Q wave	81	14	16.9 ± 3.4	8.4 ± 0.5†
Q wave	107	10	15.0 ± 1.5	7.5 ± 0.4†
Total MI	188	12	16.0 ± 1.8	7.9 ± 0.3†
Unstable angina	89	10	9.4 ± 1.1	8.0 ± 0.4
Other diagnoses	24	13	24.0 ± 7.9	10.3 ± 1.6†
Total	386	13	16.5 ± 1.4	8.5 ± 0.3†

* APACHE II scores are reported as means ± SE.
† $P < 0.01$ vs nonsurvivors.
‡ $P < 0.05$ vs nonsurvivors.

this type of analysis a value of 0.75 was observed for the total population (Figure 5). However, it predicted best for patients with congestive heart failure (0.97 ± 0.05), and worst for patients with chest pain (0.11 ± 0.07) with intermediate values for patients with myocardial infarction and arrhythmia (Table 1). Moreover, a multivariate logistic model was developed that used both diagnosis and APACHE II scores to predict mortality (Table 2). This model still needs prospective validation but does offer a potentially useful tool to assess mortality outcome in the CCU.

Acuity Systems for Unstable Angina

Our experience with APACHE II suggested little role for it in unstable angina. At present, there are two other scoring systems that have not been validated for their ability to predict mortality. The first, the

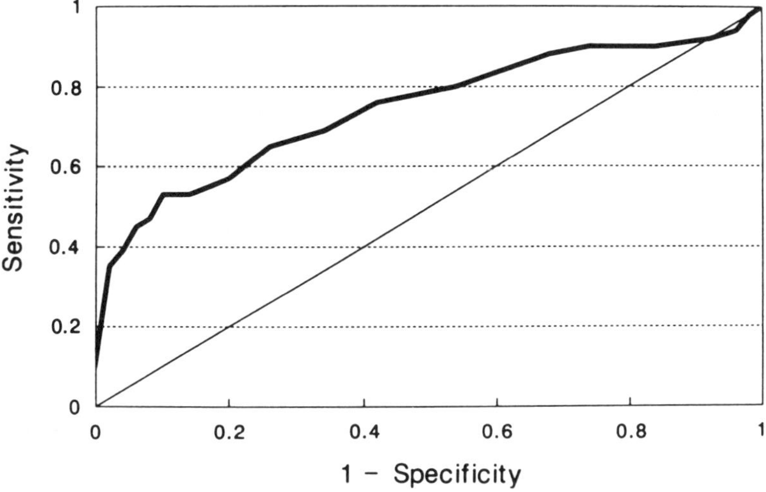

Figure 5. Receiver operating characteristic (ROC) curve for mortality as predicted by APACHE II score for all CCU admissions.

Table 2
Predicted In-hospital Mortality by Diagnosis on Admission and APACHE II score

APACHE II Score	Diagnosis*					
	Arr	CHF	CP-NYD	MI	UA	Other
0	0.03	0.01	0.04	0.02	0.02	0.01
5	0.06	0.02	0.09	0.05	0.06	0.02
10	0.12	0.04	0.20	0.11	0.12	0.04
15	0.25	0.09	0.36	0.22	0.24	0.10
20	0.44	0.19	0.57	0.39	0.43	0.20
25	0.64	0.35	0.76	0.60	0.64	0.37
30	0.81	0.56	0.88	0.78	0.80	0.58
35	0.91	0.75	0.95	0.89	0.91	0.76
40	0.96	0.87	0.98	0.95	0.96	0.88
45	0.98	0.94	0.99	0.98	0.98	0.95
50	0.99	0.97	1.00	0.99	0.99	0.98

* Arr = arrhythmias (including out-of-hospital cardiac arrest); CHF = congestive heart failure; CP-NYD = undiagnosed chest pain; MI = myocardial infarction; UA = unstable angina.

Canadian Cardiovascular Society classification (Table 3) is really a scoring system for angina based on functional capacity.[23] It does not take into account the progressive nature of systems, but merely the severity of the functional limitation. Class IV is characterized by the inability to carry on any physical activity without discomfort and symptoms may be present at rest. Recognizing these limitations, the Revascularization Panel and Consensus Methods Group in Ontario devised a priority system for coronary revascularization that further subcategorized Class IV patients as follows:

Class IV A—Unstable angina stabilized on oral therapy

Class IV B—Unstable angina with symptoms improved on oral therapy but angina present on minimal provocation

Class IV C—Unstable angina, symptoms not manageable on oral therapy, requiring coronary care monitoring and parenteral medication

Using this classification and the anatomical severity of disease, this panel suggested guidelines for the timeliness of revascularization. The utility of this revision still has not been validated.

In 1988, Braunwald proposed a classification of angina that to date has not been prospectively evaluated. This classification (Table 4) characterizes the severity and the clinical circumstances of the patients' presentation. Severity distinguished among progressive angina, angina at rest beyond 48 hours, and rest angina within 48 hours. The clinical circumstances distinguished among extracardiac precipitating factors

Table 3
Method of Assessing Cardiovascular Disability

Class	Canadian Cardiovascular Society Functional Classification
I	Ordinary physical activity, such as walking and climbing stairs, does not cause angina. Angina with strenuous or rapid or prolonged exertion at work or recreation.
II	Slight limitation of ordinary activity. Walking or climbing stairs rapidly, walking uphill, walking or stair climbing after meals, in cold, in wind, or when under emotional stress, or only during the few hours after awakening. Walking more than two blocks on the level and climbing more than one flight of ordinary stairs at a normal pace and in normal conditions.
III	Marked limitation of ordinary physical activity. Walking one to two blocks on the level and climbing more than one flight in normal conditions.
IV	Inability to carry on any physical activity without discomfort—anginal syndrome may be present at rest.

Table 4
Classification of Unstable Angina

Severity	Clinical Circumstances: A. Develops in Presence of Extracardiac Condition That Intensifies Myocardial Ischemia (Secondary UA)	B. Develops in Absence of Extracardiac Condition (Primary UA)	C. Develops Within 2 Week after AMI (Postinfarction UA)
I. New onset of severe angina or accelerated angina; no rest pain	IA	IB	IC
II. Angina at rest within past month but not within preceding 48 hr (Angina at rest, subacute)	IIA	IIB3	IIC
III. Angina at rest within 4 hr (Angina at rest, acute)	IIIA	IIIB	IIIC

occur early after myocardial infarction and the absence of these factors (primary unstable angina). While intuitively this appears logical, its utility in case management and auditing is untested.

Activities of This Unit

No longer are patients merely observed or monitored in the CCU for life-threatening arrhythmia or shock. Because of technological advances both in the treatment of ischemic heart disease and arrhythmia and evaluation of left ventricular function, the activities have radically expanded and can be summarized by the recent experience observed at Rush-Presbyterian-St. Luke's Medical Center (Figure 6). In addition to heavy uses of intravenous vasodilators and heparin, at least 11% of patients receive right heart catheterization and 4% are ventilated. Coronary angiography is used in 27% of patients while in the CCU with 9% of patients undergoing percutaneous transluminal coronary angioplasty (PTCA) and 12% coronary artery bypass surgery. With these activities, the CCU mortality for all patients is currently 4%.

Quality Assurance

Quality assurance is gaining more and more attention in this age of spiralling health care costs and increasing malpractice claims. Specific

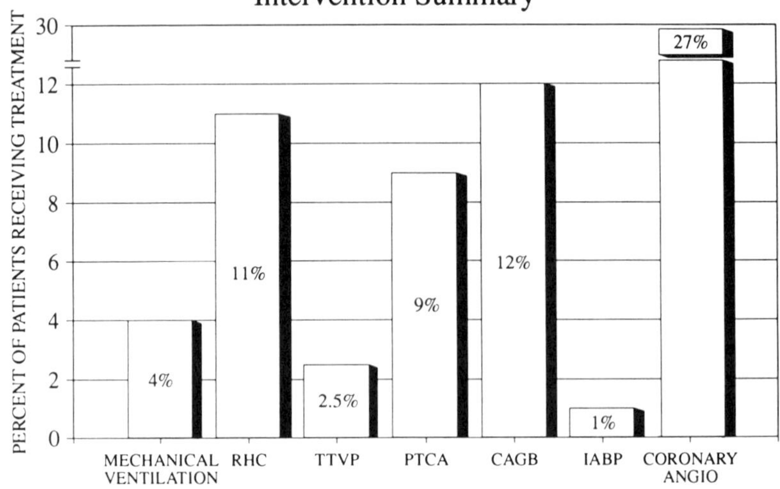

Figure 6. Treatment activities at Rush-Presbyterian-St. Luke's Medical Center CCU.

indicators reflecting structure (i.e., both physical plant and administrative organization), process and outcomes are necessary. A general outline for each of these is shown in Table 5.

Physical plant guidelines are well laid out by governments and professional societies and are reviewed elsewhere.[24–26] Administrative indicators must reflect a mission statement and require the existence of specific job descriptions, credentialling, staffing, and activity levels.

Process indicators involve the existence of policies and procedures that govern activities, admission, and discharge criteria and case management guidelines. As well acuity scoring systems and workload indicators are very important in analyzing the activities and outcomes of the unit.

By modeling the CCU as a system, an analysis of: (1) input variables such as human, technological, pharmaceutical, and physical plant resources; (2) activities and processes supporting diagnosis and treatment of critically ill cardiac patients; and (3) outcomes can be made. Data collection and analysis is the foundation for the systems' evaluative feedback loop, which is necessary for both outcome review and management (Figure 7). This allows analysis of the effectiveness of both the processes of the limits and the adequacy of there sources. Planning based on this analysis would be expected to improve outcomes. These elements represent the essential tools for front-line managers to perform their job.

Table 5
Necessary Indicators for Quality Review and Management

Structural Indicators:	
a) Physical Plant Guidelines	b) Administrative
Size of unit (Federal Guidelines exist)	Departmental philosophy/mission
	Job descriptions
Environmental control	Credentialling
Lighting	Role and responsibilities
Power source/supply	Staffing requirements
Security	Hours of operation
Planned preventive maintenance	Role of ancillary services
	Activity levels (occupancy rates)
	Case mix
	Turnover rates
	Absenteeism indicators
Process Indicators:	
Rules/regulations	
Professional guidelines (i.e., Nursing, Respiratory Therapy Medical Staff, etc.)	
Admission/discharge criteria	
Case management guidelines (treatment assessment, evaluation, etc.)	
Transfer guidelines (to and from Critical Care Units)	
Investigation guidelines (i.e., routine order formats)	
Acuity scoring systems/workload management	
Outcome Indicators:	
Mortality/morbidity	
Timeliness of diagnosis and treatment	
Quality of life (levels improved, maintained, deteriorated)	

How to Assess Quality and Manage Outcomes

Deming Re-Visited

Quality assessment requires measurement of important indicators of the quality of the processes of the system. The most common outcome measurement is mortality but other indicators of process such as morbidity, cost, and length of stay are also important.

W. Edwards Deming has been called the Father of the New Industrial Age and the Founder of the New Economics Era. His visits to Japan in 1950 have had tremendous influences upon the importance of quality and the application of statistical principles to assess it. Although this approach has been most widely applied to manufacturing in post-war

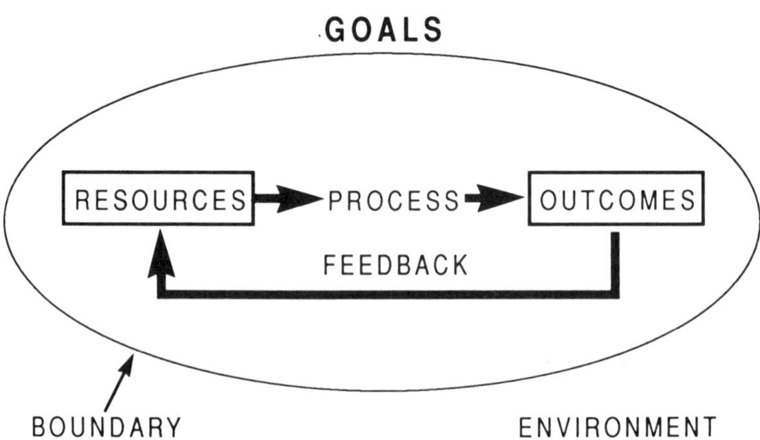

Figure 7. Schematic framework of CCU modeled as a system.

Japan, it is being more commonly practiced in North America in the last decade. Although the principles Deming[27,28] espoused were developed in particular for manufacturing, they can be easily applied to health care.

Deming's approach focused less upon managing and rewarding by results and more upon improving quality of the product and the manufacturing processes. In health care, the product really is "a process" leading to a favorable outcome and, therefore, the quality and cost effectiveness of patient care can be analyzed using statistical techniques that Deming espouses.

The basic principle of the statistical approach to quality assessment is to assess variation in outcome measurements that are felt to be meaningful. Variation can be of two varieties: (1) common causes; and (2) special causes. Common cause variation reflects the overall sum of small variations inherent to the process and determines the limits and capabilities of current operation. As an example, measurement of length of stay can be summarized for a given diagnosis each quarter. This summary provides an average number of days that are inherent for treating a specific condition and its standard deviation. If the length of stay, in general, is too long, independent of time period, common causes of variation must be sought out and analyzed so that it can be reduced.

Large variability suggested by a large standard deviation is readily identified as a problem requiring analysis of its causation.

In contrast, a large difference in complication rates between time periods may indicate special causes of variations that are not part of the process all the time. A large increase in the incidence of hemorrhage, for instance, may indicate a new resident's lack of understanding of the indications, contraindications, or pharmacology of heparin therapy. These types of problems can be resolved by addressing their special causes rather than the overall process of care delivery itself.

In Figure 8 we have summarized how one can analyze mortality for both common and special causes of variation hypothetically. For the diagnosis of myocardial infarction, the hypothetical average mortality rate is 7.2 ± 1.5% (mean ± SD) There are two observations using such analysis. First, the overall mortality rate can be compared to currently published mortality rates for myocardial infarction. If our overall mortality is consistent or better than currently accepted mortalities, the level of care is probably acceptable. Common causes of variation can be related to a number of issues such as a low rate of thrombolytic administration, low nurse to patient ratios, use of old technology, or a lack of cardiac catheterization or cardiac surgical facilities, which can be assessed.

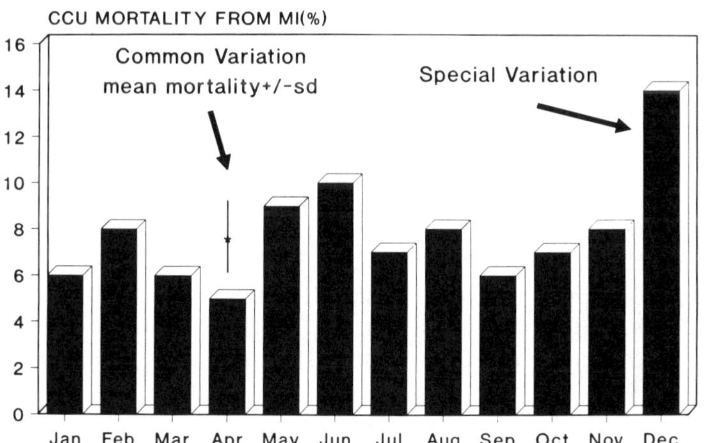

Figure 8. Identification of common and special causes of variation in the diagnoses of myocardial infarction.

Their potential causes can be addressed using a more systematic approach. On the other hand, if the variability is large and particularly if the occurrence became an unusually high rate in one time period, a special cause of variation should be sought out, identified, and corrected. Special causes of variation could represent excessive patient acuity, higher complication rates, and changes or breaches in policy or procedure, all of which should be sought out.

An Example of How to Develop Process Indicators

A common admitting diagnosis to the CCU is unstable angina and provides a useful example of how to develop process indicators. There are many problems encountered analyzing the quality of care in this condition. First, the definition is ambiguous because of multiple forms of presentation. Acuity scales have not been tested. Only recently have medical therapies like heparin[7] and ASA[29] been proven beneficial and the role of surgery seems limited to patients with either poor left ventricular function, refractory symptoms, or left main coronary artery disease.[30] The role of PTCA has not been fully evaluated.

In this context, analysis of care would appear to be fraught with difficulty. But an understanding of process (Figure 9) does provide help.[31] Our understanding of the proposed Braunwald classification allows us to stratify patients. The presence of ECG change and pain recurrence dictates a more aggressive approach. The absence of these occurrences indicate a more conservative style. Although one could debate in which patients a conservative approach could be deployed, the time interval before performing coronary angiography and the time interval before subsequent revascularization can be assessed. Using guidelines suggested by Naylor et al.,[32] these times could be assessed and serve as indicators of the process of managing unstable angina over and above mortality and morbidity. Long and inappropriate delays could be identified and addressed. Also, additional tests that don't contribute to the management strategy could be minimized. Such a process would reduce length of stay and reduce cost. Determining whether indicated medical treatments are being used is also an important indicator of process. Although this may leave open the questions of whether surgery is better than PTCA or medicine, it does provide clarity in managing the necessary processes that are not in dispute.

This general approach can be applied to any disease process or physiological problem that presents to the unit. The choice of problem is dictated by the demographics of the unit, the cost implications, and

THE PATIENT WITH UNSTABLE ANGINA
UNDERSTANDING THE PROCESS

Clinical	ECG on Presentation	Initial Treatment	Pain Recurrent within 48 hrs.	Test by 48 hrs.	Advisable time to Intervention (Naylor, et al)
		ASA NTG HEP			
Rest pain <48 hrs.	↗ + ECG	Y Y Y	Y	C	<24-72 hrs.
			N	C	
	↘ - ECG	Y Y Y	Y	C	
			N	T	
Rest pain >48 hrs.	↗ + ECG	Y ? Y	Y	C	<24 hrs. - LM >2-6 wks. - SVD
			N	C	
	↘ - ECG	Y ? ?	Y	C	
			N	T	
Progressive Angina	↗ + ECG	Y ? ?	Y	C	Within 1-6 wks.
			N	C	
	↘ - ECG	Y ? ?	Y	C	
			N	T	

Time to test 48 hrs; time to intervention would depend on anatomy; C = Coronary angiogram; T = Treadmill stress test; Y = Yes; N = No; LM = Left main, SVD = Single vessel disease; ASA = Aspirin; NTG = nitroglycerin; HEP = heparin

Figure 9. Charting the process of diagnosing and treating unstable angina.

the problem's implications for survival and quality of living. Each unit has to assess this issue in their own right. But once a problem has been identified, the related activities and processes must be delineated before good indicators can be chosen.

Outcome Management

Once causes of variation in process indicators or outcome indicators have been ascertained and analyzed, improvement must follow. This requires certain organizational structure, policies, and procedures. In the case of medical outcomes it is generally the role of the medical director as part of his job description to first measure the outcomes and analyze the processes involved. Once analysis has been completed, some recommendations should follow. The use of a Conclusions, Recommendations, Action, and Evaluation report provides the structure and documentation in this process. Completion of all four sections provides a powerful tool for both quality assessment, management, and improvement.

The next question is the reporting structure within the hospital. As an example, the reporting structure at Rush-Presbyterian-St. Luke's

QUALITY MANAGEMENT STRUCTURE FOR CCU AND MICU

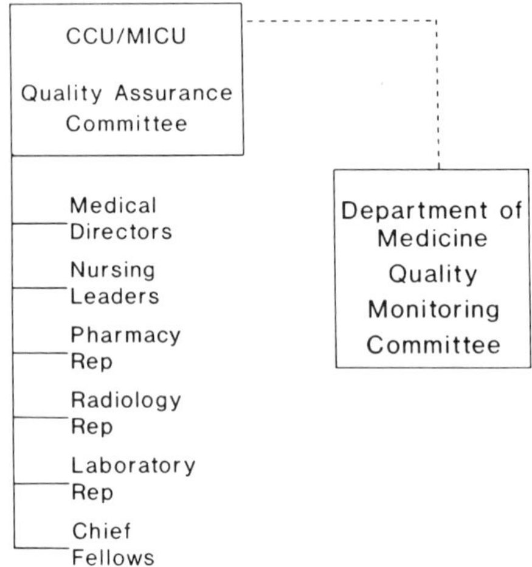

Figure 10. Organizational chart for quality assurance in critical care.

Medical Center is depicted in Figure 10. The director of both ICU and CCU report to a Critical Care Quality Assurance Committee (CCQAC), which is multidisciplinary and involves the leadership of critical care. Most issues can be resolved at this level. The CCQAC also reports to a departmental Quality Monitoring Committee to ensure adequate documentation and follow-up. These reporting structures are indeed important. They provide the communication necessary for improvement by formalizing linkages to general medical staff, the responsible hospital departments and to other stakeholders. Without this type of communication, it would be impossible to effect change when it is indicated.

Although this structure is an example, it does give an overview that acknowledges that the unit is not isolated, but part of a larger entity and it is that understanding and awareness that facilitates improvement.

Summary

The CCU of the 1990s is quite different from that envisioned in the mid-1960s. The case mix is broader and interventional therapy is utilized at lower acuity. Understanding the processes by which care is provided in the CCU allows measurement of variation in the process and outcome. This can be analyzed using statistical techniques. Improvement in outcome and lowering of cost can result by utilizing such strategies.

References

1. Lee TH, Goldman L: The coronary care unit turns 25: Historical trends and future directions. Ann Intern Med 1988;108:887.
2. Lown B, Fakhro AM, Hood WB Jr, et al: The coronary care unit: New perspectives and directions. JAMA 1967;199:188.
3. Gruppo Italiano Per Lo Studio Della Streptochi-Nasi Nell 'Infarto Miocardico (GISSI): Long-term effects of intravenous thrombolysis in acute myocardial infarction: Final report of the GISSI study. Lancet 1987;2(2):871.
4. International Study of Infarct Survival Collaborative Group (ISIS): Randomised trial of intravenous streptokinase, oral aspirin, both, or neither among 17187 cases of suspected acute myocardial infarction: ISIS-2. Lancet 1988;2(1):349.
5. Lee L, Erbel R, Brown T, et al: Multicenter registry of angioplasty therapy of cardiogenic shock: Initial and long-term survival. J Am Coll Cardiol 1991; 17(3):599.
6. Parisi AF, Folland ED, Hartigan P: A comparison of angioplasty with medical therapy in the treatment of single-vessel coronary artery disease. N Engl J Med 1992;326:10.
7. Theroux P, Ouimet H, McCans J, et al: Aspirin, heparin, or both to treat acute unstable angina. N Engl J Med 1988;319(17):1105.
8. Antman EM, Lau J, Kupelnick B, et al: A comparison of results of meta-analyses of randomized control trials and recommendations of clinical experts: Treatments for myocardial infarction. JAMA 1992;268:240.
9. Fedullo AJ, Swinburne AJ, Wahl GW, et al: Acute cardiogenic pulmonary edema treated with mechanical ventilation. Factors determining in-hospital mortality. Chest 1991;99(5):1220.
10. McEnany MT, Kay HR, Buckley MJ, et al: Clinical experience with intraaortic balloon pump support in 728 patients. Circulation 1978;58(Suppl 3):I-124.
11. DeWood MA, Notske RN, Hensley GR, et al: Intra-aortic balloon counterpulsation with and without reperfusion for myocardial infarction shock. Circulation 1980;61:1105.
12. Wampler RK, Frazier OH, Lansing AM, et al: Treatment of cardiogenic shock with the Hemopump left ventricular assist device. Ann Thorac Surg 1991;52(3):506.
13. Rose DM, Connolly M, Cunningham JN Jr, et al: Technique and results with a roller pump left and right heart assist device. Ann Thorac Surg 1989; 47(1):124.
14. Kanter KR, McBride LR, Pennington DG, et al: Bridging to cardiac trans-

plantation with pulsatile ventricular assist devices. Ann Thorac Surg 1988; 46(2):134.

15. Pennington DG, Kanter KR, McBride LR, et al: Seven years' experience with the Pierce-Donachy ventricular assist device. J Thorac Cardiovasc Surg 1988;96(6):901.
16. Fragomeni LS, Bonser RS, Kaye MP: Clinical results of heart and heart-lung transplantation. Prog Cardiovasc Dis 1990;33(2):97.
17. Killip T, Kimball JT: Treatment of myocardial infarction in a coronary care unit. Am J Cardiol 1967;20:457.
18. Norris RM, Brandt PWT, Caughey DE, et al: A new coronary prognostic index. Lancet 1969;1:274.
19. Forrester JS, Diamond G, Chatterjee K, et al: Medical therapy of acute myocardial infarction by application of hemodynamic subsets. N Engl J Med 1976;295:1356.
20. Teskey RJ, Calvin JE, McPhail I: Disease severity in the coronary care unit. Chest 1991;100:1637.
21. Knaus WA, Draper EA, Wagner DP, et al: APACHE II: A severity of disease classification system. Crit Care Med 1985;13:818.
22. Hanley JA, McNeil BJ: The meaning and use of the area under a receiver operating characteristic (ROC) curve. Diag Rad 1982;143:29.
23. Campeau L: Grading of angina pectoris [Letter]. Circulation 1976;54:522.
24. Calvin JE, and the Technology Subcommittee of the Working Group in Critical Care: Hemodynamic monitoring: A technology assessment. Can Med Assoc J 1991;145:114.
25. Subcommittee on Institutional Program Guidelines: Cardiovascular Services in Hospitals. Ottawa, Ontario, Health and Welfare Canada, 1986.
26. Task Force on Guidelines. Society of Critical Care Medicine: Recommendations for critical care unit design. Crit Care Med 1988;16(8):796.
27. Kume H: Statistical Methods for Quality Improvement. Tokyo, Japan, The Association for Overseas Technical Scholarship, 1985.
28. Gitlow H, Gitlow S: The Deming Guide to Quality and Competitive Position. Englewood Cliffs, NJ, Prentice-Hall, 1987.
29. Cairns JA, Gent M, Singer J, et al: Aspirin, sulfinpyrazone, or both in unstable angina. Results of a Canadian multicenter trial. N Engl J Med 1985; 313:1369.
30. Sharma GVRK, Deupree RH, Khuri SF, et al: Coronary bypass surgery improves survival in high-risk unstable angina: Results of a Veterans Administration Cooperative Study with an 8-year follow-up. Circulation 1991; 84(Suppl III):III-260.
31. Scholtes PR: The Team Handbook. How to Use Teams to Improve Quality. Madison, WI, Joiner Associates, Inc, 1988.
32. Naylor CD, Baigrie RS, Goldman BS, et al: Assessment of priority for coronary revascularisation procedures. Lancet 1990;335:1070.

Index

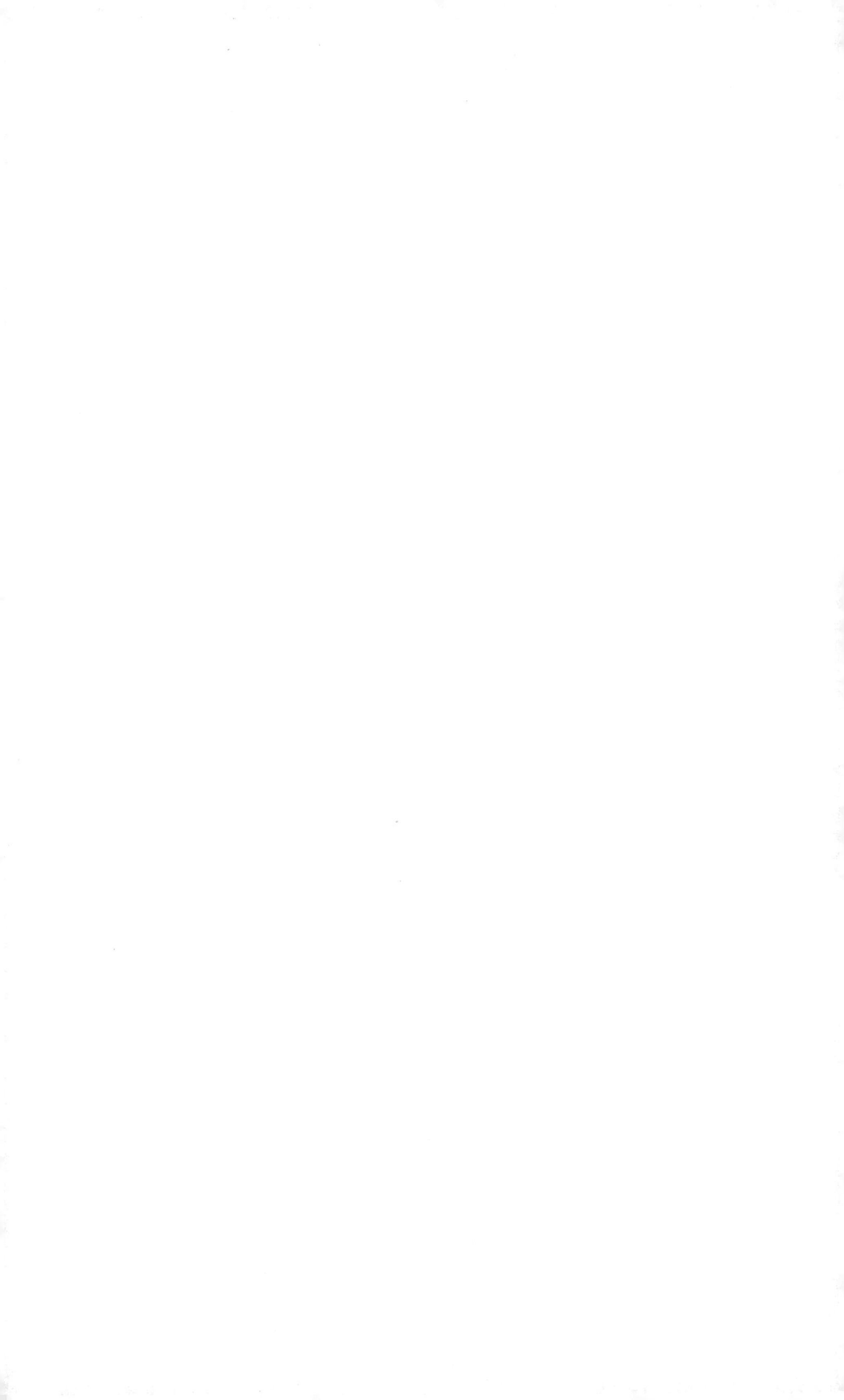